ADVANCES IN QUALITY OF LIFE RESEARCH 2001

Social Indicators Research Series

Volume 17

This new series aims to provide a public forum for single treatises and collections of papers on social indicators research that are too long to be published in our journal *Social Indicators Research*. Like the journal, the book series deals with statistical assessments of the quality of life from a broad perspective. It welcomes the research on a wide variety of substantive areas, including health, crime, housing, education, family life, leisure activities, transportation, mobility, economics, work, religion and environmental issues. These areas of research will focus on the impact of key issues such as health on the overall quality of life and vice versa. An international review board, consisting of Ruut Veenhoven, Joachim Vogel, Ed Diener, Torbjorn Moum and Wolfgang Glatzer, will ensure the high quality of the series as a whole.

The titles published in this series are listed at the end of this volume.

ADVANCES IN QUALITY OF LIFE RESEARCH 2001

Edited by

BRUNO D. ZUMBO
University of British Columbia, Vancouver, Canada

Reprinted from *Social Indicators Research*, Volume 60, Nos. 1–3 (December 2002)

KLUWER ACADEMIC PUBLISHERS
DORDRECHT / BOSTON / LONDON

A C.I.P. Catalogue record for this book is available from the Library of Congress.

ISBN 14020-1100-8

Published by Kluwer Academic Publishers,
P.O. Box 17, 3300 AA Dordrecht, The Netherlands.

Sold and distributed in North, Central and South America
by Kluwer Academic Publishers,
101 Philip Drive, Norwell, MA 02061, U.S.A.

In all other countries, sold and distributed
by Kluwer Academic Publishers,
P.O. Box 322, 3300 AH Dordrecht, The Netherlands.

Printed on acid-free paper

Printed and bound in the Netherlands.

CONTENTS

Section III. Determinants and Correlates of Well-Being and Quality of Life

BRUNO D. ZUMBO

EDITORIAL

The knowledge base in the domains of quality of life, well-being, and subjective well-being is continuing to grow at a rapid rate. In light of this growth, and the interest it reflects on the part of scholars, practitioners, and policy makers internationally, the International Socicty for Quality of Life Studies (ISQOLS) plays an important role in promoting and encouraging research in the field of quality-of-life (QOL) studies, broadly construed to involve all of the social and health sciences. In December 1998 scholars from around the world gathered in Williamsburg, Virginia, for the Second Annual ISQOLS organized Conference. The papers herein reflect much of that exchange.

This volume has much to offer the reader. The papers reflect a diversity of disciplinary and methodological perspectives. In an attempt to organize the diverse themes and yet reflect current thinking the papers are organized into three sections. Although I recognize that this organization is somewhat arbitrary, not to cluster the papers would leave them without a thread of interconnectedness. The first section contains papers issues surrounding the monitoring, assessing, and modeling of quality of life. The second section is loosely organized around matters of policy, finance, marketing, and business. And finally, the third section is devoted to some determinants and correlates of well- being and quality of life.

Finally, it is with gratitude that I acknowledge the hard work of exceptional group of reviewers who handled at least one paper.

Bryant J., Australia	Duxbury L., Carleton University
Fischer D., University of Saskatchewan	Frankish J., Vancouver
Tousignant M., Quebec	Greenwood M., Prince George
Kishor N., Vancouver	Lee J., Boston
Lehrer R., Moncton	Lindsay A., Arkansas

University of British Columbia
Scarfe Building, 2125 Main Hall
Measurement, Evaluation, and Research Methodology
Vancouver, BC V6T 1Z4
Canada

SECTION I

MONITORING, ASSESSING, AND MODELING QUALITY OF LIFE

PEGGY SCHYNS

WEALTH OF NATIONS, INDIVIDUAL INCOME AND LIFE SATISFACTION IN 42 COUNTRIES: A MULTILEVEL APPROACH *

ABSTRACT. In this study, individual and contextual determinants of life satisfaction in 42 countries were examined. The question was addressed whether income at the individual level and wealth at the national level affect life satisfaction of individuals. In addition, the hypothesis was tested whether the relationship between income and life satisfaction is stronger in poor countries than in more prosperous ones. Multilevel modeling allows differentiating between main and interaction effects of group and individual level variables on the dependent variable. It was used to explore a possible multilevel structure in the data, in which individuals are viewed as micro observations and countries as macro observations. The results showed that, in addition to and independent of individual income, the economic prosperity of a nation contributed to a person's life satisfaction level. Also, the hypothesized cross-level interaction between wealth and income was tested and found significant: poor people living in poor countries were less satisfied with their lives than poor people living in affluent countries. Moreover, complex variation in life satisfaction was found at the within-nation level: poor individuals varied more in their life satisfaction than rich individuals.

1. INTRODUCTION

In the literature on Quality of Life (QoL), many studies have replicated the finding that within nations, the relation between income and subjective well-being is positive but weak (Ahuvia and Friedman, 1998; Diener and Oishi, 2000; Schyns, 2000; Diener and Biswas-Diener, 1999). Although richer people are found to be more satisfied with their lives than poor people, correlations usually only lie between the range of 0.10 and 0.25.

---

* This article is an adapted version of a paper presented at the ISA XIV World Congress of Sociology in Montréal, Canada, July 26–August 1, 1998, and the Second ISQOLS Conference in Williamsburg, Virginia, United States, December 3–6, 1998.

Social Indicators Research **60:** 5–40, 2002.

However, between-nation data show a much stronger relationship between the wealth of a nation and the average subjective well-being. Diener et al. (1995), for example, found a correlation of 0.59 in their sample; Veenhoven (1995) reported a correlation of 0.55 in a university students sample and 0.69 in a general sample; Schyns (1998) found a correlation of 0.64. It means that in wealthier countries people are, on average, more satisfied with their lives than people in poor countries.

This discrepancy in outcomes between the two levels has puzzled several researchers. One explanation for the difference in strength of the correlations is a methodological one. Aggregation of data to the level of countries implies that the error term at the individual level is averaged out, so that national values of life satisfaction reflect only mean between-nation differences. Individual level characteristics like personality and temperament can have a substantial influence on well-being at the individual level, but they are averaged out at the national level, which results in higher correlations (Diener and Oishi, 2000: p. 198).

To give an example, Diener and Oishi found in the World Values Survey II a mean correlation between income and life satisfaction of 0.24. Aggregation of these individuals into 10 separate income groups resulted, however, in a correlation between the 1 to 10 income categories and mean life satisfaction within those categories of 0.99. Effects of income did, of course, not grow any stronger, but were being considered in the light of a different error term (*ibid.*, p. 200).

A more substantial explanation is that a correlation found at the individual level does not necessarily mean the same as a correlation at the national level. Two well-known fallacies are the ecological fallacy – also called the "Robinson effect" after Robinson (1950) – which is the interpretation of aggregated data at the individual level, and the atomistic fallacy, which is the interpretation of micro-level data at the aggregated level (Hox, 1995: p. 5). Both fallacies stem from incorrect interpretation of mono-level data. Applied to the example in this study, it is very well possible that separate effects take place at different levels at the same time: it may be the case that at the country level, wealthier countries "produce" a higher *average* level of life satisfaction, but also that at the within-country level, household income is only modestly correlated with *individual* life satisfaction.

This explanation lies at the core of a multilevel problem, which will be the topic of the present study. A multilevel problem is "a problem that concerns the relationships between variables that are measured at a number of different hierarchical levels" (*ibid.*, p. 5). It is interesting to not only know what the possible effects of economic objective indicators on subjective well-being are at each level (the macro level and micro level),[1] but also how variables of both levels simultaneously relate to the response variable at the individual level.

In other words, it is also interesting to detect the effects of nation level characteristics such as the wealth of a nation on life satisfaction, in addition to individual level characteristics such as income, or – one step further – to see whether this national characteristic influences the relationship between income and life satisfaction.[2] These steps are seldom undertaken, and will be the main focus of this study.

The World Values Survey II data offer an opportunity to link nation level variables to individual level variables. Since the sample design of the World Values Survey is individuals within countries, and the main focus of this study is the impact of contextual and individual variables on life satisfaction, as well as cross-level interaction effects, the use of a multilevel approach is called for.

The main research question was: what is the effect of economic prosperity at the nation level and income at the individual level on life satisfaction? In addition to these main effects, it is also interesting to see if there are any interaction effects between the nation level and the individual level. Hence, the second question was: does the relationship between income and life satisfaction differ depending on the wealth of a nation?

The statistical programs MLn and MlwiN[3] were used to analyze these relationships between and within 42 countries of the World Values Survey II (Woodhouse, 1995).

The following section 2 illustrates a typical multilevel example and briefly reviews multilevel modeling in general in the first part, and then focuses on multilevel theory and its application in the Quality of Life domain in the second part. At the end of the section, hypotheses concerning the relationship wealth (nation level), income[4] (individual level), and life satisfaction are formulated. Section 3 describes the data. In section 4, the multilevel model and results are presented, and in section 5 conclusions and some thoughts for discussion are presented.

2.1 MULTILEVEL EXAMPLE AND OVERVIEW OF MULTILEVEL MODELING

Before turning to a short historical overview of multilevel modeling, I will briefly describe a typical multilevel example in the QoL field. Several studies have shown that at the individual level people who are unemployed have lower subjective well-being than people who are employed, an outcome that is rather intuitive (Clark et al., 1999). At the level of nations, Di Tella et al. (2000), for example, found that people were on average happier when inflation and unemployment in a country were low.

Both findings are mono-level findings: they concern either the individual level (i.e., within-nation) or the group (i.e., between-nation) level. However, since people do not live in a social vacuum, it is also interesting to study the effect of a higher level phenomenon on an individual's subjective well-being. This is called a contextual analysis: the effect of a higher level variable on an individual level variable is assessed. An interesting study in this regard was carried out by Clark (1999), who examined, among other things, the effect of the unemployment rate of the region and the effect of the unemployment of members of the household on the well-being of individuals. Individual well-being was shown to be negatively correlated with both regional unemployment and the unemployment of other household members (Clark, 1999: p. 3).

One could go even one step further: perhaps the relationship between the employment status of an individual and their well-being may differ depending on a certain value of the group variable. For example, there could be a strong negative relationship between an individual's employment status (0 being employed, 1 being unemployed) and subjective well-being if the other household members are employed (employment status at the household level), whereas the relation may be far less negative, and even zero or positive in the extreme, if the household has only unemployed members. Indeed, closer examination of the data revealed that the unemployment of relevant others (household level) mostly reduced the well-being of the employed, but had a strong positive effect on the well-being of the unemployed, whereas the opposite was the case if the household had only employed members. This portrays a cross-level interaction statement: the group level variable (unemployment rate of the household) interacts with the micro-level relationship between employment status and subjective well-being.

Let us now turn to a brief overview of multilevel modeling. In the past, whenever researchers were interested in combining context or macro-level variables with micro-level variables to explain a certain phenomenon at the micro level, they had to analyze variables from both levels either at the macro level or at the micro level.[5] In this way, the two levels were artificially reduced to one level, which – if a researcher was not careful – could result either in the already mentioned ecological fallacy (interpretation at individual level of a macro-level analysis) or the atomistic fallacy (interpretation at macro level whilst analyzing at the individual level).

In addition to these conceptual problems, there were also some statistical problems. To give an example of a traditional contextual analysis, if one was interested in group effects on individual level variables, e.g., the effect of the wealth of a nation or of a region's unemployment rate on individual life satisfaction, each individual would receive the country's score on wealth or the region's score on unemployment, hence transforming a context variable into a "context variable ascribed to an individual" (Tacq, 1994). This means that a few data values from a small number of group units are artificially " 'blown up' into values for a much larger number of subunits, [. . .] which leads to significance tests that reject the null-hypothesis far more often than the nominal alpha level suggests" (Hox, 1995: p. 4–5). That is, a large number of spuriously "significant" results are found.

Later on, "two step" or "slopes as outcomes" analyses were developed. For an overview see, for example, Tacq (1994) and Kreft and De Leeuw (1998). Applying a two step analysis to the income or (un)employment example, the first step is for each nation or for each household to estimate separate regression coefficients for the relationship at the lowest level, and the second step is to explain these coefficients with either country level characteristics such as wealth, or household level characteristics such as the household's unemployment rate.

Although they can be seen as an improvement compared with the mono-level contextual analysis, the two step models still have some major problems, one being that most micro analyses are based on too few cases, making the analyses quite unreliable (Tacq, 1994).

For these and other technical reasons, the multilevel model[6] was developed. The idea is basically the same as that of the "two step" model, but its major advantages are, firstly, that the analysis occurs in one step (the model acknowledges a nested structure, e.g., individuals within countries or households) and, secondly, more reliable estimations of the regression coefficients can be calculated, since micro analyses in separate groups are avoided (Tacq, 1994). Or, stating it differently, "multilevel models are designed to analyze variables from different levels simultaneously, using a statistical model that includes the various dependencies" (Hox, 1995: p. 7).

Most of the multilevel research has been carried out in the educational research field (pupils within schools, e.g., Aitkin and Longford, 1986). In other fields, for example, organizational research with individuals nested in organizations (e.g., Rosenfeld, 1992), and recently in longitudinal research, the model has also been applied (several measurement occasions within respondents, e.g., Hox, 1995).

2.2 MULTILEVEL THEORY AND MODELS IN QUALITY OF LIFE RESEARCH

Compared to the above mentioned fields, multilevel analysis in the field of QoL research is still in its infancy. Some studies have been carried out in the social welfare field, e.g., a study by Van der Poel on the effects of an egocentric network on the individual's well-being (Van der Poel, 1993). In the field of QoL research, there is a study by Fernandez and Kulik (1981) on the neighborhood effects on life satisfaction; a study in Norway by Mastekaasa and Moum (1984),[7] concerning contextual effects of counties on life satisfaction; a study by Rampichini and Schifini d'Andrea (1998), in which they determined the individual and contextual factors that contribute to life satisfaction in Italy;[8] and, finally, a study by Oishi et al. (1999), who tested for cross-cultural differences in predictors of life satisfaction. All in all, however, multilevel studies in the life satisfaction field are not really overwhelming.

One reason for the small number of statistical multilevel methods in QoL research might be that often not enough cases (e.g., too few countries) are available at the group level to allow a multilevel analysis. Although there are no strict rules as to how many cases each level should contain, as a rule of thumb, cases at the group level should not drop below 25 (Jones et al., 1992: p. 357).

Another explanation might be that many researchers are still not really convinced of the advantages of multilevel model over the more "old-fashioned" models. Nevertheless, it is not really a matter of taste but of necessity, since using "two step" models or contextual analysis instead of multilevel models can lead to substantially different outcomes (see Snijders and Bosker, 1997: p. 39).

Moreover, using a multilevel model rather than a standard mono-level regression procedure also has the major advantage that several effects can be separated: it is possible to differentiate in one model between the main effects of context or group level variables on life satisfaction, the main effects of individual level variables on life satisfaction, and the possible interaction effects between the two levels, something which cannot be done in the traditional regression models.

Another advantage is that it is a technique that can deal with complex variation at both levels. In other words, it does not treat individuals or nations as having the same error variance, but can explicitly model differences in variance at both levels. This is important since higher level variation can be mistakenly confused for lower level variation. In brief, multilevel modeling assigns variability to the appropriate level (Jones and Duncan, 1998: p. 116).

In the QoL field, there are several theories that describe the relationship between objective QoL indicators and subjective life satisfaction. They are usually restricted to either the individual level or the national level. Examples of the former are need theory, comparison theory, and personality theory (for a discussion see Diener et al., 1995; Veenhoven, 1991, 1995). Examples of the latter are livability theory and national character theory[9] (Veenhoven, 1995; Inkeles, 1997). Theories that explicitly try to connect both the impact of social contexts and individual level factors on life satisfaction are, however, seldom encountered.[10]

Here, some first steps are made towards the formulation of a multilevel theory. The theory will elaborate on need theory at the individual level and livability theory at the nation level. Comparison theory and personality or national character theory are not considered at this stage, since robust indicators to test these theories – theories which are sometimes not yet fully developed – are still lacking (see Ahuvia and Friedman, 1998).

What does need theory state at the individual level? Elsewhere, I have described the theory in more detail (Schyns, 1998). Here, only the main points are mentioned. Its ideas are based on Maslow's needs pyramid. According to need theory, in order to function as a human being certain minimal demands need to be fulfilled. These are the need for food, clothes, shelter, and security. The amount of need-satisfaction determines largely the way we feel and think about our lives. Physiological and safety needs especially are deemed essential for the mere survival of an individual (Maslow, 1970).

In addition to these basic needs, Maslow distinguishes love needs, esteem needs, and self-actualization needs respectively. According to Maslow, the satisfaction of these higher needs is almost unlimited (*ibid.*, p. 100). Satisfaction of physiological and safety needs has, however, a certain point of diminishing marginal utility; too much food (e.g., obesity) and too much safety (e.g., overprotection) could, in the long run, even have negative effects on a person's well-being (see Maslow, 1987: p. 39; Schor, 1991).[11]

In need theory, income can be seen as a means of satisfying needs. Directly, money buys food and, in a more indirect way, it also buys safety. A basic or higher level of income is also needed to satisfy at least some of Maslow's higher needs. However, some argue that above a certain level, income does not have an extra effect on life satisfaction, since basic needs have been fulfilled and income has no real utility beyond that (Schor, 1991; Veenhoven, 1991; Ahuvia and Friedman, 1998; Lane, 1998). A second approach states, on the contrary, that even very high levels of income can still produce greater happiness since activities such as traveling abroad, sailing, and mountaineering, which help people to satisfy their self-actualization needs, might only be available to those with high levels of income (Diener et al., 1985; Diener and Oishi, 2000). As previous studies have found effects on subjective well-being even beyond a basic income, the notion of no extra effect after a certain threshold is rejected in this study.

Let us now turn to livability theory, in which the concept of livability refers to a macro-level characteristic. According to Veenhoven, "the livability of one's society is the degree to which collective provisions and demands fit with individual needs and capacities" (Veenhoven, 1995: p. 36). Human societies can be seen as collective arrangements to gratify these needs. If a country is economically more prosperous, in the sense that people can pursue the life they want to lead, it is better able to fulfil the above described needs of individual citizens, hence, the mean satisfaction level will be higher. The better the living conditions in a country, the more satisfied its citizens will be (*ibid.*, pp. 35–36).[12]

When stating which country characteristics are connected to individual characteristics, one needs to define a mechanism through which this process of direct and indirect influence takes place. It can be stated that people living in the same country share some basic common socio-economic and political conditions (e.g., education system, wealth, health care, infrastructure, and political climate); it is a context within which people shape their lives and draw satisfaction from life. Although the same context can have different effects on different people, and not all people have equal access to these collective provisions, one can also assert that the availability of certain basic goods and services in a country provides some main base line which can contribute to an individual's life satisfaction, assuming that structural nation characteristics precede individual life satisfaction.[13] A contextual variable in this study then can be viewed as a proxy of economic factors that vary over the different countries and that have direct and indirect effects on life satisfaction levels.

Also here – in line with the reasoning at the individual level – beyond a certain level of wealth, some argue that the effect of this macro variable on life satisfaction will decrease, according to the law of diminishing marginal utility (Veenhoven, 1995). A more radical viewpoint holds that too much wealth has harmful effects, such as consumerism and materialism,[14] which are detrimental to life satisfaction (Kuper and Kuper, 1996: p. 226; La Barbera and Gurhan, 1997). Since few researchers have found a negative relationship between wealth and life satisfaction, only the possibility of a diminishing extra effect is taken into account here.

The above mentioned theories all describe hypothesized *main* effects of individual and contextual variables on life satisfaction. An interesting step in multilevel theory is to find possible cross-level interactions between explanatory group level variables and individual level variables; that is, to theorize what effect macro variables might have on the micro-level *relationship* between income and life satisfaction.

Here, both theories are combined in order to make some statements concerning cross-level interactions. First of all, within each country a positive relationship exists between income and life satisfaction. This relationship might, however, not be a fixed relationship over all countries, fixed meaning that it does not vary over countries. Since it was also stated that wealth at the country level contributes to an individual's life satisfaction, it follows from the different levels of wealth between countries that some countries are better providers of these objective living conditions than others.

All else being equal, in relatively poor countries it is plausible to expect to find a different relationship between income and life satisfaction than in relatively wealthy countries. In poorer countries, income can be a stronger determinant of life satisfaction, since having an income can literally be a matter of life or death. The possession of income is more important in countries where basic needs are not being met for the whole or the majority of the population. It is a "scarce resource", and people are more dependent on it. In wealthy countries, in contrast, there might be provisions such as health care, social security, education, etc., that function as a safety-net in the case of loss of income or a major drop in income, and which, in turn, might cushion the decline in life satisfaction. In other words, for economically prosperous people, where they live matters less in terms of life satisfaction, since they have their own income to fall back on, and they possibly have a greater chance of benefiting from the living conditions in a country, even if these conditions are poor.

Finally, in addition to estimating fixed (main and interaction) effects as described above, multilevel modeling is also a powerful tool for modeling variance in the dependent variable. Much quantitative modeling, such as traditional regression analysis, usually assumes homogeneity of the data, i.e., that there is the same variance in life satisfaction within and between nations. However, in the empirical world, heterogeneity is usually the norm (Bullen et al., 1997: p. 585; Jones and Duncan, 1998: p. 107). The hypothesized cross-level interaction effect already presumed complex variability at the country level intercepts and slopes were allowed to vary – but it is also important to check for complex variability at the within-nation level, since both levels might be confounded. Therefore, in this study, it is expected that individuals within nations will differ with regard to variation in life satisfaction, and heterogeneity between individuals will be explicitly modeled.

In sum, the following hypotheses are stated:

Hypotheses

∗ Individual level

1. Income and life satisfaction are weakly but positively correlated.

   1.1 Beyond a certain income, the relation will become curvilinear: more income adds less to extra life satisfaction, but it does not approach zero.

∗ Country level

2. Wealth of nations and life satisfaction are positively correlated.

   2.1 The relation between wealth and life satisfaction is a curvilinear one, that is, beyond a certain level of wealth, wealth produces less effect on life satisfaction according to the law of diminishing marginal returns (again no zero or negative relation assumed).

∗ Cross-level interaction

3. In poor countries, the relationship between income and life satisfaction is stronger than in rich countries.

Figure 1 summarizes the hypotheses in a graphical way.

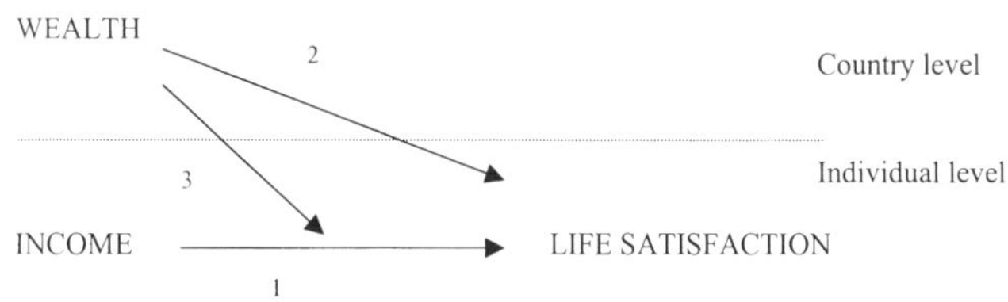

Figure 1. Micro (= 1), Macro (= 2), and cross-level interaction (= 3) effects on life satisfaction.

2. DATA

Data from the 1990 World Values Survey II were arranged to allow modeling on two levels: the individual (un)satisfied person, and the geographical country.[15] For Australia and Iceland, data from the 1980 World Values Survey I were used, since relevant variables were missing in the 1990 wave.[16] Analyses are based on 50,046 individual respondents over 42 countries. Not only are individuals treated as a sample coming from a distribution, so are countries. This is an important difference between multilevel modeling and mono-level modeling: in multilevel modeling, the higher-level units (i.e., countries) are treated as random, whereas in mono-level modeling they are treated as fixed (Jones and Duncan, 1998: p. 111). Consequently, it is assumed that outcomes can be generalized to a wider population of world countries.[17]

The sample size within each country ranged from 727 respondents in Argentina to 3,279 in Spain. This meets with the recommendation of Patterson and Goldstein, that a data structure should have at least 25 respondents in each of 25 higher-level units (see Jones et al., 1992: p. 357). It poses, however, another problem, namely, that most results will be highly significant because of the large *N*. Therefore, it is important to look at the relevance of the variables.

The dependent variable in this study was life satisfaction. Life satisfaction can be defined as the degree to which an individual judges the overall quality of his or her life-as-a-whole favorably (Veenhoven, 1984: p. 22). It was measured by asking people directly how satisfied they are with their lives. The following question was asked in the survey: "All things considered, how satisfied are you with your life as a whole these days?" Respondents could rate themselves on a scale from 1 (dissatisfied) to 10 (satisfied). Although in a strict sense, this scale is only ordinal, studies that used both measures have shown that treating the variable either as ordinal or as metric leads to approximately the same results (e.g., Diener et al., 1995: p. 861). Here the dependent variable will be depicted as an interval variable.

In order to model life satisfaction, a number of predictor variables from both the within-nation level and between-nation level were included. The most important predictor at the within-nation level was household income. Unfortunately, in the World Values Survey, this variable was not measured on a metric scale (allowing each respondent to give an exact household income per year), but on an ordinal scale. Respondents were asked to rate their household income (wages, salaries, pensions, and other incomes, before taxes and other deductions) in a certain category. Most countries used ten income-categories, each in their own respective currency unit, ranging from the lowest income-group (1) to the highest (10).

However, since the 1–10 income scale was not used in every country, the income variable was transformed in two ways. First, income-quartiles were computed, putting respondents who earned up to 25% of the total income-scale in the first category (Income Low), 25–49% in the second (Income MedLow), 50–74% in the third (Income MedHigh), and 75% and higher in the last category (Income High). This resulted in the creation of three dummy-coded variables, with the poorest income category as the reference group. Second, the income-scale was standardized in z-scores, resulting in a "metric" scale of income. Although, strictly speaking, this is not correct, this measure was only used to show the effects in a graphic way later on. To test whether income had a curvilinear effect on life satisfaction, one can look at the relative size of the coefficients of the dummy variables. If the size declines, it points to a curvilinear effect.

In addition to income, age, sex and marital status were included as control variables at the individual level.[18] While the majority of studies have shown that the relationship between life satisfaction and age is positive, there is evidence in some studies for a non-linear relation, with the young and old more satisfied than the middle-aged (Mastekaasa and Moum, 1984; Rampichini and Schifini d'Andrea, 1998). Although sex usually shows no relationship with life satisfaction (Headey and Wearing, 1992), it was included because some studies found a conditioning effect on the relationship between other variables and well-being (Schyns, 1996; Rampichini and Schifini d'Andrea, 1998). Finally, married people clearly rate higher on life satisfaction than singles, whereas separated and divorced people show the lowest levels (Fernandez and Kulik, 1981; Mastekaasa and Moum, 1984; Headey and Wearing, 1992; Schyns, 1996; Diener et al., 1999).

Age is a continuous variable, and both age and age-squared were included in the model to account for the curvilinear effect of age on life satisfaction. Sex and marital status were coded as dummy variables. For sex, males are the reference group. Marital status consists of three dummy variables: being married, being widowed, and being divorced, leaving the single person category as the reference group. In Table I, the mean life satisfaction level and standard deviation is shown for each country. In Table II, the mean life satisfaction scores and the standard deviation over the different categories are presented for the whole sample.

In addition to individual level data, the set also contained contextual data, namely the country's real Gross Domestic Product (real GDP) per capita in US Dollars (in $1000) in 1990, drawn from the 1993 United Nations Development Programme (UNDP) Human Development Report (HDR). The advantage of a "real" GDP – also called Purchasing Power Parity (PPP) – over a normal GDP is that it tells more about the purchasing power of people than the normal GDP. Real GDP per capita expresses "the number of units of that currency required to purchase the same representative basket of goods and services that a US dollar would buy in the United States (or a similar basket of goods and services)" (United Nations Development Programme, 1996: p. 223). Based on earlier research, the variable has shown strong correlations with mean life satisfaction (Diener et al., 1995; Schyns, 1998).

TABLE I

Mean Life Satisfaction and Standard Deviation in 42 Countries

	Mean LS	SD		Mean LS	SD
France	6.80	1.99	Brazil	7.38	2.40
W. Germany	7.30	1.90	Nigeria	6.51	2.60
Italy	7.29	2.09	Chile	7.57	2.20
Netherlands	7.80	1.48	Belarus	5.53	2.25
Denmark	8.18	1.86	India	6.69	2.27
Belgium	7.67	1.86	Czechslov.	6.31	2.14
Spain	7.17	1.90	E. Germany	6.80	1.95
Ireland	7.90	1.92	Slovenia	6.29	2.22
USA	7.76	1.81	Bulgaria	5.05	2.24
Canada	7.90	1.72	Romania	5.87	2.33
Japan	6.59	1.72	China	7.31	2.09
Mexico	7.41	2.12	Portugal	7.06	2.14
S. Africa	6.73	2.71	Austria	6.51	3.41
Hungary	6.03	2.46	Turkey	6.42	2.46
Norway	7.72	1.72	Lithuania	6.08	2.33
Sweden	7.99	1.69	Latvia	5.80	2.38
Argentina	7.21	2.05	Estonia	5.98	2.13
Finland	7.74	1.85	Russia	5.46	2.37
S. Korea	6.74	2.38	UK	7.57	1.90
Poland	6.67	2.34	Australia 81	7.91	1.72
Switzerland	8.33	1.71	Iceland 81	8.11	1.58

Note: OLS regression based on 50,046 respondents in total.

3. MULTILEVEL MODEL

The multilevel model that was tested in this study is illustrated in Figure 2.[19]

It shows a fully random model where, in addition to the intercepts (i.e., average life satisfaction in a given country), the slopes (i.e., the relationship between income and life satisfaction in a given country) are allowed to vary over countries. On the vertical axis, individual life satisfaction is displayed; on the horizontal axis, household income.[20] The upper lines denote the wealthy countries, and the lower lines show the poor ones.

The hypothesized cross-level interaction effect between wealth, income, and life satisfaction can also – more indirectly – be derived

TABLE II

Mean Life Satisfaction and Standard Deviation for Categories

	Mean LS	SD		Mean LS	SD
Income			Age		
Income Low	6.57	2.55	18–24	7.00	2.20
Income MedLow	7.02	2.26	25–34	7.04	2.21
Income MedHigh	7.12	2.17	35–44	6.97	2.25
Income High	7.31	2.04	45–54	6.90	2.30
Marital status			55–64	7.03	2.38
Married/Living as	7.13	2.24	65+	7.09	2.45
Divorced/Separ.	6.31	2.49	Sex		
Widowed	6.56	2.57	Male	7.05	2.24
Single	6.90	2.24	Female	6.96	2.32

Note: OLS regression based on 50,046 respondents in total.

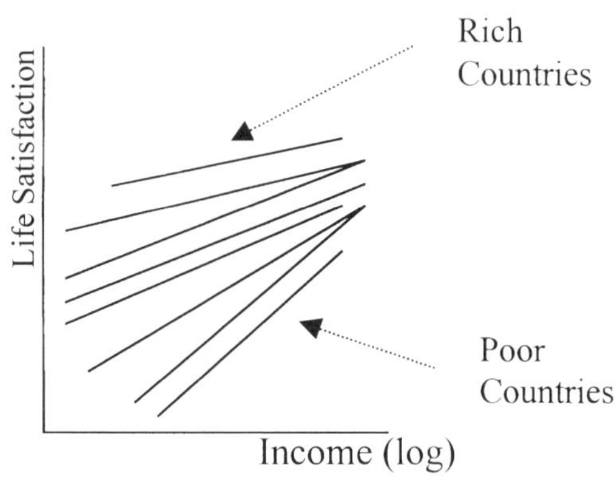

Figure 2. Fully Random Model, large negative covariance between slope and intercept.

from the figure: the relation between income and life satisfaction is weaker in economically more prosperous countries (flat lines at the top), whereas the opposite is the case in poorer countries (steeper lines at the bottom).

Model Estimation

At the individual level, for every individual i in nation j, the level of life satisfaction was predicted from income, age, age-squared, marital status and sex. At the level of nations, one variable was added to predict life satisfaction, namely wealth of a nation. To see whether the relation between income and life satisfaction varied between nations, the slopes of the income dummy variables were allowed to vary over countries (random slopes model). In order to model the hypothesized cross-level interaction effects, product terms of wealth and income were included.

Inserting all variables in the model resulted in the following equation:[21]

$$\begin{aligned} LS_{ij} = {} & \gamma_{00} + \gamma_{10}\text{IncMedLow}_{ij} + \gamma_{20}\text{IncMedHigh}_{ij} + \\ & \gamma_{30}\text{IncHigh}_{ij} + \gamma_{40}\text{Age}_{ij} + \gamma_{50}\text{AgeSquared}_{ij} + \\ & \gamma_{60}\text{Divorced}_{ij} + \gamma_{70}\text{Widowed}_{ij} + \gamma_{80}\text{Married}_{ij} + \\ & \gamma_{90}\text{Sex}_{ij} + \gamma_{01}\text{RealGDP}_{j} + \gamma_{11}\text{IncMedLow}_{ij} * \\ & \text{RealGDP}_{j} + \gamma_{21}\text{IncMedHigh}_{ij} * \text{RealGDP}_{j} + \\ & \gamma_{31}\text{IncHigh}_{ij} * \text{RealGDP}_{j} + (\mu_{pj}X_{pij} + \mu_{0j} + \varepsilon_{ij}) \end{aligned} \quad (1)$$

It can be read that life satisfaction for every individual i in nation j is a function of income, age, age-squared, marital status, and sex at the individual level, of wealth at the nation level, and of a cross-level interaction between income and wealth. All the variables in the model with γ-coefficients are referred to as the fixed part of the model. The remainder of the model is called the random part, and it contains the μ_{pj} X_{pij}, μ_{0j} and ε_{ij} random terms.[22] This is the part where a multilevel model differs from traditional regression models. The ε_{ij} random term is familiar from the regression models, and is the usual residual error term. The difference lies in the error terms at the group level: μ_{pj} X_{pij} and μ_{0j}. Since the error term μ_{pj} is multiplied by the explanatory variables X_{pij}, the resulting total error will be different for different values of explanatory variables at the individual level (heteroscedasticity). In normal regression modeling, however, homoscedasticity is assumed, which is one of the reasons why a multilevel model does not work very well with a normal regression program (Hox, 1995: p. 14). As stated before, in this study, heterogeneity was explicitly modeled at both levels.

Finally, the used estimators are Maximum Likelihood (ML) estimators, which, stated simply, "maximize the probability of finding the sample data that we have actually found" (*ibid.*, p. 17).

4. RESULTS

In multilevel modeling one must first estimate a baseline, called the null model or intercept only model, to see whether there is any country variation at all, and whether a multilevel model is justified:

$$LS_{ij} = \gamma_{00} + \mu_{0j} + \varepsilon_{ij} \tag{2}$$

The results can be found in Table III, model 1. The estimated null model presents a significant country variance component of 0.666. The estimated intra-class correlation[23] – the population estimate of the variance explained by the grouping structure (*ibid.*, p. 15) – is $(\sigma^2_{\mu 0}/(\sigma^2_{\mu 0} + \sigma^2_{\varepsilon})) = (0.666/(0.666 + 4.635)) = 12.6\%$. The model of equation (2) does not explain any variance, it just decomposes the variance into variance at the group level and variance at the individual level (*ibid.*, p. 15). Thus, on the basis of the estimated model, 12.6% of the total unexplained variation in life satisfaction level is due to the different country of residence, while the remaining 87.4% is due to individual characteristics. It indicates that individuals differ more from each other than do countries (Kreft and De Leeuw, 1998: p. 64).

The overall average life satisfaction in the 42 countries is 6.979. To see whether this two-level model fits the data better than an OLS model with only one level (not shown), the difference in deviance (defined as minus twice the natural logarithm of the likelihood) of both models was computed. The difference in deviance has a Chi-square distribution and it shows, compared to the degree of freedom lost, if one model is a significant improvement on another (*ibid.*, p. 65). The difference of 5625 (224619 – 218994) is highly significant (df = 1, critical $\chi^2 = 3.84$) and thus a two level model is preferred.

In the second step, a model with all lower level explanatory variables fixed will be analyzed. This means that the corresponding variance components of the slopes of the lower level variables are fixed at zero. The contribution of each individual explanatory variable is assessed. The following individual level variables were included in the model: income (3 dummy variables, lowest income group is reference group), marital status (3 dummy variables, single persons are reference group), and age and age-squared. The latter two variables were entered as centered variables in order to give substantial meaning to the intercept.[24] Sex was not significant and was deleted from the final model. The reference person hence became a single, low income person of average age.

The results are shown in Table III, model 2. The improvement of the final model chosen in this step can be tested again by looking at the difference between the deviance of this model and the intercept only model. The degrees of freedom equal the number of variables added in the second model, which is 8. The critical value of the Chi-square variate with 8 degrees of freedom and $p < 0.05$ is 15.51. The difference in deviance of 1363 is larger and hence the model is an improvement compared to the first model.

If we look at the unstandardized coefficients, the interpretation is much like that of an OLS regression analysis. People are more satisfied with their lives if their income category is higher than the lowest group, and if they are married (compared to single). They are less satisfied if they are widowed and most dissatisfied if they are divorced. Age and age-squared were both significant. They indicate that younger and older people are slightly more satisfied with their lives than middle-aged people. These results are in line with earlier findings (see Fernandez and Kulik, 1981; Mastekaasa and Moum, 1984; Headey and Wearing, 1992; Rampichini and Schifini d'Andrea, 1998; Diener et al., 1999).

A possible curvilinear effect of income on life satisfaction can be witnessed by inspecting the relative size of the coefficients of the dummy variables. If one moves up from the reference group to the higher income groups, a declining effect can be seen. This would point in the direction of a curvilinear effect of the income-groups on life satisfaction. Hence, both hypothesis 1 and 1.1 were confirmed.

The R^2 of this model at the individual level is 2.7% ((4.635 – 4.511)/4.635), and at the nation level R^2 is –0.8% ((0.666 – 0.671)/0.666).[25] If the unexplained variance at the group level increases after introducing individual explanatory variables, this usually points to the omission of important explanatory variables at the group level. Unfortunately, this is not a rare phenomenon in multilevel analysis; introduction of lower level variables can cause a rise in the variance at a higher level.

As stated before, an important feature of multilevel modeling is that it allows for modeling both means and variances. That is, in

TABLE III

Coefficients of the 5 Multilevel Models (Unstandardized, Standard Error in Brackets)

	Model 1		Model 2		Model 3		Model 4		Model 5		Model 5
	Coefficient	SE	Coefficient	SE	Coefficient	SE	Coefficient	SE	Coefficient	SE	Standardized Coefficient β
FIXED PART											
Individual effect											
Constant	6.979	(0.126)	6.248	(0.131)	6.273	(0.156)	6.271	(0.128)	6.270	(0.124)	
IncMedLow			0.315	(0.028)	0.288	(0.051)	0.289	(0.054)	0.289	(0.052)	0.055
IncMedHigh			0.550	(0.028)	0.511	(0.084)	0.512	(0.084)	0.512	(0.078)	0.096
IncHigh			0.702	(0.028)	0.672	(0.091)	0.673	(0.091)	0.673	(0.085)	0.128
Age			–0.002	(0.001)	–0.002	(0.001)	–0.002	(0.001)	–0.002	(0.001)	–0.014
Age-squared			0.0004	(0.0000)	0.0004	(0.0000)	0.0004	(0.0000)	0.0004	(0.0000)	0.053
Divorced			–0.315	(0.028)	–0.327	(0.051)	–0.327	(0.051)	–0.481	(0.049)	–0.046
Widowed			–0.174	(0.051)	–0.186	(0.051)	–0.187	(0.052)	–0.228	(0.051)	–0.024
Married			0.378	(0.029)	0.375	(0.029)	0.374	(0.029)	0.243	(0.027)	0.050
Group effect											
Real GDP (/1000)							0.070	(0.016)	0.104	(0.008)	0.284
Interaction effect											
IncML∗Rgdp (/1000)									–0.014	(0.008)	–0.019
IncMH∗Rgdp (/1000)									–0.034	(0.013)	–0.046
IncHigh∗Rgdp (/1000)									–0.035	(0.014)	–0.047

TABLE III

Continued

	Model 1		Model 2		Model 3		Model 4		Model 5		Model 5
	Coefficient	SE	Coefficient	SE	Coefficient	SE	Coefficient	SE	Coefficient	SE	Standardized Coefficient β
RANDOM PART											
Level 2											
Var Cons	0.666	(0.146)	0.671	(0.148)	0.996	(0.221)	0.630	(0.143)	0.589	(0.134)	
Cov Cons-IncML					–0.156	(0.060)	–0.120	(0.048)	–0.102	(0.044)	
Var IncMedLow					0.082	(0.026)	0.081	(0.026)	0.074	(0.024)	
Cov Cons-IncMH					–0.342	(0.101)	–0.247	(0.079)	–0.210	(0.070)	
Cov IncML-IncMH					0.139	(0.038)	0.139	(0.038)	0.120	(0.034)	
Var IncMedHigh					0.259	(0.064)	0.256	(0.064)	0.214	(0.055)	
Cov Cons-IncH					–0.372	(0.110)	–0.276	(0.086)	–0.233	(0.077)	
Cov IncML-IncH					0.154	(0.041)	0.154	(0.041)	0.135	(0.037)	
Cov IncMH-IncH					0.281	(0.068)	0.279	(0.068)	0.237	(0.058)	
Var IncHigh					0.313	(0.076)	0.310	(0.075)	0.265	(0.065)	
Level 1											
Var Cons	4.635	(0.029)	4.511	(0.029)	5.527	(0.069)	5.526	(0.069)	5.527	(0.069)	
"Cov" Cons-IncML					–0.515	(0.045)	–0.515	(0.045)	–0.515	(0.045)	
"Cov" Cons-IncMH					–0.675	(0.044)	–0.675	(0.044)	–0.675	(0.044)	
"Cov" IncL-IncH					–0.974	(0.041)	–0.974	(0.041)	–0.974	(0.041)	
Deviance		218994		217631		216465		215451		216443	
Deviance difference		5625		1363		1166		14		9	
Df difference		1		8		13		1		3	

Note: N = 50,046 individuals in 42 countries. Age, age-squared and real GDP are entered as centered variables.

TABLE IV

Variance of Life Satisfaction at Level 1 and Level 2 for Model 3, 4, and 5

	Model 3		Model 4	Model 5
Income Group	Level 1 Variance	Level 2 Variance	Level 2 Variance	Level 2 Variance
Income Low	5.527	0.996	0.630	0.589
Income MedLow	4.497	0.765	0.473	0.459
Income MedHigh	4.177	0.572	0.392	0.390
Income High	3.579	0.565	0.388	0.388

Note: Level 1 Variance does not change in Model 4 and 5.

addition to modeling differences in average life satisfaction between income categories (the fixed part of the model), it is also possible to model differences in variances in life satisfaction between nations and between individuals (the random part of the model). The model in this study anticipates complex between-nation and between-individual heterogeneity. In other words, it is expected that not only nations but also individuals differ with regard to variance in life satisfaction.

It is important to consider both levels of heterogeneity simultaneously in a model, since one might be mistaken for the other: what may appear as between-nation heterogeneity can in reality be between-individual heterogeneity (Bullen et al., 1997: p. 585; Jones and Duncan, 1998: p. 107). In the next step, the coefficients of the dummy variables of income were made random at the individual level and at the nation level. Since income is a categorical predictor in the model, contrast-coding was employed to estimate the (co)variances at both levels.[26] Results are shown in model 3, Table III.

In order to see more clearly how the variance in life satisfaction at level 1 and 2 for model 3 changes as the income rises, in Table IV variances for each income group are presented:[27] both at the between-nation and the within-nation level, the variation in life satisfaction between the four income groups declines as the income rises. The greatest variation in life satisfaction *between nations* remains for the lowest income group, while the highest two income groups have the smallest remaining variation. At the *within-nation*

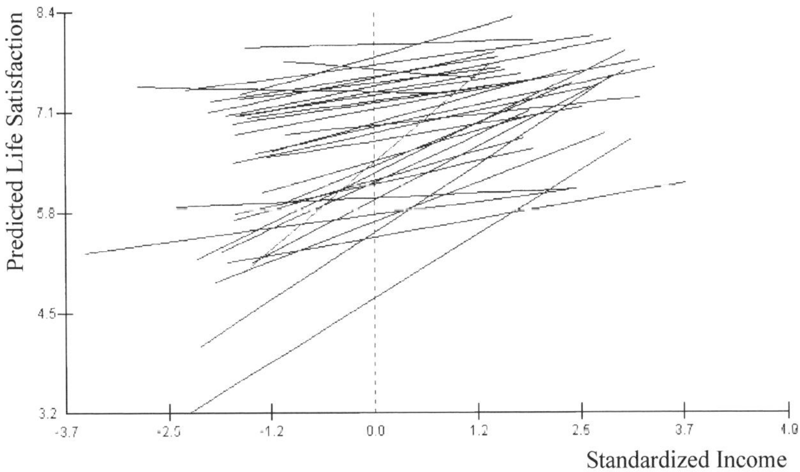

Figure 3. Country variation in life satisfaction: 42 regression lines between income and life satisfaction.

level, the lowest income category is the most variable in life satisfaction, while the highest category is the most consistent. It can also be seen that the between-nation variation is relatively small compared to the between-individual variation.

The Chi-square test shows that this model is an improvement compared to the previous model. The difference in deviance is 1166, which, compared to a critical value of 22.36 (df = 13, $p < 0.05$) is significant. The fully random model can be visualized by plotting the 42 different regression lines between income and predicted life satisfaction, as shown in Figure 3.[28] It can be seen that this figure is rather similar to Figure 2.

In the following model, an explanatory variable of the highest level was included to explain between-nation variability in life satisfaction: real GDP per capita in 1990 (in $1000). The variable was entered as a centered variable. The average respondent in the model hence became a low income, single person, of average age, living in an average wealthy nation. To test a possible curvilinear relationship between wealth and life satisfaction, in addition to the normal real GDP, the quadratic term of real GDP was also included (not shown). However, the effect of real GDP-squared was not significant and was therefore not included in the model.

As can be seen in Table III, model 4, the wealth of a nation is positively related to life satisfaction, even after taking a range of individual level variables into account. It suggests that individuals who live in economically more prosperous countries witness a higher life satisfaction irrespective of their individual characteristics. These results confirmed hypothesis 2, but did not confirm hypothesis 2.1.

The introduction of real GDP reduced the proportion of unexplained variance due to country variation quite substantially (see Table IV, model 4). Nevertheless, the variance component is still significantly different from zero, which means that the nation variable introduced in this model cannot explain all the between-nation variability in life satisfaction.

Compared to the model with only lower level explanatory variables, this model is an improvement. The difference in deviance is 14 (216465–216451), which, compared to the critical value of 3.84 ($df = 1; p < 0.05$), is significant.

In sum, in the previous models, firstly, the main effects of the individual level explanatory variables were shown. Income at the individual level was positively (curvilinearly) related to life satisfaction, even when controlling for the other variables. Secondly, complex variation at level 2 and level 1 was found: between nations, the lowest income group had the greatest remaining variation in life satisfaction, and within nations, life satisfaction varied greater among poor individuals than among rich. Thirdly, at the nation level, real GDP was included to explain between-nation variability in life satisfaction. It was positively (linearly) related to life satisfaction and its inclusion resulted in a reduction of country level variance to quite an extent.

Finally, interaction-terms between real GDP and the three income dummy variables were added to the model. It was hypothesized that in wealthier countries the relationship between income and life satisfaction is weaker than in poor countries. The economic prosperity of a nation acts as a moderator variable for the relationship between income and life satisfaction. This resulted in the fully specified multilevel model in Table III, model 5.

All three cross-level interaction effects were significant (although just barely) and negative. At first, this might seem counterintuitive, since one would expect richer countries and richer individuals to be more satisfied with their lives. To get a better impression of the

TABLE V

Estimated Values of Life Satisfaction, as a Function of the Individual's Income Group and the Nation's Score on Real GDP

Income Group	Min. Real GDP	Mean Real GDP	Max. Real GDP
Income Low	5.29	6.27	7.41
Income MedLow	5.71	6.56	7.55
Income MedHigh	6.13	6.78	7.55
Income High	6.29	6.94	7.70

Note: Values of the "average" respondent (single, average age) are shown in the table.

substantive content of the interaction effects, estimated life satisfaction scores were computed for some combinations. Since real GDP was centered, the minimum value (poorest nation), mean value (average nation) and maximum value (richest nation) were used for each income category (reference group to highest income group). Results are shown in Table V.

What is obvious from the table is that in the poorest nation, differences between the life satisfaction scores of the low-income individual and the highest-income individual are largest, whereas in the richest nation these differences are much smaller. Put differently, poor persons who live in a poor nation are less satisfied with their lives than poor persons who live in an affluent nation (difference of 2.12), whereas this difference in life satisfaction is less for the highest income-group (difference of 1.41). This result is in accordance with the hypothesized relation between wealth of a nation and the relation between income and life satisfaction: the relation between income and life satisfaction is weaker in rich nations than in poor nations (hypothesis 3). The introduction of the cross-level interaction effects reduced the proportion of unexplained between-nation variance only marginally, as can be seen in Table IV, model 5. This final model is an improvement over model 4 (difference in deviance 9, critical value 7.81 with 3 degrees of freedom, $p < 0.05$).

However, the effects are just barely significant, and definitely need to be confirmed in other data sets. Interaction effects are visually presented in Figure 4. In addition, this figure shows more clearly

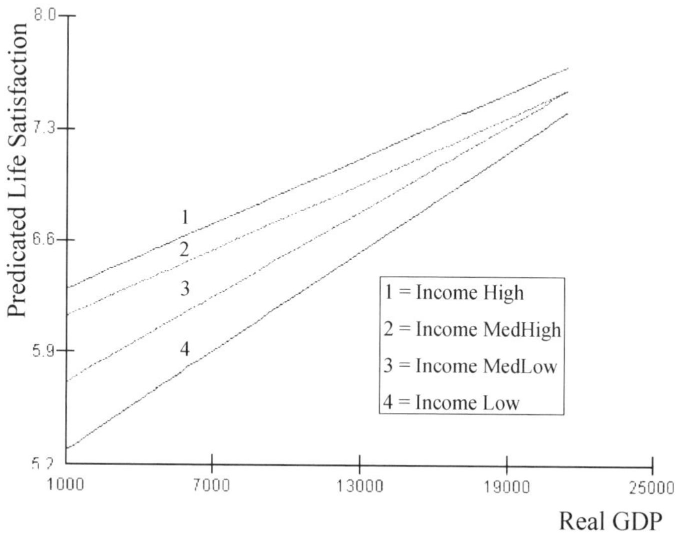

Figure 4. Cross-level interaction effect: Wealth of nations, income and life satisfaction.

than Table V that differences in life satisfaction between the income quartile groups become smaller as a nation's wealth grows.

Finally, since it is standard practice in multilevel modeling to present only the unstandardized coefficients, it is difficult to compare the impact of the different effects. For example, real GDP is measured on a different scale than household income, so in order to compare the effects in the final model, beta coefficients were computed manually. This is shown in the last column of Table III. The strongest effect can be witnessed for wealth of a nation, 0.284, as compared to the relatively low effects of income, the control variables, and the interaction-effects. This means that the macro-level variable wealth of a nation is a stronger predictor of life satisfaction than the micro-level variables.

5. CONCLUSION AND DISCUSSION

The starting point of this study was a multilevel design in which, in addition to individual characteristics, country characteristics were assumed to be related to life satisfaction at the individual level. Two theories that are not usually directly connected, since they are tested at one level only, were now combined in one multilevel theory and the implications were translated into five hypotheses. The last hypothesis concerned a cross-level interaction effect between the individual and the context level.

The first question was: what are the effects of economic prosperity at the nation level and income at the individual level on life satisfaction? At the individual level, a positive but weak relationship between income and life satisfaction was found: people in higher income groups were more satisfied with their lives, even when marital status and age were taken into account. The curvilinear hypothesis that income has a diminishing marginal utility was confirmed in the sense that the coefficients of the dummies showed a drop in their relative size. However, although there was a declining effect, their size was still large enough to refute the argument that there is no extra effect at all. Introduced variables at this level only accounted for 2.7% of the explained variance at the individual level.

At the level of nations, one variable was deemed important to increase a person's life satisfaction, namely the wealth of a nation. Real GDP was positively correlated with life satisfaction, and it reduced the variance at the level of nations to quite some extent. The hypothesized curvilinear relationship between wealth of countries and life satisfaction was, however, not confirmed by the data, that is, beyond a certain level of wealth, no declining effect on life satisfaction was witnessed. Nevertheless, the between-nation variance was still significantly different from zero, which means that variables other than those introduced in this study are needed to explain between-nation differences in life satisfaction.

The second question was whether, in addition to these main effects, there is a cross-level interaction effect of a nation level variable on the relationship between individual level variables. It was hypothesized that the relationship between income and life satisfaction differs depending on the wealth of a nation: in poor countries this relationship is stronger than in rich countries. The interaction effects were significant, although weak, and confirmed the hypothesis. Poor persons living in a poor nation were less satisfied with their lives than poor persons living in a rich nation: the difference in life satisfaction was on average 2.12 points on a 10 point-scale. In more general terms: in countries with low real GDP, there are quite some differences in life satisfaction between the income categories, however, in countries with high real GDP, these differences disappear, and all people are happier.

Moreover, it was found that individuals with low incomes vary more in life satisfaction than individuals with high incomes. This resulted from explicitly modeling heterogeneity at the within-nation level. It emphasizes even more the importance of having a sufficient income to satisfy basic needs for people in the lower income ranges.

This study was a first step towards a multilevel theory and model in the QoL field. Several things need to be improved. First of all, missing values need to be studied in order to determine if a particular group of respondents is systematically missing. It is known, for example, from several panel studies, that people who are missing on the income variable usually belong to the lower income groups and the most affluent groups. This could mean that the sample that was used for this analysis is skewed towards the mean or modal income groups. Moreover, the income variable in the World Values Survey was not measured perfectly either. More precise indicators (on a ratio-scale, and including, for example, savings, property (e.g., housing), information on household composition, etc.) of income improve the quality of the data.

Second, in order to make general statements, a better sample of the world population is needed. Although the World Values Survey II contains several economically less prosperous countries, it is still skewed towards the richer Western nations. In this sense, the 42 countries are not a perfect random sample coming from a distribution, hampering a generalization to the world population. Replicating the model on a bigger and more varied data set (e.g., the World Values Survey III with 54 nations)[29] will make the results found in this study more robust.

It is also known from other studies (e.g., Schyns, 2000) that income-satisfaction is an important intermediary variable connecting income and life satisfaction. Future models should take this variable into account as well.

As stated earlier, it would also be interesting to include other variables at the between-nation level that might affect life satisfaction, for example, income inequality and cultural factors such as freedom or individualism. Some critics claim that it is not absolute wealth that matters to people, but relative wealth. Stated simply, in countries in which wealth is unequally distributed, those below the average income-line are less satisfied with their lives, and those above the line are more satisfied (see, for example, Easterlin, 1995; Wilkinson, 1996).

At the level of nations, results concerning the effect of income (in)equality on subjective well-being are, however, not unambiguous: several studies found a positive relationship between income equality and subjective well-being, which sometimes disappeared after the effect of wealth was taken into account, whereas for income *in*equality, some studies found nonsignificant effects for the zero order correlation, but positive effects after having controlled for wealth (for an overview see Diener and Oishi, 2000).[30]

In the present study, some preliminary analyses including the Gini coefficient for 40 countries of the World Values Survey in the multilevel model, showed a small significant positive correlation between income *in*equality at the country level and life satisfaction at the individual level. Although replication of the findings on a larger sample of nations is needed before any firm conclusions can be drawn, the results suggest that income equality is not necessarily a requirement for a higher subjective well-being, nor does it appear to be a more important factor in contributing to a person's life satisfaction than absolute wealth of a nation.

Concerning the inclusion of a cultural variable, other problems were encountered. Variables such as political rights, individualism, and the emancipation of women correlated highly with the wealth of a nation, making it impossible to disentangle the different effects on life satisfaction in one model.[31] For practical reasons also, adding many variables to the model – especially at the higher level with only a small N – should be avoided, and a parsimonious model is preferred.

These outcomes teach us that at the level of formulation of theories (especially concerning social comparison), and at the level of finding robust indicators a lot of work still has to be done.

Nevertheless, the multilevel approach is a powerful tool and has several advantages over the more traditional ways of analyzing effects on subjective well-being, such as the nation level study or individual level study (mono-level studies) mentioned in the introduction.

Compared to the traditional "two step" models, on which the multilevel model is conceptually based, the multilevel model has the technical advantage of connecting regressions within groups and between groups in one model, resulting in more reliable estimations (Kreft and De Leeuw, 1998: p. 2).

Moreover, the multilevel method allows for differentiating between three separate effects: main effects at the individual level, main effects at the group level, and cross-level interaction effects on life satisfaction. In mono-level studies, no conclusions can be drawn at another level, since this would imply committing one of the famous fallacies. Using multilevel modeling, however, resulted in the finding of an independent, larger effect of wealth of the nation on life satisfaction in addition to a small positive effect of income on life satisfaction. This is an important contribution to the discussion, since it reveals that the social context in which people live can have an independent effect on life satisfaction. Also, in the earlier mentioned multilevel studies, similar context effects were found at the neighborhood, country, and regional level (Fernandez and Kulik, 1981; Mastekaasa and Moum, 1984; Rampichini and Schifini d'Andrea, 1998). After all, the idea that individuals respond to their social contexts is a major claim of the sociological discipline (DiPrete and Forristal, 1994).

Finally, multilevel modeling is an instrument that does not take differences between individuals and nations for granted, but can explicitly model these variances. It is not only important to estimate averages, but also to take differences between nations and people into account. This study is one of the first studies that has shown that people with low income vary more in their life satisfaction than people with high income.

All in all, the multilevel approach is a fruitful one, if one is interested in combining several levels theoretically as well as empirically. It definitely deserves more attention from QoL researchers in the future.

ACKNOWLEDGEMENTS

I would like to thank the following people for their helpful comments on earlier drafts and/or the final version: Aaron Ahuvia,

Andrew Clark, Bob Cummins, Kelvyn Jones, Paul Nieuwbeerta, Ruut Veenhoven, Bruno Zumbo, and two anonymous reviewers.

NOTES

[1] The terms macro level, group level, and (between-)nation level will be used interchangeably to denote the level of nations/countries, whereas the terms micro level, individual level and within-nation level will be reserved for the level of individuals.

[2] It should be noted that although causal language is employed throughout this article, multilevel modeling – as is true for most statistical modeling techniques – produces at best only correlational output. It is up to the researcher to build an a priori causal theory, in which causal paths are explicitly mentioned. However, there is empirical evidence that suggests that a causal path leads from income to subjective well-being (Diener and Oishi, 2000: p. 197). If the causal chain is reversed, the effects of happiness on income are not large (*ibid.*, p. 198).

[3] For graphical displays, the programme MlwiN – MLn's windows version – was used.

[4] Here the term "wealth" or "economic prosperity" will be reserved for the economic variable at the country level, and "income" or "household income" for the economic variable at the individual level.

[5] This is called, respectively, aggregation and disaggregation of the data (Hox, 1995: p. 4).

[6] Other names for the models are hierarchical (mixed) linear model, bayesian linear model, and random coefficients model (DiPrete and Forristal, 1994: p. 333).

[7] Apparently, they did not use a hierarchical model, but a "two step" model.

[8] Rampichini and Schifini D'Andrea used a hierarchical probit model for their analysis.

[9] Although these theories are formulated at the country level, they are "hidden" multilevel theories since they connect country characteristics such as wealth and national character to life satisfaction, which is a micro-level characteristic. It can be added that national character theory in the sense of "modal personality" of a country (as defined by, for example, Inkeles (1997)) is a macro-level theory derived from the micro level.

[10] Exceptions are the earlier mentioned studies by Fernandez and Kulik (1981), Mastekaasa and Moum (1984), Rampichini and Schifini d'Andrea (1998), and Oishi et al. (1999).

[11] Maslow portrays a somewhat ambiguous view on the (over)satisfaction of love and esteem needs: on the one hand he admits the needs' unlimited nature of satisfaction, but on the other hand he acknowledges pathological problems associated with being loved and adored too much.

[12] Livability has a broader connotation than economic prosperity alone. One could also think of livability in terms of economic inequality, or cultural factors such as political freedom or individualism. However, due to theoretical and

empirical problems (e.g., conceptual ambiguity, multicolinearity, lack of clear indicators for 42 countries), in this study, livability will be confined to the area of economic prosperity. See also the discussion.

[13] Individuals can also affect group level variables, but in this study only effects of higher level variables on the lower were studied.

[14] La Barbera and Gurhan (1997) found in their study a negative correlation between materialism and happiness.

[15] Most surveys were held in 1990. Some countries collected their data at a different point in time, ranging from winter 1988 (Switzerland) to spring 1993 (Romania).

[16] Australia was not included in the 1990 wave, and Iceland lacked the income variable in 1990. According to Headey, life satisfaction in Australia did not change much in the 1980s and disposable income inequality was about the same in 1990 as in 1980 (e-mail communication, November 2000). Hence, using the 1980 data instead of 1990 data can bc justified. Life satisfaction in Iceland remained approximately the same as well (mean life satisfaction of 8.06 in 1981, and 8.02 in 1990; standard deviation of 1.61 in 1981, and 1.60 in 1990). Unfortunately, figures on, for example, changing Gini coefficients could not be found, but it seems reasonable to assume that income inequality has not changed dramatically either over these 10 years in Iceland.

[17] It has to be noted that, although countries included in the World Values Survey are much more representative of the world than past surveys, nevertheless, extremely poor countries, as well as small nations, remain underrepresented.

[18] Unfortunately, education – which is often used as a background variable as well – was missing for quite some countries in the World Values Survey, and hence not included in the analyses.

[19] Adapted from Jones et al. (1992).

[20] Since the relationship between income and life satisfaction is presumed to be curvilinear, here the log of income is displayed on the horizontal axis. In the analysis, however, no log transformation was carried out, since the relative size of the coefficients of the income dummy variables already shows a possible curvilinear effect.

[21] *Technical note*: For the interested reader, a description is provided of the derivation of the formula. The difference with the usual regression model is that here we assume that each country is characterized by a different intercept coefficient β_{0j} and also a different slope coefficient β_{1j} (Hox, 1995: p. 11). For each country, assuming for reasons of simplicity only one explanatory variable X, the general equation would be: (i) $Y_{ij} = \beta_{0j} + \beta_{1j}X_{ij} + \varepsilon_{ij}$.

In this example, Y_{ij} is the level of life satisfaction of individual i in country j. The model can be decomposed into a systematic part and a random part. The systematic part consists of the level of life satisfaction of an average income individual in country j (β_{0j}) plus the change in life satisfaction for a unit increase in income in country j ($\beta_{1j}X_{ij}$). The random part consists of the residual variation for each individual (ε_{ij}).

Since the coefficients are allowed to vary over countries, the next step in the multilevel model is to predict the variation of the regression coefficient β_{0j} and β_{1j} by introducing variable Z at the country level. This results in the two following equations:

(ii) $\beta_{0j} = \gamma_{00} + \gamma_{01}Z_j + \mu_{0j}$, and
(iii) $\beta_{1j} = \gamma_{10} + \gamma_{11}Z_j + \mu_{1j}$,

where, in this example, β_{0j} is life satisfaction of a person of average income in country j, γ_{00} is the overall intercept, that is, the average life satisfaction of a person of average income everywhere, $\gamma_{01}Z_j$ is the effect of wealth of countries, and μ_{0j} is the differential intercept for country j. β_{1j} is the relationship between life satisfaction and income in country j, γ_{10} is the overall slope, representing the relationship between life satisfaction and income everywhere, $\gamma_{11}Z_j$ is the effect of wealth of countries, and μ_{1j} is the differential slope for country j. In equation (ii) and (iii), μ_{0j} and μ_{1j} are the random residual error terms at the country level. If one rearranges the terms and inserts all the variables, equation (1) will follow.

[22] Here the complete random part is not fully written out in order to keep the model readable. X_{pij} stands for p lower level explanatory variables; nine in this model.

[23] The intra-class correlation is the variance at the group level divided by the total variance. At the level of countries, the error variance is 0.666, whereas at the level of individuals the variance of errors is 4.635. Individuals vary much more with regard to life satisfaction than do countries.

[24] The intercept is the value of the response variable when all explanatory variables are zero. Since neither age nor age-squared have meaningful zeros (the minimum age is 18), centering the variables results in a meaningful intercept. That is, the intercept reflects the life satisfaction of an average aged, single, low income person.

[25] In normal regression modeling, it is impossible for the multiple correlation R^2 to get smaller after adding explanatory variables. Since in a multilevel model variances at two levels are present, R^2 does not have the same meaning anymore, hence it is better to speak of a pseudo R^2. For a discussion, see Kreft and De Leeuw (1998).

[26] For a more detailed description of the techniques of contrast-coding and separate coding with categorical variables, see Bullen et al. (1997).

[27] The variances were calculated as follows at the between-nation level: variance for the reference category (lowest income group) = $\sigma^2_{\mu 0}$; variance second income quartile = $\sigma^2_{\mu 0} + 2\sigma_{\mu 0 \mu 1} + \sigma^2_{\mu 1}$; variance third quartile = $\sigma^2_{\mu 0} + 2\sigma_{\mu 0 \mu 2} + \sigma^2_{\mu 2}$; variance fourth quartile = $\sigma^2_{\mu 0} + 2\sigma_{\mu 0 \mu 3} + \sigma^2_{\mu 3}$. At the within-nation level: variance reference group = $\sigma^2_{\varepsilon 0}$; second income quartile = $\sigma^2_{\varepsilon 0} + 2\sigma_{\varepsilon 0 \varepsilon 1}$; third income quartile = $\sigma^2_{\varepsilon 0} + 2\sigma_{\varepsilon 0 \varepsilon 2}$; fourth income quartile = $\sigma^2_{\varepsilon 0} + 2\sigma_{\varepsilon 0 \varepsilon 3}$.

[28] The z-income instead of the three dummy variables was used to show the slopes between income and life satisfaction. As stated before, it was only used for demonstration purposes.

[29] Unfortunately, at the time of analyzing the data, the WVS III were not yet publicly available.
[30] According to Diener and Oishi, this unexpected positive correlation probably occurred because in some Latin American nations subjective well-being is higher than would be predicted based on income, but income equality is low, and some Eastern European nations have relatively high income equality versus a low subjective well-being (Diener and Oishi, 2000: p. 206).
[31] Because of multicolinearity, in MLn two models were run separately, each with one of the group level variable (real GDP or political rights) included at a time. Real GDP turned out to be the most significant variable.

REFERENCES

Ahuvia, A. C. and D. C. Friedman: 1998, 'Income, consumption, and subjective well-being: toward a composite macromarketing model', Journal of Macromarketing 18(2), pp. 153–168.

Aitkin, M. A. and N. T. Longford: 1986, 'Statistical modeling issues in school effectiveness studies', Journal of the Royal Statistical Society A 149, pp. 1–43.

Bullen, N., K. Jones and C. Duncan: 1997, 'Modelling complexity: analysing between-individual and between-place variation – a multilevel tutorial', Environment and Planning A 29, pp. 585–609.

Clark, A.: 1999, Unemployment as a social norm: psychological evidence from panel data (Document de Recherche).

Clark, A., Y. Georgellis and P. Sanfrey: 1999, Scarring: the psychological impact of past unemployment (Document de Recherche).

Diener, E., M. Diener and C. Diener: 1995, 'Factors predicting the subjective well-being of nations', Journal of Personality and Social Psychology 5, pp. 851–864.

Diener, E., J. Horwitz and R. Emmons: 1985, 'Happiness of the very wealthy', Social Indicators Research 16, pp. 263–274.

Diener, E. and S. Oishi: 2000, 'Money and happiness: income and subjective well-being across nations', in E. Diener and E. M. Suh (eds.), Subjective Well-Being across Cultures (MIT Press, Cambridge MA).

Diener, E., E. M. Suh, R. E. Lucas and H. L. Smith: 1999, 'Subjective well-being: three decades of progress', Psychological Bulletin 125, pp. 276–302.

DiPrete, E. and R. Biswas-Diener: 1999, Income and Subjective Well-being: Will Money Make Us Happy? (Unpublished paper).

DiPrete, T. A. and J. D. Forristal: 1994, 'Multilevel models: methods and substance', Annual Review Sociology 20, pp. 331–357.

Di Tella, R., R. J. MacCulloch and A. J. Oswald: 2000, 'Preferences over inflation and unemployment: evidence from surveys of happiness', Forthcoming in American Economic Review.

Easterlin, R. A.: 1995, 'Will raising the income of all increase the happiness of all?', Journal of Economic Behaviour and Organisation 27, pp. 35–47.

Fernandez, R. M. and J. C. Kulik: 1981, 'A multilevel model of life satisfaction: effects of individual characteristics and neighborhood composition', American Sociological Review 46, pp. 840–850.

Headey, B. and A. Wearing: 1992, Understanding Happiness, A Theory of Subjective Well-being (Longman Cheshire, Melbourne).

Hox, J. J.: 1995, Applied Multilevel Analysis (TT-Publikaties, Amsterdam).

Hüttner, H. J. M.: 1995, 'Marginaal: Onderzoeken op niveau', Sociologische Gids, jg. XLII, juli/okt., pp. 272–284.

Inkeles, A.: 1997, National Character, A Psycho-Social Perspective (Transaction Publishers, New Brunswick).

Jones, K. and C. Duncan: 1998, 'Modelling context and heterogeneity: applying multilevel models', in E. Scarborough and E. Tanenbaum (eds.), Research Strategies in the Social Sciences: A Guide to New Approaches (Oxford University Press, Oxford).

Jones, K., R. J. Johnston and C. J. Pattie: 1992, 'People, places and regions: exploring the use of multi-level modelling in the analysis of electoral data', British Journal of Political Science 22: pp. 343–380.

Kreft, I. and J. De Leeuw: 1998, Introducing Multilevel Modeling (Sage Publications, London).

Kuper, A. and J. Kuper: 1996, The Social Science Encyclopedia (Routledge, New York).

La Barbera, P. and Z. Gurhan: 1997, 'The role of materialism, religiosity and demographics in subjective well-being', Psychology and Marketing 14, pp. 71–97.

Lane, R. E.: 1996, The Joyless Market Economy. Paper presented at the Conference on Economics, Values, and Organization (Yale University, New Haven, CT), April.

Maslow, A. H.: 1970, Motivation and Personality, 2nd edition (Harper & Row Publishers, New York).

Maslow, A. H.: 1987, Motivation and Personality, 3rd edition (Longman Publishers, New York).

Mastekaasa, A. and T. Moum: 1984, 'The perceived quality of life in Norway: regional variations and contextual effects', Social Indicators Research 14, pp. 385–419.

Oishi, S., E. Diener, R. Lucas and E. Suh: 1999, 'Cross-Cultural variations in predictors of life satisfaction: perspectives from needs and values', Personality and Social Psychology Bulletin 25(8), pp. 980–990.

Poel, van der, M. G. M.: 1993, Personal Networks: A Rational Choice Explanation of Their Size And Composition (Swets & Zeitlinger, Lisse).

Rampichini, C. and S. Schifini d'Andrea: 1998, 'A hierarchical ordinal probit model for the analysis of life satisfaction in Italy', Social Indicators Research 44, pp. 41–69.

Robinson, W. S.: 1950, 'Ecological correlations and the behavior of individuals', American Sociological Review 15, pp. 351–357.

Rosenfeld, R.: 1992, 'Job mobility and career processes', Annual Review of Sociology 18, pp. 39–61.

Saris, W. and A. Andreenkova: 1997, 'Study of the effect of individual income changes on satisfaction in Russia', in W. Saris, R. Veenhoven, R. Scherpenzeel and B. Bunting (eds.), A Comparative Study of Satisfaction with Life in Europe (Eötvos University Press, Budapest).

Schor, J. B.: 1991, The Overworked American, The Unexpected Decline of Leisure (Basic Books, New York).

Schyns, P.: 1996, Gender en geluk. Paper presented at the Young Researcher's Day, SISWO, November 22, Amsterdam.

Schyns, P.: 1998, 'Crossnational differences in happiness: economic and cultural factors explored', Social Indicators Research 43, pp. 3–26.

Schyns, P.: 2000, 'The relationship between income, change in income and life satisfaction in West Germany and the Russian Federation: absolute, relative or a combination of both?', in E. Diener and D. Rahtz (eds.), Advances in Quality of Life Theory and Research (Kluwer, Dordrecht).

Snijders, T. and R. J. Bosker: 1997, The Introduction to Multilevel Analysis, reader, March.

Tacq, J. J. A.: 1994, 'Vragen aan Jacques', Facta, Sociaal Wetenschappelijk Magazine, vol.2 (issue 5), pp. 32–37 (3).

United Nations Development Programme: 1993, Human Development Report 1993 (Oxford University Press, New York).

United Nations Development Programme: 1996, Human Development Report 1996 (Oxford University Press, New York).

Veenhoven, R.: 1991, 'Is happiness relative?', Social Indicators Research 24, pp. 1–34.

Veenhoven, R.: 1995, 'The cross-national pattern of happiness: test of predictions implied in three theories of happiness', Social Indicators Research 34, pp. 33–68.

Wilkinson, R. G.: 1996, Unhealthy Societies, The Afflictions of Inequality (Routledge, London).

Woodhouse, G. (ed.): 1995, A Guide to MLn for New Users (Institute of Education, University of London).

World Values Study Group: 1994, World Values Survey (Codebook), 1981–1984 and 1990–1993 (ICPSR version, ICPSR, Ann Arbor, Michigan).

SHEREEN T. ISMAEL

A PAR APPROACH TO QUALITY OF LIFE: MODELING HEALTH THROUGH PARTICIPATION

Health is a fundamental component of quality of life. How one defines what constitutes health affects the extent to which we understand its impacts on quality of life in communities. In this paper an expanded model of health which uses a participatory action approach will be proposed. This will be accomplished by: (1) briefly outlining the Canadian government's changing vision of health; (2) examining core concepts related to participatory action research; (3) using a case example of a First Nation community in Northern Alberta to demonstrate the importance of the interrelationship between research and action in understanding the determinants of health and quality of life.

In examining the Canadian Federal Government's health policies, it is concluded that Canada has evolved a new vision of health. Canada's approach to health can be seen to have gone through three phases, each expanding on what constitutes health. The first phase (or model) is a narrow biomedical focus pathologizing the individual person (regardless of gender) on the basis of biology. The second phase of the evolution involved the recognition of women as being separate and distinct in terms of medical needs (e.g., epidemiological research of breast cancer). Phase three involved the expansion of the medical model to recognize the relevance of social factors as related to health. This phase identified broad social categories such as class and gender as being relevant to health. These categories tended to be examined as discrete variables without consideration of how they interacted with each other. Recently, there has been an interest in the area of Population Health to consider how these variables interact.

Understanding the relationship and the interaction of social, economic, political and environmental variables in communities is essential when attempting to explain the determinants of health.

Social Indicators Research **60:** 41–54, 2002.

From a feminist perspective the research has tended to focus on women as a discrete group. For example, recently the senior advisor on the status of women at Health and Welfare Canada, Frieda Paltiel (Paltiel, 1993), argued that women's health can be understood to be affected by several "interlocking" variables:

- absolute-relative poverty or the threat thereof;
- gender-based violence;
- a support gap wherein women give far more care and support than men or than they receive;
- reproductive tasks of pregnancy, childbirth and breastfeeding;
- greater longevity than men;
- discrimination/sexism

The feminist approach taken by Paltiel and others regarding women's health is a first step in developing a more comprehensive definition of health. I argue that it is essential to address **all** members of communities in the context of race, class and gender in exploring the interrelationship of the variables – social, economic, political, and environmental – to fully understand the determinants of health. Furthermore, I maintain that it is essential to understand how a community experiences health and health care services.

CORE CONCEPTS

Fundamental to this model of health is the incorporation of a process known as participatory action research (PAR). PAR is a style of research which sees **process** as the integral link between research and action. The approach is based on the intersection of the core concepts of: (1) participatory action; (2) needs assessment; and (3) emancipatory practice. If we are to maximize health and overall quality of life of individuals, communities and society, then a research process that involves collective social investigation and education is critical.

1. *Participatory Action*

PAR is a form of action research and has many variations in both theory and practice. These variations reflect differing epistemological traditions. A generic definition that addresses the phenomenological dimensions defines PAR as

> ... a process of systematic inquiry, in which those who are experiencing a problematic situation in a community ... participate collaboratively with trained researchers as subjects, in deciding the focus of knowledge generation, in collecting and analyzing information, and in taking action to manage, improve, or solve their problem situation (Deshler and Ewart, 1995).

There are a set of values common to the various theoretical traditions that embrace PAR.

These include:

1. the democratization of knowledge
2. production and use of ethical fairness in the benefits of knowledge generation process
3. an ecological stance toward society and nature
4. appreciation of the capacity of humans to reflect, learn and change and
5. a commitment to nonviolent social change (House et al., 1995)

2. *Needs Assessment*

Like the definitions of participatory action, there are many approaches to needs assessments in theory and practice. The definitions vary on epistemological and phenomenological dimensions. Summers sums this up by noting that needs assessment may be described as a methodology "that integrates ideas from political theories of democracy with practices flowing from the mainstream of social science research" (Summers, 1987: p. 3). Rothman's typology of needs provides a framework for understanding epistemological variation. He identifies four types of needs: (1) normative need, in which standards of service or living standards are compared to an established standard; (2) comparative need, in which the standard of comparison is another group; (3) felt need, which is need as determined by those experiencing the problem, and (4) expressed need, which is need inferred from requests for service (Rothman and Gant, 1987: pp. 35–43). Community health needs assessment has developed into an important tool for the identification of health service needs in the context of health status. "Health status refers to the present state of wellness or illness in a community and is defined by measures of good and poor health practices, rates of death and disease (chronic and infectious), and the prevalence of symptoms/conditions of illness and wellness" (Deprez and Horton, 1996).

3. *Emancipatory Practice*

Emancipatory practice is a concept that expresses a kind of professional human service practice that focuses on outcomes rather than processes. Specifically, the outcome of emancipation is the point of practice. Webster's dictionary defines emancipation as "a setting free or being set free from servitude, bondage, or restraint". This is not to imply that we are arguing that the end justifies the means. Rather, we argue that means are the ends (two sides of the same coin or two coins of the same side). In the framework of emancipatory practice, in other words, the process must be emancipatory, and therefore is an end in itself.

While the works of Pablo Friere (1990) and Franz Fanon (1967) laid the intellectual foundations for the concept of emancipatory practice, the works of Mullaly and Bishop provided the framework for its application to social work practice. Mullaly defined his approach as structural social work and explained it accordingly:

> The approach to social welfare system emanates from the radical humanist school of thought. This approach is based on the belief that changing people by personal consciousness-raising on a massive scale is a prerequisite for changing society. This consciousness-raising, which is carried out by structural social workers with service users and with co-workers focuses on raising people's awareness of how capitalist society shapes, limits, and dominates their experiences, thus alienating them from social structures, from each other, and from their true selves. Only by becoming aware of how others define us to suit their own interests and by understanding how ideological hegemony makes our subjugation appear acceptable can we become free to regain control over our lives and our destiny (Mullaly, 1993: p. 154).

Utilizing the core concepts: (1) participatory action; (2) needs assessments; and (3) emancipatory practice, removes the separation between research (knowing) and action (doing). Furthermore, PAR removes a dichotomy between knower and known. This empowers those involved in the research process to improve their health and quality of life. In summary, quality of life research needs to move beyond the description and interpretation of determinants of social dynamics and needs to empower individuals and communities and enable them to develop strategies that address social contradictions and inequities. I will apply the participatory action approach to a model of health using a case example of a First Nation Community in Northern Alberta.

THE HEALTH MODEL

As we have noted, we argue that a broader definition of health which considers the interrelationship of a wide variety of social, economic, political and environmental factors is essential in ensuring a model of health that addresses communities and all their constituents. One of the key benefits of such a model is that it conceives of health as an integral component of quality of life and an outcome of social, economic, political and environmental interaction. Also, inherent in this model of health is a degree of flexibility to accommodate the diversity of individuals and communities in Canada.

Given these requirements, we utilize an expanded version of the health model developed by the Ottawa Charter of Health Promotion (1986) that states:

> The fundamental conditions and resources for health are peace, shelter, education, food, income, a stable eco-system, sustainable resources, social justice and equity. Improvement in health requires a secure foundation in these basic prerequisites (Canadian Public Health Association, 1986).

Core to this model are the following:

- education
- employment and level of income
- housing
- water
- waste disposal
- transportation of dangerous goods and hazardous waste disposal

- climate
- external programs and services: doctor, dentist and community health nurse . . .
- existing human resources: Community Health Representatives, NNADAP workers, nursing services, . . .

The model of health requires a process that has both action and research as outcomes. I argue that PAR offers the best framework to enable us to do this. This can be achieved utilizing the following steps, as will be demonstrated in the case example:

1. Establishing a working group to collect community information, establish community involvement and develop a strategic plan (action).
2. Develop, design and collect research that identified important health issues.
3. Strategic planing is a disciplined program of understanding the health issues, needs and concerns of the community, outlining a vision and mission to be considered, preparation of direction setting statements and options that involves all key stakeholders who will be instrumental in the success of any new "health services" or administration.

WHY A FIRST NATION CASE EXAMPLE

In February 1997, the Royal Commission on Aboriginal Peoples released its mammoth multi volume report. Examining the health conditions of Aboriginal people, the report noted:

> The health status of Aboriginal people in Canada today is both a tragedy and a crisis. Illness of almost every kind occurs more often among Aboriginal people than among other Canadians.
>
> - Registered Indians (for whom we have the best data) can expect to die to 8 years younger than other Canadians. This difference in life expectancy has two major causes: a higher rate of death among Aboriginal babies (twice the national average), and a higher rate of injury and accidental death among Aboriginal children, youth and young adults.
> - Twenty-five years of effort by local, provincial and national health caregivers have raised Aboriginal health status from the lows to which it had sunk by mid-century. Still, the results fall far short of the goal of equal health outcomes for all Canadians.

Aboriginal people urgently need resources to help them reduce infant mortality, tuberculosis, diabetes, heart disease and other illnesses. But they know that curing diseases of the body alone cannot restore well-being. What they are looking for is more fundamental and more transformative. They are trying to bring balance and vitality to body, mind, emotions and spirit – as ends in themselves and as preconditions for balance and vitality in their societies. In short, they are looking for whole health (Royal Commission on Aboriginal Peoples, 1997, http://www.inac.gc.ca/rcap/report/look.html).

Months before the release of the Royal Commission report, but in effect reflecting the same spirit, a Northern Alberta First Nation community embarked on a community health needs assessment. In May 1996 the community negotiated an agreement with the Medical Services Branch of Health and Welfare Canada to undertake a community health needs assessment as part of the pre-transfer planning process for community health programs. I was brought in as a needs assessment consultant.

CASE EXAMPLE

A Snapshot of the Community (1997)

The community comprises a population of approximately 335 people. It is considered rural but not remote. The nearest full facility town is approximately 250 km away. The road that leads to the community is gravel. Few services and facilities exist. There is no bank (no bank machine), no shelved/stocked store, no pharmacy, no laundry mat, no formal childcare facility. The community does have a school that houses grades k–9. Any further schooling beyond this requires moving (relocating) to a larger centre (the nearest one being approximately 2.5 hours by vehicle). Not surprisingly education levels are low, approximately 50% of the adult community has an elementary education (k–6) and the remaining 50% have the equivalent of a secondary school education (7–9). There are insufficient, almost non existent, community recreational activities. The community has no hospital, no resident doctor, no resident dentist, no resident nurse. The nearest hospital is again approximately 2.5 hours away by vehicle. There are few employment opportunities, approximately 45% of the community is unemployed. The average income ($13 500 per year) of adult community members falls close to the poverty line. For approximately 82% of the adult community, English is not their first language, neither is it the language spoken in their home. Approximately 58 percent of the adult community does not have running water in either their kitchen or washroom; 76 percent of the adult community do not have drinkable tap water (it is not considered suitable for consumption and residents have found fecal matter in samples). Many of the homes use either propane or wood as fuel for heating homes. Eight months of the year are lived in winter conditions and the temperatures range from –15 degrees Celsius to –45 degrees Celsius (not including wind chill factors). Clearly the community is faced with a number of problems: physical impairments, poor nutrition, alcohol or drug abuse, unsanitary conditions in the community, poor housing conditions, accidents and injuries, incidence of violence, and mental health problems.

Step 1: Establishing a Working Group

In forming a working group, the community Chief and Council were approached. They, in conjunction with the facilitators, appointed individuals to the working group. Appointments were made using several criteria including: knowledge of community health issues, commitment to the project/process, and their central role as caregivers in the community. A ten-member community-working group was formed for this process. There was broad representation of the community to establish the credibility of the process and to ensure that the survey methods were comprehensive and inclusive. A facilitator external to the community was contracted to guide and manage the project to ensure objectivity. This working group comprised all women, which is not surprising given that women in this community are the formal and informal providers of health services. Women are considered the mothers of "their communities" and thus all issues affect and can be affected by women. If women can reclaim ownership over quality of life issues, the success of future generations is enhanced.

Step 2: Develop, Design and Collect Research that Identified Important Health Issues

The needs assessment was seen as an effective way to measure what community members and professionals were thinking and how they perceived community health needs. While the working group anticipated that the findings of the needs assessment would be valuable, the process of gathering the information was considered just as important. Specifically, this process allowed the community members to:

- collect information about citizens' attitudes and opinions regarding precisely defined issues, problems or opportunities;
- analyze the data to better understand how citizens ranked issues, problems and opportunities in order of importance and urgency;
- provide community members with a voice in determining policy, goals, and priorities;
- determine community support for initiatives;
- evaluate current programs; and
- end speculation about what people are thinking and establish what people want.

The working group envisioned the health needs assessment as a process for the community to record and understand the health needs of all members. The information gathered could then be used to examine the existing health care system and resources of the community they could then determine whether or not there were sufficient resources, and if there were, whether or not they are being used appropriately. The information coming from the health needs assessment could also assist the community to develop a health system and resources which can take care of future needs. Thus the objectives of the needs assessment were specified as follows:

1. To examine the delivery of health and social services offered to the community.
2. To examine the physical, social, and emotional health of individuals in the community.
3. To identify environmental hazards which affect the community's health.

4. To understand how community members view the current delivery of health services.

Two broad questions provided a frame of reference to developing various methods necessary to collect data relevant to meet the above objectives:

1. Who do we need to collect information from to properly assess community health needs?
2. What methods of data collection are appropriate for each of these groups?

To ensure that data was collected from as many sources as possible, four methods were established to collect information on community health needs. These included:

1. **Background portfolios** – the portfolios were created and distributed by the consultant, the goal being to establish the participatory base of the needs assessment process and to ensure:

   - community ownership,
   - enhancement of research skills for working group,
   - an introduction to the necessary components of a health needs assessment,
   - establishment of participation as a key component of the needs assessment process.

Topics covered were:

(a) education
(b) employment and level of income
(c) housing
(d) water
(e) waste disposal
(f) transportation of dangerous goods and hazardous waste disposal
(g) climate
(h) external programs and services: doctor, dentist and community health nurse . . .
(i) existing human resources: Community Health Representative, NNADAP workers, nursing services, . . .

Essentially, each working group member researched a series of questions in the above areas.

2. **Door-to-Door questionnaire** – it was agreed that the goal would be to develop a questionnaire that:
   - covered pubic health and social welfare domains,
   - was 15 minutes maximum to deliver (approximately 55 questions),
   - was translatable into community mother tongue with relative ease,
   - promoted broader community participation in data collection, and
   - disseminated information on the needs assessment process to community members.

Six committee members received formal data collection training. Ninety-five percent of the adult population in the community were successfully accessed to answer the questionnaire.

3. **Elder interviews** – Several community elders were identified as key respondents. Seven open-ended questions formed the basis for the interview. These interviews were conducted primarily through a translator.
4. **Key informant interviews** – This was done by a mail-out questionnaire composed of ten questions relating to professional services delivered in the community (e.g. doctor, dentist . . .)

The utilization of four different methods ensured that the significant stakeholders where involved in the process. The perspectives on community needs were solicited from each group.

Step 3: Strategic Planning

The needs assessment provided the data necessary for forming an integrated plan of action to address health issues within the community. The needs assessment data guided the specification of goals, objectives, strategies and tasks. "Friendly neighbors, good schools, green spaces, quality health care, high-wage jobs, smooth streets . . ." The community saw itself at a crossroads of challenge and opportunity as the community identified a unified vision, a common purpose, and finally, a plan of action for managing the future.

A series of vital or core recommendations were developed by taking stock of current conditions and health services. Core strategies were developed to close the gap between the ideal (the vision) and the real (needs assessment results). Recommendations became the organizing principles, a framework for everyone, to set goals and a foundation for action/change. The primary recommendations were as follows:

1. That the community take greater control of health services.
2. That Council establish a health committee, health department, and recruit a health administrator.
3. That Council accept the following list of health programs as priorities:
   - disease control
   - maternal and child health
   - environmental health and safety
   - mental health
   - dental health
   - education, promotion and prevention
   - disaster planning and prevention
   - geriatric health
   - substance abuse
   - family violence
   - injury prevention
   - treatment services – orthodontic, chiropractic, optometric
   - healthy lifestyle
   - home nursing

We conclude with a vision statement that the working group developed which substantiated their view on what is quality of life in their community.

> Our community will become a modern, dynamic community and the strongest community in the region. Through active participation of all its members, our community will provide the leadership and direction to develop a Christian aboriginal community that meets the needs of its members and residents. We see a community that is economically strong, offers opportunities to learn and earn, respects and practices traditional skills and crafts, is healthy and safe, and provides a full range of health, educational, recreational and social activities for all. It is a place that will always be "home" for its members, where people can thrive, dream, prosper and enjoy life.

CONCLUSION

In terms of the Rothman typology, the Report of the Royal Commission on Aboriginal People addresses both normative need and comparative need with respect to social needs in general and community health needs in particular. It also addresses the need for community empowerment as an overriding issue in addressing these needs. The complex and technical nature of health care has effectively disempowered the non-expert from participation in health needs research and assessment. In addressing the question of "what makes a community health?", people's answers reflect their understanding of the complexity of the problem, and this very complexity in effect obviates the possibility or potential of PAR:

> It's not just doctors and hospitals, skilled medical professionals, the right drugs and the right machines, though these things certainly help a lot. People live longer and healthier lives if they eat a good diet, are well housed, secure from war, crime, and domestic violence, not deranged by drugs or alcohol, if they have plenty of clean water for drinking and washing, if they can breathe clean air, if they have access to basic vaccines and antibiotics, if they can exercise some sense of choice in their lives, and if they have friends and family to give life meaning (Flower, 1993: p. 2).

It is our contention that health needs assessment must be based on PAR as the first step in the re-empowerment of a community over their health. While the concepts of PAR and needs assessment address the epistemological basis for this contention, the concept of emancipatory practice addresses its ontological basis. Health is a fundamental component of quality of life. In this paper we proposed a model of health and assessment which uses a participatory action model. A participatory action model represents an attractive alternative research method for examining quality of life.

REFERENCES

Bishop, A.: 1994, Becoming an Ally: Breaking the Cycle of Oppression (Fernwood Publishing, Halifax).

Canadian Public Health Association: 1986, Ottawa Charter for Health Promotion (Canadian Public Health Association, Ottawa).

Deprez, R. and S. Horton: 1996, 'Community health status and service needs assessment: an analytical tool in a changing health care delivery system',

Journal of Hospital Marketing 10(2), pp. 117–128 [on-line]. Available: http://auburn.maine.com/people/phrg/mnifsto.htm.
Deshler, D. and M. Ewart: 1995, Participatory Action Research: Traditions and Major Assumptions [on-line]. Available: http://www.parnet.org/tools/tools_1.cfm#evaluation.
Fanon, F.: 1967, Black Skin, White Mask (Grove Press, Inc., New York).
Flower, J.: 1993, 'Healthier communities: a compendium of best practices', Health Care Forum Journal 36(3), pp. 1–38.
Freire, P.: 1990, Education for Critical Consciousness (The Continuum Publishing Company, New York).
Freire, P.: 1990, Pedagogy of the Oppressed (2nd ed.) (The Continuum Publishing Company, New York).
Grundy, S.: 1992, 'Three modes of action research', in Kemmis and McTaggart (eds.), The Action Research Reader (Deakin University Press, Geelong).
House, E., M. Patton, M. Scriven and N. Uphoff: 1995, Participatory Action Research: Traditions and Major Assumptions [on-line]. Available: http://www.parnet.org/tools/tools_1.cfm#evaluation.
Mullaly, R.: 1993, Structural Social Work Ideology, Theory, and Practice (McClelland & Stewart Inc., Toronto).
Paltiel, F.: 1993, 'Canadian women's health issues in the 1990s', The Canadian Journal of Ob/Gyn and Women's Health Care, November 5, pp. 510–513.
Rothman, J. and L. Gant: 1987, 'Approaches and models of community interventions', in D. Johnson, L. Miller and G. Summers (eds.), Needs Assessment: Theory and Methods (Iowa State University Press, Ames, Iowa), pp. 350–344.
Royal Commission on Aboriginal Peoples: 1997, Report of the Royal Commission on Aboriginal Peoples (Government of Canada, Ottawa) [on-line]. Available: http://www.inac.gc.ca/rcap/reprot/look.html.
Summers, G.: 1987, 'Democratic governance', in D. Johnson, L. Miller and G. Summers (eds.), Needs Assessment: Theory and Methods (Iowa State University Press, Ames, Iowa), pp. 3–19.

College of Arts, Social and Health Sciences
University of Northern British Columbia
3333 University Way
Prince George, BC V2N 4Z9
Canada
E-mail: ismaels@unbc.ca

ALESSANDRA PETRUCCI and SILVANA SCHIFINI D'ANDREA

QUALITY OF LIFE IN EUROPE: OBJECTIVE AND SUBJECTIVE INDICATORS

A Spatial Analysis Using Classification Techniques

1. INTRODUCTION

Here we will present the preliminary results of a geographical study[1] among the regions in Europe. It is an exploratory comparative analysis among the regions in Europe that represents the first phase in a larger analysis which aims to study quality of life at the European level.[2]

Our aim here is to show that, in Europe, it is the region (a subnational administrative unit) that is taking on a much more important significance than that of the nation in the study of quality of life.[3] The well-known contribution by Inglehart and Rabier (1984) on the importance of "nationality" in the determination of individual satisfaction is losing its initial significance. Europe, in fact, is going through a phase of profound transformation that would have been unthinkable only decades ago. In a Europe in which the futures of the various populations will have ever more in common, it is very important to have available as much comparative information as possible.

It is our opinion that quality of life studied at a "macro" level,[4] that is at the country level, must be the result of an ensemble of factors referred both to the objective reality of the area under study and also to the evaluations expressed by individuals living within the area itself. Thus, the basic unit of territorial observation takes on an increasingly important role.

Social Indicators Research **60:** 55–88, 2002.

2. THE DATA

The statistical sources[5] of the study are:

- Eurostat Yearbook, EU (Regions) in which one finds economic, social and demographic information at three levels of territorial groupings (Nuts 0, Nuts 1, Nuts 2, and Nuts 3);
- Eurobarometer Survey (n. 42, 1994).

Problems were encountered in attempting to unite these two separate statistical sources at the same territorial level as there are two European International Agencies that produce these two sources.[6] Our comparison deals with a geographic situation that is a merger of different territorial levels, and our data is at times at a high level of detail, at others intermediate, and, occasionally, is even at the national level. The comparison is made on 115 European observations, but we hope, with the help of appropriate agencies, to pursue further research. We must, in fact, underline the need for improvement in the quality and comparability of European statistics, particularly considering the ever increasing need for comparison in this area. In addition, while Eurobarometer is a questionnaire-based survey that has already been tested and in use for many years, the data published by Eurostat have an aim that is more geared to diffusing information than to promoting scientific research and a comparison between the two presents some substantial difficulties. Some difficulties are connected to the definition of the character surveyed, and others pertain to content, while still others are of a technical nature if we use, as in this case, printed data. Here are some examples. *Definitional problems*: measurement of the infant mortality rate implies a definition of stillbirths, on which an important indicator for the individuation of demographic unease is based, but the definition of "stillbirth" is not the same across the board. This same type of problem applies also to the definition of "unemployed"; *contextual problems*: educational structures differ in the various countries of Europe, be it with respect to length of mandatory schooling or to the structure of the various school levels. Specific rates of scholarization cannot therefore be measured while if we calculate generic rates (educated population as a ratio of total population) the ratio reflects the age structure of the population and loses its comparative significance; *technical problems*: certain phenomena are measured by means of published indicators[7] with a structure that is so generic as to render territorial differences practically invisible.

2.1. *The Indicators*

2.2. *Objective indicators*

A first evaluation of the quality of life was done considering just the objective component. The selected objective indicators refer to the reality of the considered territorial units and are indicators of the "environment" where people lives. So, it's possible to compare societies using indices that summarize a varicty of important objective social indicators. The indicators are chosen on the basis of the social unease for stressing the most difficult and problematic realities inside the countries of the European Union.

A number of objective indicators were selected that were made comparable by a reproportioning in which minimum and maximum values are represented by two extremes corresponding to two actual regions. Since our objective is focused, above all, on the outlining of areas of "unease," the observational unit that assumes a higher value than the indicator is that which presents greater unease in that category.

Thus, we have aggregated reproportioned data and obtained 11 indicators. Some of these correspond to the initial indicator (ex: GDP/pop.; suicide rate); others are the result of an aggregation (death/pop. for environmental reasons) so as to obtain a synthetic indicator. The lack of information in some cases prevented further probing. Indicators of unease:

- Demographic unease (demographic aging – low birth rate – migratory discount) [IDEM]
- Economic unease (complement of per capita GDP.) [ECO]
- Employment unease (unemployment of youth, adults, women) [OCC]
- Gender Disequilibrium (among the working and unemployed populations) [SEX]
- Unease in the healthcare system (beds/pop.; doctors/pop.) [SAN]
- Percentage growth of agricultural population [AGR]

- Low percentage of population in industry [IND]
- Low percentage of population in the service sector [TER]
- Lack of roads infrastructure (highways/sqkm – cars/pop.) [AUTO]
- Social unease (rates of suicides) [SUI]
- Deaths for environmental causes (cardiovascular deaths, tumors) [AMB]

2.3. *Subjective indicators*

The subjective evaluations of the persons interviewed are reported for the same territorial units used to calculate the objective indicators.

The following 6 subjective indicators were selected and are expressed across 18 types of responses (ex: life satisfaction is composed of 4 types of responses: Very satisfied, Fairly satisfied, not very satisfied, not at all satisfied):

- Life satisfaction [MSOD-ASOD-AINSOD-MINSOD]
- Definition of oneself as religious or not [REL-NOREL]
- The economic optimist/pessimist index (ECO) is constructed on the basis of the assessment of the changes in the Nuts's economic situation over the past 12 months and over the next 12 months. The index represents the individual evaluation of the general economic situation of the country [ECOPES-ECONEU-ECOOTT]
- The financial situation optimist/pessimist index (FIN) is constructed on the basis of the assessment of the changes in the financial situation of an individual household over the past 12 months and over the next 12 months. The index represents the individual evaluation of the financial situation of the family [FINPES-FINNEU-FINOTT]
- Social class to which the subject evaluated belongs [COPERAI-CMEINF-CMESUP]
- European Social Grade (7-point scale) based on the recommendation of the European Society for Opinion and Marketing Research (ESOMAR) to harmonize the measurement of social grade across borders and elaborated upon by Eurobarometer [MAXESG-NEUESG-MINESG]

We consider these indicators for the two following levels of the analysis. At the first step we consider all the listed subjective indicators. These indicators express jointly the individual evaluation of quality of live, the individual evaluation of the economic situation of the country, the financial situation of the family and the evaluation the individual social class.

At a more detailed level, using only the first four indicators listed, we express the quality of life in terms of social well-being (SWB). The expressions noted show how the individuals evaluate theirs lives, in terms of global satisfaction, but also in terms of waits and expectations of theirs future. Individualism is a cultural variable. Referring the SWB to the territorial units which are very different for history, tradition, religion, language, habits, etc. we try to identify the contribution of the affective reaction (moods and emotions) component to the quality of life over the territory.

3. RESULTS

Cluster analysis is a very interesting kind of explorative analysis in geographic studies. In our case, it allowed for the evaluation of various levels of aggregations of the European regions. Depending on the level at which a similarity occurred a number of different clusters were formed. Obviously, the number of clusters is higher when there is greater similarity. In this case, small very specific clusters formed in which only very similar regions were grouped together. As similarity progressively decreased also the number of clusters decreased and more numerous groups were formed with less specific characteristics in common. Ward's method was used.[8]

3.1. *Objective Quality of Life*

We have considered the first level of aggregation to be that of 82.43% similarity corresponding to the formation of 75 clusters (of which 47 are unitary). This point signals the beginning of a fusion among regions of different nations. We are, therefore, at a high level of detail that we consider only in order to put together this particular aspect of the analysis.

At a level of aggregation with similarity so high many regions remain isolated and constitute clusters with just one observation.

Clearly the first aggregations are formed by a limited number of observations. It is important to note that the first aggregations form within the nations themselves and that they are made up of areas that are already clearly delineated, oftentimes, by a joining of adjacent areas. These first clusters show the strongest ties that each nation has internally and in many cases one senses historical and cultural ties that characterize many areas in Europe. The indicators used are objective and thus the aggregations represent areas that are homogenous from an economic, social and demographic point of view.

At a slightly lower level of similarity (80%) two clusters have formed between regions in different nations: the first region that joins another in a different country is Antwerp (Belgium) with Hessen (Germany); the next is the North-West region of the UK which joins with Lisbon (Portugal).

It should be noted that, in these first aggregations, all the capitals (or capital regions), with the exception of Lisbon, remain isolated and do not present any similarities either among themselves or with other regions.

Table I (see appendix) shows the scheme of evolution of the cluster formations over successive stages of aggregation that we indicate with the number of the clusters that form (4-7-16-20).

Increasing the size of the clusters, the differences between the value of intermediate values declines because different realities merge. However, even an extreme that would divide Europe into two, three or four parts, can be interesting. For example, dividing Europe into only four typologies leads to the exact reconstitution of the national territory in the cases of France, the Netherlands and the UK. Other countries show either similarities with bordering states (France-Belgium) or distinct internal divisions (Italy) that lead to the formation of groupings with other countries. Italy is noticeably divided into two typologies, one which aligns with Germany, the other with Spain, with the exception of Rome (region: Lazio) that joins with the region of Madrid.

Our objective, however, is not that of recreating nations. On the contrary, it is of singling out small areas within countries that display homogeneity with areas in other countries. Thus, it is more inter-

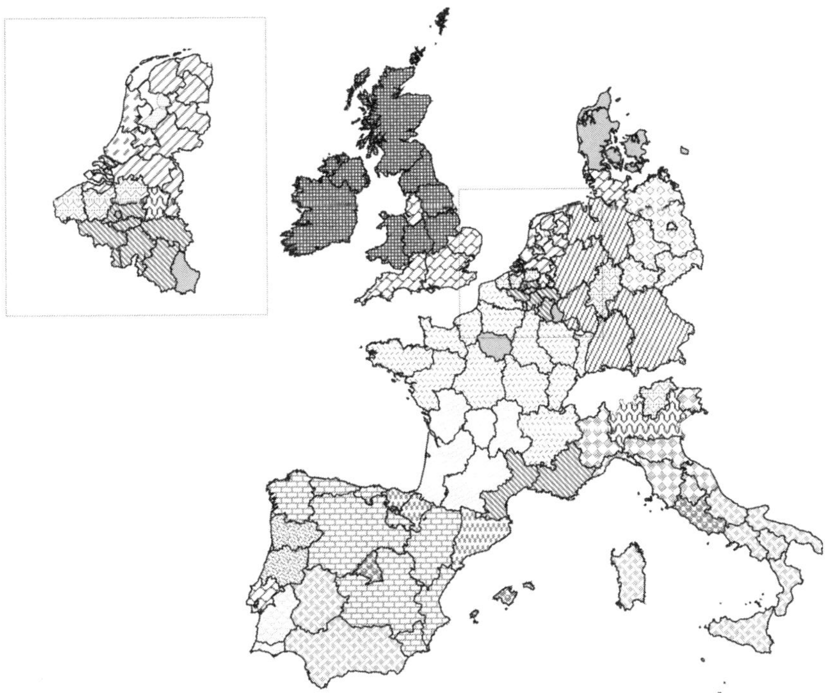

Figure 1. Objective indicators: cutting the clustering tree at 20.

esting to analyze the typologies at a higher level of similarity with the formation of a greater number of clusters.

Table II (see appendix) contains average values of the indicators at various levels of cluster size (4-7-16-20) selected by using a tree clustering analysis.

In order to compare the transformations that take place at the successive levels of cluster formation, we have placed the values obtained on the map of Europe.

In this presentation we proceed, however, to the examination of only the typologies that it form at the level of 20 European areas (Figure 1) and we compare them with the final situation represented by the four larger clusters shown in Figure 2.

The maps should be interpreted together with the outline in Table I (see appendix) and the average values in Table II (see appendix).

Figure 2 points out well defined areas that do not correspond in any way to national boundaries; in fact, they outline areas that are common to two or more countries.

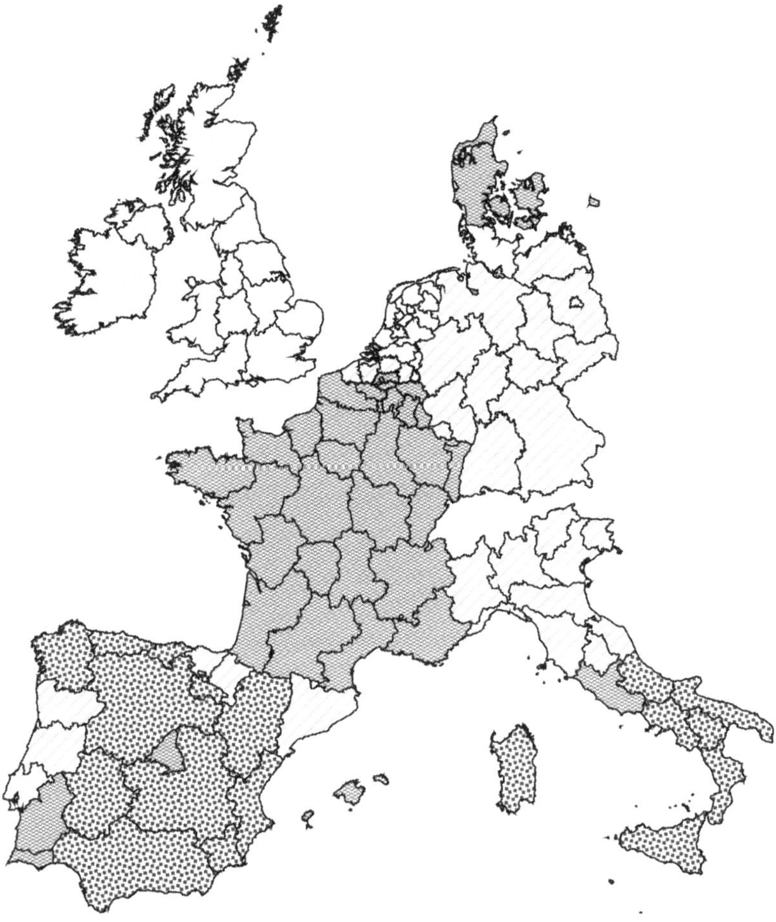

Figure 2. Objective indicators: cutting the clustering tree at 4.

The first larger cluster is comprised of 37 observations that exactly recreate the territorial boundaries of France, show a formation of some adjacent regions in Belgium (including Brussels) and two European capitals (Lazio, which includes Rome, and Madrid). This larger cluster has an average level of aging, a low level of industrial development, a good environmental level, but a high level of suicide.

At a more detailed level of observation, we see that one cluster (1.20.10)[9] unites two capitals in southern Europe; another (1.20.1) unites Brussels, Paris, two big cities such as Hamburg and Bremen and the nations of Denmark and Luxembourg. These two clusters have an analogous process of demographic aging and of service sector activity, but the first cluster shows greater economic, employment, and health unease and a gender disequilibrium; the second has greater social and environmental unease. A great portion of France remains compact and very stable (1.20.12). Here economic unease is stronger than employment unease (there is a high percentage of agricultural population); in addition, there is a high level of social unease that, together with cluster (1.20.13), joins other regions in France and reaches the highest level in all Europe. Two regions in Southern France group instead with Belgian regions (1.20.4). The second larger cluster, comprised of 32 observations, has a high level of demographic unease with aging process and low birth rate each as strong factors. Economic unease is intermediate, industrial activity is high and health and environmental unease is medium-high. Various Italian regions are included in this group, among which the north-central region which forms a compact and stable group (2.20.15) characterized by the strongest aging process in all of Europe.

One cluster (2.20.7) exactly unifies all the German regions of the eastern area where economic and environmental unease are very high. In fact, only the central-north area of Portugal (2.20.19) has a higher level of economic unease, with the difference that the Portuguese area has the highest percentage of agricultural population in Europe and, thus, does not have a high level of unemployment.

The third larger cluster, comprised of 27 observations, extends across the whole of northern Europe to which is joined also Lisbon. This cluster has a higher level of demographic development, with a minimum employment unease, a low level of gender disequilibrium and a better healthcare situation. At the detailed level, Lisbon initially joins with Berlin and some English regions among which is also the area of London (3.20.5), creating a cluster with a minimum of gender disequilibrium and a minimum of employment unease. There is a cluster comprised of only Dutch regions (3.20.16) that is demographically young, with a stronger level of economic than employment unease, a good environmental situation and an excellent healthcare situation.

The fourth larger cluster, made up of 19 observations, remains separated from the rest of Europe over an extended period of time and only at a very low level of similarity does it join to the preceding larger clusters. It is a cluster with a fairly high level of aging and with a strong unease extended across all fields. However, with respect to the others, it has a better environmental situation and a situation of social unease that is worse.

Cluster 4.20.8 unites all the regions of southern Italy to two regions in the south of Spain; cluster 4.20.9 joins only Spanish regions. A comparison of the two clusters indicates that the first has a lower level of demographic aging, a greater level of gender and healthcare system disequilibrium, a lower level of industrialization but also greater unease in the service sector and a higher suicide rate. The two clusters have a high percentage of agricultural population. It should also be pointed out that the first nuclei of similarity to come from the cut of the tree at the 82.43% similarity level already joined together two initial groups of Spanish regions (Aragon-La Rioja and Cantabria-Castilla) and two Italian regions (Campania-Sicilia and Puglia-Basilicata-Sardegna) which represent the first nuclei of the two groupings.

3.2. *Subjective Quality of Life*

If we apply once again the same procedure of cluster analysis using only subjective indicators, taken from Eurobarometer, the situation changes greatly. The first level of aggregation that signals the beginning of a fusion among regions of different nations is at 88.24% level of similarity. That is an aggregation which occurs earlier than with objective data.

From a first glance taken from the examination of the redivision of Europe into 4 larger clusters, the countries that resulted as being more delineated by the objective data (France, Germany, and the UK[10]), now show a greater internal heterogeneity. On the contrary, we see a more defined reality among the Mediterranean countries. In the case of Spain and Portugal, we observe a greater internal homogeneity and a higher level of similarity between the two countries. Italy becomes almost entirely aggregated leaving two regions isolated (Tables III and IV, see appendix).

Let us compare the redivision set out in 20 clusters in which greater heterogeneity becomes evident, with that of the more aggregated level formed by the 4 larger clusters.

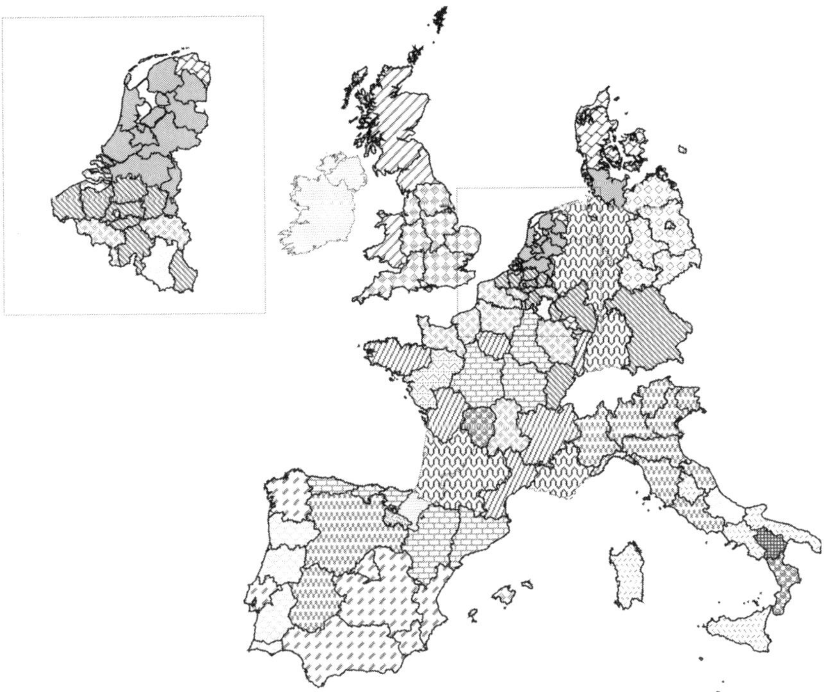

Figure 3. Subjective indicators: cutting the clustering tree at 20.

With 20 clusters we can see common aspects among individual regions or among groupings of regions which are often adjacent to one another though they often belong to different countries (Figure 3).

The highest life satisfaction is seen in Denmark which joins to a Dutch region (Groningen) and a German one (Saarland) (cluster 1.20.5); followed by Ireland and Northern Ireland which, according to this profile, join together (cluster 2.20.17). The greatest dissatisfaction is found in Portugal (cluster 4.20.20) followed by certain regions in the north-center of France (cluster 3.20.8) and Spain (cluster 4.20.18).

Even zones in the south of Italy also have a widespread level of dissatisfaction, though they show a less categorical response, as there is a higher percentage value found for the response "fairly dissatisfied" (cluster 2.20.12).

The most pessimistic view of a population towards its own country's economic situation is found in certain regions of the UK (cluster 3.20.16); the most optimistic, apart from two small moun-

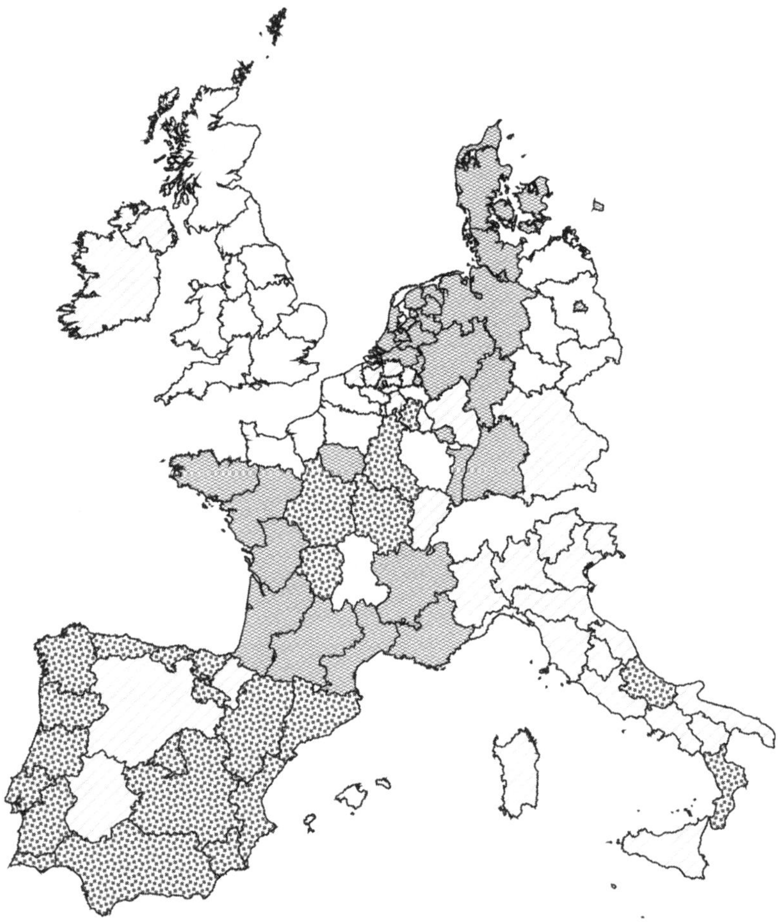

Figure 4. Subjective indicators: cutting the clustering tree at 4.

tain regions, one in Italy (Basilicata), the other in Spain (Navarra), is found in Ireland and Northern Ireland (cluster 2.20.17), in Denmark joined to the Dutch region of Groningen and the German region of the Saarland (cluster 1.20.5). Oddly, not far behind there is also the aggregate of southern Italy (cluster 4.20.12). Even the evaluation of the financial situation of one's family, thus narrowing the scope of the indicator to the direct personal financial situation, reconfirms pessimism for numerous regions in the UK, followed by an area that is economically developed such as Hamburg, Bremen and the Pays de la Loire. It should be added that the highest European Social Grade is reached by these last three regions and by all the Dutch regions that join in one cluster, with the exception of Zeeland

(1.20.1). The lowest level of this indicator is found in Portugal and in some mountain regions of various countries: Calabria (IT); Limousin (FR), and La Rioja (ES).

The evolution of the clusters examined in the successive phases, that is progressively considering a smaller number of clusters, reinforces the presence of typologies internal to the nations that are repeated also in other nations.

Comparing these results with the groups formed with the preceding objective data, reconfirms that the objective situation is much more defined and traceable to national boundaries than the subjective situation. With the objective indicators cutting the clustering tree at 16, some national uniformities emerge that were not seen with subjective indicators. Nations are better defined with objective data at higher levels of aggregation (8 and 4 clusters). Subjective data reconfirms subnational area divisions.

The most glaring example is France: a real puzzle at the subjective level, and a compact unit at the objective level.

Portugal represents an exception as with objective data it is fragmented, something that with subjective data is not seen at all. In part this also occurs for Italy which, with subjective data, it is more uniform though separate regions can be seen.

3.3. *Social Well-Being*

If we represent the quality of life just on the basis of the individual evaluation expressed as the life satisfaction index plus the optimist/pessimist of the future life indices we obtain a possible evaluation of the SWB. Adding the evaluation component due to the religious sense that in other studies on the Italian and European regions[11] showed his importance as decisive element of life satisfaction. The SWB map shows a extreme fragmentation that is free from the national borders and much more marked than obtained before. The national borders are fuzzy with the exception of the former Germany and partly of the United Kindom which are the only areas showing a solid territorial identity (Figure 5).

Many nations can be ideally divided in small areas which are the result of the process of aggregation of regions characterized by similar individual cultural level. In our country, Italy, some clusters of regions reflect the historical and cultural factors of great interest

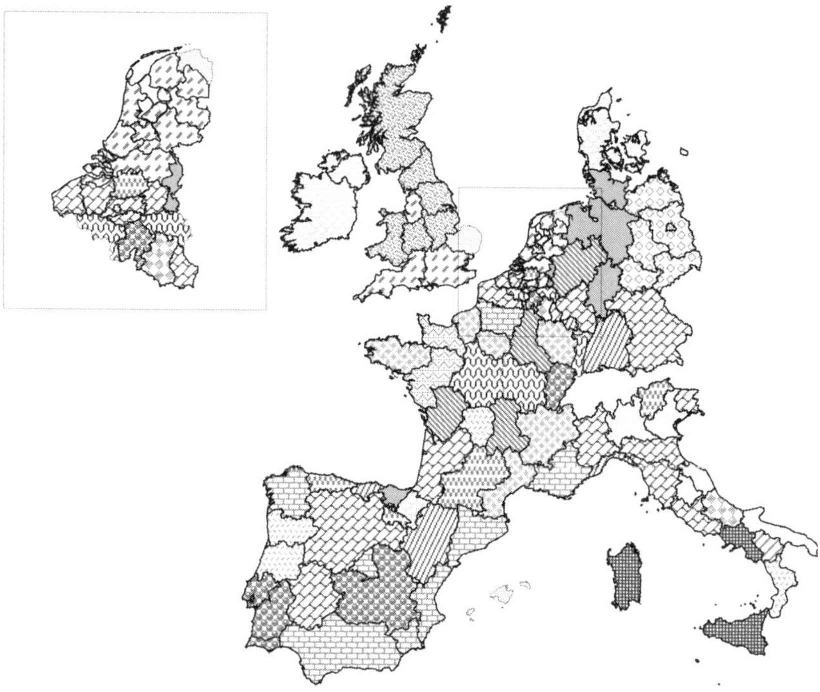

Figure 5. Subjective well-being indicators: cutting the clustering tree at 20.

for many fields of research. According to the previous subjective map which included economic and professional indicators, the differences are more evident.

The passage from the details of 20 clusters to the partition in 4 cluster unify areas defined through the nation (Table V, see appendix). Their definition is less clear than the definition of those obtained through objective or subjective (including social classes) indicators.

It is interesting to observe clustering according to the same criteria in Italy and in Spain. It seems that there are overnational criteria, these are capable to overcome the national borders and individuate similar patterns in different countries. France has now cultural relations with Italy and Spain, even if the geographical distribution of the subjective indicators shows clear borders between France and each of the two near countries.

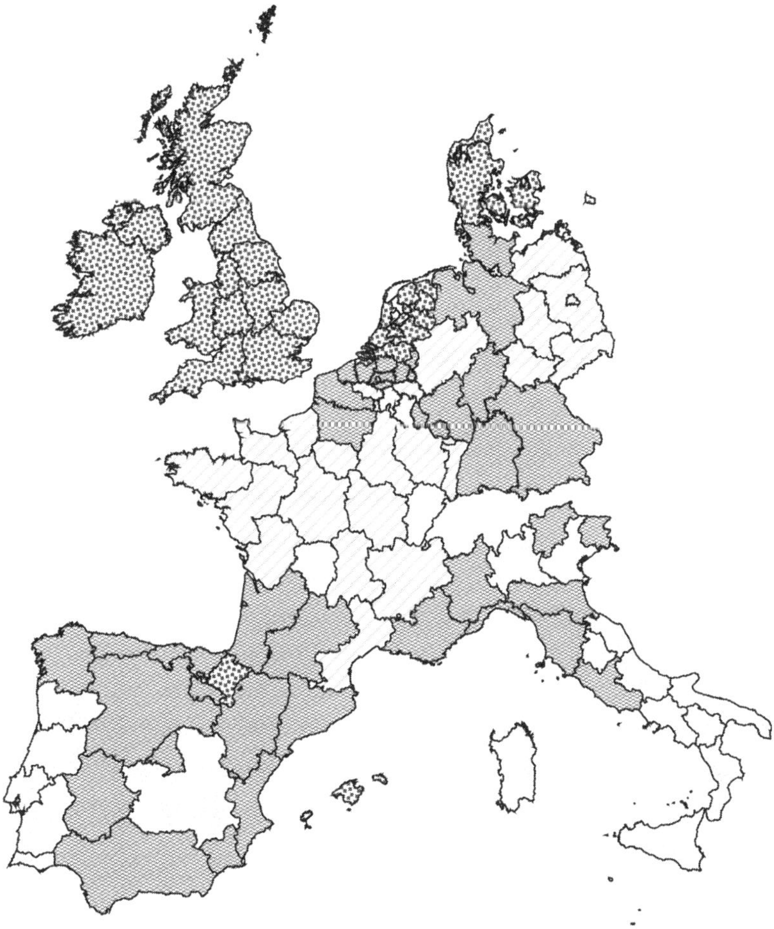

Figure 6. Subjective well-being indicators: cutting the clustering tree at 4.

3.4. *Quality of Life with Objective-Subjective Indicators*

The results obtained can lead to some difficulty in their interpretation, but at the same time, they cause us to reflect on the importance of the individual evaluative components.

Objective indicators reflect the socio-economic situation, the objective well-being of a country. For example, the main economic indicators, even at a disaggregated level within the country, reflect the overall national political and economic situation.

Subjective indicators express sensations, expectations, hopes and disappointments of a population, aspects that are often connected to the local situation. The subjective indicators are affected by cultural and historical factors, tradition, habit and, in some cases, "resignation" that lead to a different perception of seemingly entrenched situations. The European reality differentiates itself more under the subjective profile than it does under the objective one.

To intervene on the subjective aspect is much more difficult though it is important to comprehend the subjective reality. It is to this end than we emphasize the usefulness of Eurobarometer information.

The definition of "quality of life" we have set forth in the introduction, alongside the results we have obtained with the large differences between subjective and objective indicators, leads us to consider the two types of indicators together. Social Indicators and Subjective well-being measures are complementary.

In this presentation, the analysis of the formation and transformation of the various groups is by necessity synthetic, but our research is progressing with more recent data and greater territorial detail.

Let us consider the formation of groups at successive levels of similarity , cutting the clustering tree at the different levels (20-16-8-4) (Tables IV and VI, see appendix). As for the two preceding applications we begin with the 4 cluster case and look at from what "kernels" the more detailed groupings are derived (Figure 7).

Larger cluster n.1: The is the first among the 4 clusters to form and thus is the most homogeneous. It is formed by 24 observations which include Germany (former West Germany), all of central-north Italy (excluding Abruzzi and Molise), some Belgian regions, Luxemburg and Denmark. As far as Italy and Germany are concerned, initially the regions of the respective countries group together, though Italy remains separate until cluster n.8.

Larger cluster n.2: formed by 32 observations, includes all of the Netherlands, the UK, and Ireland, some important urban areas in Germany (Berlin, Bremen, and Hamburg) and in France (l'Ile de France, Provence, Alpes et Cote d'Azur, Languedoc-Roussillon) and Brussels. It is a cluster that is centered in northern Europe with the exception of the French Mediterranean regions. Among the 6 different realities at the outset only that relative to a part of the UK (North, Yorkshire, East and West Midlands, Wales and Scotland) remain separate for an extended period.

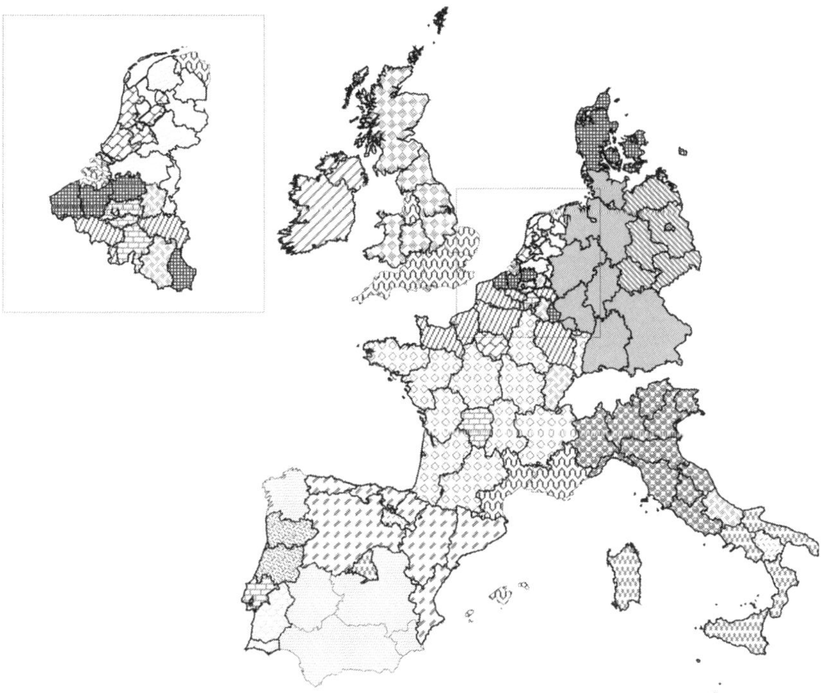

Figure 7. Objective and subjective indicators: cutting the clustering tree at 20.

Larger cluster n.3: formed by 23 observations, this cluster includes Germany (former East Germany), most of the French regions and the two Belgian regions of Liegi and Hainaut. This cluster originates as three clusters from which that which reunited the German regions remains separate for an extended period (3.20.4).

Larger cluster n.4: formed by 36 observations including all of Spain, Portugal, southern Italy and some French and Belgian regions, and the Dutch region of Limburg. The greatest uniformity is seen in the Iberian Peninsula where Spain and Portugal form a single vast area that unites to southern Italy and the two French regions (Franche-Compte and Limousin).

Larger cluster 4 remains separate from the other three for a long time and only at a very low level of similarity does it join with the three other, already formed, aggregates.

The origin of this cluster emerges from 8 highly characteristic initial kernel. Contrary to what may appear to be the case, they are not only groupings within single countries. Table VI

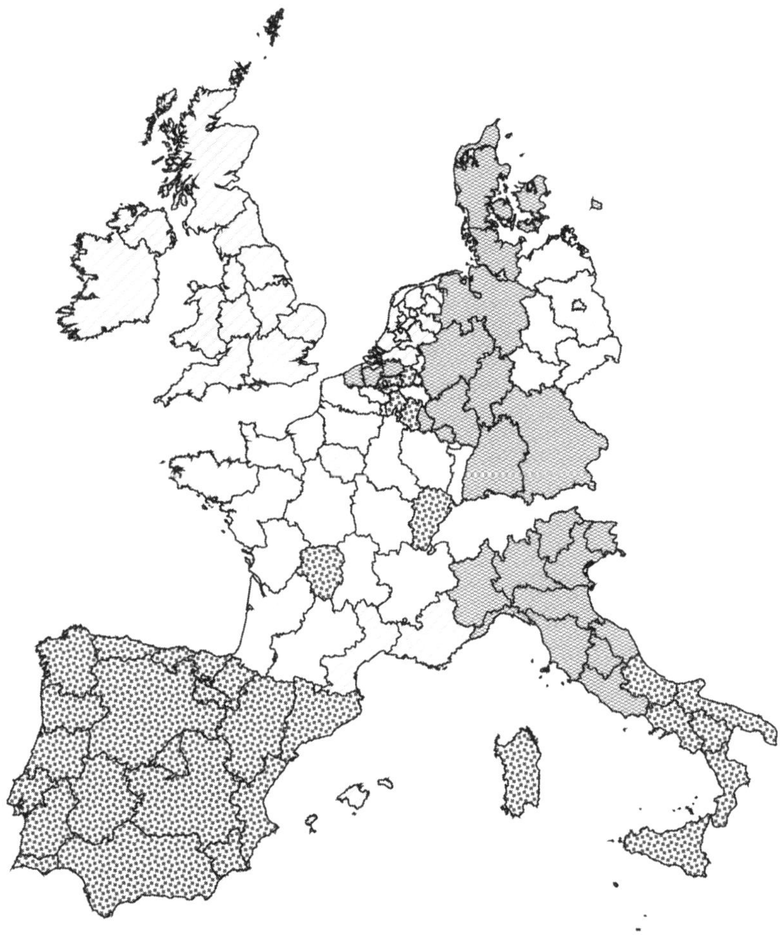

Figure 8. Objective and subjective indicators: cutting the clustering tree at 4.

shows very heterogeneous groupings which form large compact areas only when the distances are increased. For example, one can observe a cluster formed by Limousin, Brabant, Namur, and Lisbon (4.20.9), another formed by many regions in southern Italy together with Madrid (4.20.11); two small mountain regions join together: Basilicata (IT) and La Rioja (ES). The other clusters are within the countries of Portugal and Spain.

It is worth noting that cluster n.4 is not very homogenous. In fact, the two clusters: Spain and southern Italy and Portugal, the French and Belgian regions mentioned, aside from a single Italian region, remain markedly distinct for an extensive period of time.

4. CONCLUSIONS

The results obtained show the different territorial aggregations obtained by the separate use of objective indicators, subjective indicators and the two types of indicator together. From the results we deduce that the use of "nation" (France, Germany, The Netherlands, Italy, etc.) as a standard unit of observation in Europe is losing its significance and can no longer be considered an exhaustive unit of measurement. In order to study quality of life, the unit of "region" (a subnational administrative unit) is taking on a much more important and complete significance than that of "nation."

Looking at the internal situation within each nation, we can see that there are zones characterized by their economic, social, and cultural uniformity, joined together by similar behavior and similar life satisfaction, which do not correspond to national borders but which, instead, are more similar to areas outside their national boundaries and, indeed, to quite distant areas. Our analysis was carried out with three successive lists of indicators: objective data, subjective data, and both objective and subjective data together. The whole of the variables that act on a collective level and those that act on an individual level determined by differentiated interests, internal to the nations, that would be lost with just a single nation-level observation.

As far as availability of disaggregated data, we have noted the difficulty that is encountered in the outlining of comparable territorial units using simultaneously objective and subjective statistical sources. In this phase of research, we feel it premature to set out "typologies" of quality of life in the European areas formed by a grouping together of the territorial unit "region." We have circumscribed our results in an introductory framework.

This is, however, an ideal time to underline the need and the opportunity to orient studies on the quality of life in Europe towards a more analytical territorial level, because the results we have obtained indicate that it is often small areas internal to countries that demonstrate greater similarity with areas in other nations.

APPENDIX

TABLE I

Objective indicators: cutting the clustering tree at the different levels (20-16- 7-4)

CLUSTERS 20		CLUSTERS 16		CLUSTERS 7		CLUSTERS 4 (Larger Clusters)		
Brabant (Wallon+Vlaams)	1.20.4*	Brabant (Wallon+Vlaams)	1.16.4	Bruxelles	1.7.1	Bruxelles	BE	1
Hainaut		Hainaut		Brabant (Wallon+Vlaams)		Brabant (Wallon+Vlaam	BE	
Liege		Liege		Hainaut		Hainaut	BE	
Namur		Namur		Liege		Liege	BE	
Luxembourg		Luxembourg		Namur		Namur	BE	
Languedoc-Roussillon		Poitou-Charentes		Luxembourg		Luxembourg	BE	
Provence-Alpes-Cote d'Azur		Aquitaine		DANMARK		DANMARK	DK	
Poitou-Charentes	1.20.13	Midi-Pyrénées		Hamburg		Hamburg	DE	
Aquitaine		Limousin		Bremen		Bremen	DE	
Midi-Pyrénées		Auvergne		Baleares		Baleares	ES	
Limousin		Languedoc-Roussillon		Canarias		Canarias	ES	
Auvergne		Provence-Alpes-Cote d'Azur		Madrid		Madrid	ES	
Alentejo	1.20.20	Alentejo	1.16.16	Ile de France		Ile de France	FR	
Algarve		Algarve		Poitou-Charentes		Champagne-Ardenne	FR	
Baleares	1.20.10	Baleares	1.16.9	Aquitaine		Picardie	FR	
Canarias		Canarias		Midi-Pyrénées		Haute-Normandie	FR	
Madrid		Madrid		Limousin		Centre	FR	
Lazio		Lazio		Auvergne		Basse-Normandie	FR	
Bruxelles	1.20.1	Bruxelles	1.16.1	Languedoc-Roussillon		Bourgogne	FR	
DANMARK		DANMARK		Provence-Alpes-Cote d'Azur		Nord-pas de Calais	FR	
Hamburg		Hamburg		Lazio		Lorraine	FR	
Bremen		Bremen		LUSSEMBURGO		Alsace	FR	
Ile de France		Ile de France		Alentejo		Franche-Compté	FR	
LUSSEMBURGO		LUSSEMBURGO		Algarve		Pays de la Loire	FR	
Champagne-Ardenne	1.20.12	Champagne-Ardenne	1.16.10	Champagne-Ardenne	1.7.6	Bretagne	FR	
Picardie		Picardie		Picardie		Poitou-Charentes	FR	
Haute-Normandie		Haute-Normandie		Haute-Normandie		Aquitaine	FR	
Centre		Centre		Centre		Midi-Pyrénées	FR	
Basse-Normandie		Basse-Normandie		Basse-Normandie		Limousin	FR	
Bourgogne		Bourgogne		Bourgogne		Rhone-Alpes	FR	
Nord-pas de Calais		Nord-pas de Calais		Nord-pas de Calais		Auvergne	FR	
Lorraine		Lorraine		Lorraine		Languedoc-Roussillon	FR	
Alsace		Alsace		Alsace		Provence-Alpes-Cote d'/	FR	
Franche-Compté		Franche-Compté		Franche-Compté		Lazio	IT	
Pays de la Loire		Pays de la Loire		Pays de la Loire		LUSSEMBURGO	LU	
Bretagne		Bretagne		Bretagne		Alentejo	PT	
Rhone-Alpes		Rhone-Alpes		Rhone-Alpes		Algarve	PT	
Antwerpen	2.20.2	Antwerpen	2.16.2	Antwerpen	2.7.2	Antwerpen	BE	2
Oost-Vlaanderen		Oost-Vlaanderen		Oost-Vlaanderen		Limburg	BE	
West-Vlaanderen		West-Vlaanderen		West-Vlaanderen		Oost-Vlaanderen	BE	
Hessen		Niedersachsen		Niedersachsen		West-Vlaanderen	BE	
Trentino		Nordrhein-Westfalen		Nordrhein-Westfalen		Niedersachsen	DE	
Niedersachsen	2.20.6	Hessen		Hessen		Nordrhein-Westfalen	DE	
Nordrhein-Westfalen		Rheinland-Pfalz		Rheinland-Pfalz		Hessen	DE	
Rheinland-Pfalz		Baden Wuerttemberg		Baden Wuerttemberg		Rheinland-Pfalz	DE	
Baden Wuerttemberg		Bayern		Bayern		Baden Wuerttemberg	DE	
Bayern		Saarland		Saarland		Bayern	DE	
Saarland		Trentino		Brandeburg		Saarland	DE	
Brandeburg	2.20.7	Brandeburg	2.16.6	Macklenburg Vorpommern		Brandeburg	DE	
Macklenburg Vorpommern		Macklenburg Vorpommern		Sachsen		Macklenburg Vorpomm	DE	
Sachsen		Sachsen		Sachsen-Anhalt		Sachsen	DE	
Sachsen-Anhalt		Sachsen-Anhalt		Thuringen		Sachsen-Anhalt	DE	
Thuringen		Thuringen		Piemonte+V D'Aosta		Thuringen	DE	
Piemonte+V. D'Aosta	2.20.15	Piemonte+V D'Aosta	2.16.11	Liguria		Cataluna	ES	
Liguria		Liguria		Trentino		Navarra	ES	
Friuli V.G.		Friuli V G		Friuli V G		Pais Vasco	ES	
Emilia Romagna		Emilia Romagna		Emilia Romagna		Piemonte+V D'Aosta	IT	
Toscana		Toscana		Toscana		Liguria	IT	
Marche		Marche		Marche		Lombardia	IT	
Umbria		Umbria		Umbria		Trentino	IT	
Limburg	2.20.3	Limburg	2.16.3	Limburg	2.7.3	Veneto	IT	
Lombardia		cataluna		Cataluna		Friuli V G	IT	
Veneto		Navarra		Navarra		Emilia Romagna	IT	
Cataluna	2.20.11	Pais Vasco		Pais Vasco		Toscana	IT	
Navarra		Lombardia		Lombardia		Marche	IT	
Pais Vasco		Veneto		Veneto		Umbria	IT	
Norte	2.20.19	Norte	2.16.15	Norte		Norte	PT	
Centro		Centro		Centro		Centro	PT	
Madeira		Madeira		Madeira		Madeira	PT	

TABLE I

Continued

CLUSTERS 20		CLUSTERS 16		CLUSTERS 7		CLUSTERS 4 (Larger Clusters)		
Schleswig-Holstein	3.20.5	Schleswig-Hol	3.16.5	Schleswig-Hol	3.7.4	Schleswig-Hols	DE	3
Berlin		Berlin		Berlin		Berlin	DE	
Lisboa		IRELAND		IRELAND		IRELAND	IE	
North-West		Lisboa		Lisboa		Groningen	NL	
East Anglia		Scotland		Scotland		Friesland	NL	
South East		North		North		Dranthe	NL	
South West		Yorkshire e Humber		Yorkshire e Humber		Overijssel	NL	
IRELAND	3.20.14	North-West		North-West		Gelderland	NL	
Scotland		East Midlands		East Midlands		Flevoland	NL	
North		East Anglia		East Anglia		Utrecht	NL	
Yorkshire e Humber		West Midlands		West Midlands		Noord-Holland	NL	
East Midlands		Wales		Wales		Zuid-Holland	NL	
West Midlands		South East		South East		Zeeland	NL	
Wales		South West		South West		Noord-Brabant	NL	
Northern Ireland		Northern Ireland		Northern Ireland		Limburg	NL	
Groningen	3.20.16	Groningen	3.16.12	Groningen	3.7.7	Lisboa	PT	
Friesland		Friesland		Friesland		Scotland	UK	
Dranthe		Dranthe		Dranthe		North	UK	
Overijssel		Overijssel		Overijssel		Yorkshire e Hu	UK	
Gelderland		Gelderland		Gelderland		North-West	UK	
Zeeland		Zeeland		Flevoland		East Midlands	UK	
Noord-Brabant		Noord-Brabant		Utrecht		East Anglia	UK	
Limburg		Limburg		Noord-Holland		West Midlands	UK	
Flevoland	3.20.17	Flevoland	3.16.13	Zuid-Holland		Wales	UK	
Utrecht	3.20.18	Utrecht		Zeeland		South East	UK	
Noord-Holland		Noord-Holland		Noord-Brabant		South West	UK	
Zuid-Holland		Zuid-Holland		Limburg		Northern Irelan	UK	
Andalusia	4.20.8	Andalusia	4.16.7	Andalusia	4.7.5	Andalusia	ES	4
Extremadura		Extremadura		Aragon		Extremadura	ES	
Molise e Abruzzi		Molise e Abruzzi		Asturias		Asturias	ES	
Campania		Campania		Cantabria		Cantabria	ES	
Puglia		Puglia		Castilla leon		Castilla leon	ES	
Basilicata		Basilicata		Castilla la mancha		Castilla la manc	ES	
Calabria		Calabria		Extremadura		Extremadura	ES	
Sicilia		Sicilia		Galicia		Galicia	ES	
Sardegna		Sardegna		Murcia		Murcia	ES	
Acores		Acores		La Rioja		La Rioja	ES	
Aragon	4.20.9	Aragon	4.16.8	Pais Valenciano		Pais Valencianc	ES	
Asturias		Asturias		Molise e Abruzzi		Molise e Abruz	IT	
Cantabria		Cantabria		Campania		Campania	IT	
Castilla leon		Castilla leon		Puglia		Puglia	IT	
Castilla la mancha		Castilla la mancha		Basilicata		Basilicata	IT	
Galicia		Galicia		Calabria		Calabria	IT	
Murcia		Murcia		Sicilia		Sicilia	IT	
La Rioja		La Rioja		Sardegna		Sardegna	IT	
Pais Valenciano		Pais Valenciano		Acores		Acores	PT	

The first number is referred to the larger cluster, the second is referred to the cut of the clustering tree, the third is referred to the cluster number.

TABLE II

Objective indicators: cluster related averages at the different aggregation levels

	4 Clusters			
Indicators	1	2	3	4
DEM	60.39	72.81	54.12	67.91
ECO	61.63	64.74	67.04	85.60
OCC	33.06	22.95	15.39	65.40
SEX	20.77	34.18	15.75	60.52
SAN	59.56	68.80	31.93	75.30
AGR	19.27	18.62	12.66	50.20
IND	62.79	28.52	59.85	58.37
TER	39.86	64.16	37.05	66.35
AUTO	58.41	48.56	65.71	78.04
SUI	63.45	36.63	27.67	22.87
AMB	46.26	61.62	51.97	40.77

	7 Clusters						
Indicators	1	2	3	4	5	6	7
DEM	63.64	74.98	67.28	57.35	67.91	54.39	50.07
ECO	58.92	61.60	72.75	69.41	85.60	66.63	64.08
OCC	33.65	20.71	28.65	17.42	65.40	31.97	12.85
SEX	23.49	32.09	39.52	7.91	60.52	15.75	25.56
SAN	59.16	67.32	72.60	47.96	75.30	60.30	11.89
AGR	18.01	15.14	27.50	10.79	50.20	21.59	15.01
IND	72.70	32.53	18.25	52.27	58.37	44.50	69.33
TER	31.74	58.64	78.28	41.09	66.35	54.85	32.00
AUTO	54.89	42.42	64.27	73.47	78.04	64.91	56.00
SUI	56.56	43.14	19.98	27.83	22.87	76.18	27.48
AMB	51.61	71.07	37.48	64.57	40.77	36.37	36.23

TABLE II

Continued

16 Clusters																
Indicators	1	2	3	4	5	6	7	8	9	10	11	12	13	14	15	16
DEM	61.65	63.08	72.77	63.50	57.35	79.73	58.41	78.47	61.28	54.39	90.29	54.46	0.00	55.06	56.29	75.23
ECO	18.81	51.60	61.49	71.17	69.41	91.76	87.64	83.33	67.06	66.63	55.79	65.29	80.41	55.41	95.27	89.53
OCC	17.75	12.53	40.62	35.78	17.42	31.68	65.07	65.77	56.83	31.97	25.75	14.63	7.51	9.89	4.70	22.23
SEX	14.49	27.61	50.07	20.47	7.91	20.02	67.74	52.51	44.72	15.75	47.76	29.31	18.07	18.03	18.42	26.16
SAN	45.65	62.54	67.84	56.74	47.96	65.67	80.51	69.52	66.72	60.30	76.01	9.59	43.20	7.61	82.13	99.06
AGR	5.37	11.57	13.73	22.13	10.79	14.75	50.00	50.42	13.62	21.59	21.03	15.91	25.91	8.97	55.04	40.03
IND	70.95	29.83	12.50	70.52	52.27	29.65	69.20	46.33	76.39	44.50	38.84	57.86	90.97	92.71	29.75	83.68
TER	23.52	57.92	72.05	36.37	41.09	60.40	58.37	75.22	25.75	54.85	58.50	40.98	24.56	10.53	90.73	40.60
AUTO	44.57	39.78	57.37	56.86	73.47	61.27	71.14	85.70	53.80	64.91	33.09	65.89	0.00	48.27	78.07	76.23
SUI	56.86	43.42	26.93	67.96	27.83	58.64	19.16	27.00	15.09	76.18	31.64	26.99	20.32	31.15	6.09	70.21
AMB	57.93	61.77	35.03	52.18	64.57	82.10	40.06	41.56	28.34	36.37	77.82	40.92	0.00	35.80	42.38	75.82

20 Clusters																				
Indicators	1	2	3	4	5	6	7	8	9	10	11	12	13	14	15	16	17	18	19	20
DEM	61.65	64.03	68.94	57.72	59.53	62.28	79.73	58.41	78.47	61.28	76.61	54.39	71.59	55.45	90.29	54.46	0.00	55.06	56.29	75.23
ECO	18.81	46.08	52.48	70.85	65.15	56.19	91.76	87.64	83.33	67.06	70.50	66.63	71.62	73.14	55.79	65.29	80.41	55.41	95.27	89.53
OCC	17.75	14.59	20.45	36.84	12.67	10.81	31.68	65.07	65.77	56.83	60.79	31.97	34.29	21.57	25.75	14.63	7.51	9.89	4.70	22.23
SEX	14.49	33.69	52.09	26.10	8.80	22.54	20.02	67.74	52.51	44.72	48.06	15.75	12.59	7.13	47.76	29.31	18.07	18.03	18.42	26.16
SAN	45.65	67.15	76.14	60.62	50.27	58.69	65.67	80.51	69.52	66.72	59.53	60.30	51.31	45.93	76.01	9.59	43.20	7.61	82.13	99.06
AGR	5.37	12.89	13.29	12.64	8.54	10.47	14.75	50.00	50.42	13.62	14.18	21.59	35.42	12.75	21.03	15.91	25.91	8.97	55.04	40.03
IND	70.95	43.33	9.26	72.92	60.57	18.58	29.65	69.20	46.33	76.39	15.74	44.50	67.15	45.01	38.84	57.86	90.97	92.71	29.75	83.68
TER	23.52	49.17	74.19	27.45	33.40	65.20	60.40	58.37	75.22	25.75	69.92	54.85	48.87	47.81	58.50	40.98	24.56	10.53	90.73	40.60
AUTO	44.57	44.91	42.89	55.67	61.53	35.50	61.27	71.14	85.70	53.80	71.84	64.91	58.52	83.92	33.09	65.89	0.00	48.27	78.07	76.23
SUI	56.86	43.21	29.50	65.47	31.21	43.59	58.64	19.16	27.00	15.09	24.36	76.18	71.44	24.87	31.64	26.99	20.32	31.15	6.09	70.21
AMB	57.93	53.54	40.12	50.41	66.46	68.62	82.10	40.06	41.56	28.34	29.95	36.37	54.66	62.91	77.82	40.92	0.00	35.80	42.38	75.82

TABLE III

Subjective indicators: cutting the culstering tree at the different levels (20-16-8-4)

CLUSTERS 20	CLUSTERS 16	CLUSTERS 8	CLUSTERS 4 (Larger Clusters)
Schleswig-Holstein 1.20.1	Schleswig-Holstein	Schleswig-Holstein	Schleswig-Holstein 1
Friesland	Saarland	Niedersachsen	Hamburg
Drenthe	Groningen	Nordrhein-Westfale	Niedersachsen
Overijssel	Friesland	Hessen	Bremen
Gelderland	Drenthe	Baden Wuerttemberg	Nordrhein-Westfale
Flevoland	Overijssel	Saarland	Hessen
Noord-Brabant	Gelderland	Aquitaine	Baden Wuerttemberg
Limburg	Flevoland	Midi-Pyrénées	Saarland
Utrecht	Noord-Brabant	Provence-Alpes-Cot	Berlin
Noord-Holland	Limburg	Groningen	Ile de France
Zuid-Holland	Utrecht	Friesland	Alsace
Saarland 1.20.5	Noord-Holland	Drenthe	Pays de la Loire
Groningen	Zuid-Holland	Overijssel	Bretagne
DANMARK	DANMARK	Gelderland	Poitou-Charentes
Niedersachsen 1.20.3	Niedersachsen	Flevoland	Aquitaine
Nordrhein-Westfale	Nordrhein-Westfale	Noord-Brabant	Midi-Pyrénées
Hessen	Hessen	Limburg	Rhone-Alpes
Baden Wuerttemberg	Baden Wuerttemberg	Utrecht	Languedoc-Roussill
Aquitaine	Aquitaine	Noord-Holland	Provence-Alpes-Cot
Midi-Pyrénées	Midi-Pyrénées	Zuid-Holland	Groningen
Provence-Alpes-Cot	Provence-Alpes-Cot	DANMARK	Friesland
Hamburg 1.20.2	Hamburg	Hamburg	Drenthe
Bremen	Bremen	Bremen	Overijssel
Pays de la Loire	Berlin	Berlin	Gelderland
Berlin 1.20.6	Ile de France	Ile de France	Flevoland
Ile de France	Alsace	Alsace	Noord-Brabant
Alsace	Pays de la Loire	Pays de la Loire	Limburg
Bretagne	Bretagne	Bretagne	Utrecht
Poitou-Charentes	Poitou-Charentes	Poitou-Charentes	Noord-Holland
Rhone-Alpes	Rhone-Alpes	Rhone-Alpes	Zuid-Holland
Languedoc-Roussill	Languedoc-Roussill	Languedoc-Roussill	Bruxelles
Bruxelles	Bruxelles	Bruxelles	DANMARK
Rheinland-Pfalz 2.20.4	Rheinland-Pfalz	Rheinland-Pfalz	Rheinland-Pfalz 2
Bayern	Bayern	Bayern	Bayern
Franche-Compté	Franche-Compté	Franche-Compté	Franche-Compté
Brabant (Wallon+Vlaams)	Brabant (Wallon+Vlaams)	Brabant (Wallon+Vlaams)	Lombardia
Antwerpen	Antwerpen	Antwerpen	Emilia Romagna
Limburg	Limburg	Limburg	Lazio
Oost-Vlaanderen	Oost-Vlaanderen	Oost-Vlaanderen	Campania
West-Vlaanderen	West-Vlaanderen	West-Vlaanderen	Piemonte+V. D'Aosta
Namur	Namur	Namur	Liguria
LUSSEMBURGO	LUSSEMBURGO	LUSSEMBURGO	Trentino
NORTHERN IRELAND 2.20.17	NORTHERN IRELAND	NORTHERN IRELAND	Veneto
IRELAND	IRELAND	IRELAND	Friuli V.G.
Navarra	Navarra	Navarra	Toscana
Lombardia 2.20.11	Lombardia	Lombardia	Umbria
Emilia Romagna	Emilia Romagna	Emilia Romagna	Marche
Lazio	Lazio	Lazio	Puglia
Piemonte+V. D'Aosta	Campania	Campania	Basilicata
Liguria	Piemonte+V. D'Aosta	Piemonte+V. D'Aosta	Sicilia
Trentino	Liguria	Liguria	Sardegna
Veneto	Trentino	Trentino	Brabant (Wallon+Vlaams)
Friuli V.G.	Veneto	Veneto	Antwerpen
Toscana	Friuli V.G.	Friuli V.G.	Limburg
Marche	Toscana	Toscana	Oost-Vlaanderen
Canarias	Umbria	Umbria	West-Vlaanderen
Castilla leon	Marche	Marche	Namur
Extremadura	Puglia	Puglia	LUSSEMBURGO
Campania 2.20.12	Basilicata	Basilicata	NORTHERN IRELAND
Umbria	Sicilia	Sicilia	IRELAND
Puglia	Sardegna	Sardegna	Canarias
Sicilia	Canarias	Canarias	Navarra
Sardegna	Castilla leon	Castilla leon	Castilla leon
Basilicata 2.20.14	Extremadura	Extremadura	Extremadura

TABLE III

Continued

CLUSTER 20	CLUSTER 16	CLUSTER 8	CLUSTERS 4 (Larger Clusters)
Brandeburg 3.20.7	Brandeburg	Brandeburg	Brandeburg 3
Macklenburg Vorpom	Macklenburg Vorpom	Macklenburg Vorpom	Macklenburg Vorpom
Sachsen	Sachsen	Sachsen	Sachsen
Sachsen-Anhalt	Sachsen-Anhalt	Sachsen-Anhalt	Sachsen-Anhalt
Thuringen	Thuringen	Thuringen	Thuringen
Nord-pas de Calais 3.20.8	Nord-pas de Calais	Nord-pas de Calais	Nord-pas de Calais
Picardie	Picardie	Picardie	Picardie
Haute-Normandie	Haute-Normandie	Haute-Normandie	Haute-Normandie
Basse-Normandie	Basse-Normandie	Basse-Normandie	Basse-Normandie
Lorraine	Lorraine	Lorraine	Lorraine
Auvergne	Auvergne	Auvergne	Auvergne
Hainaut	Hainaut	Hainaut	Zeeland
Liege	Liege	Liege	Hainaut
Zeeland 3.20.15	Zeeland	Zeeland	Liege
Yorkshire Humber	Yorkshire Humber	North	North
East Midlands	East Midlands	Yorkshire Humber	Yorkshire Humber
East Anglia	East Anglia	East Midlands	East Midlands
South-East	South-East	East Anglia	East Anglia
South-West	South-West	South-East	South-East
West Midlands	West Midlands	South-West	South-West
North-West	North-West	West Midlands	West Midlands
Baleares	Baleares	North-West	North-West
North 3.20.16	North	Wales	Wales
Wales	Wales	Scotland	Scotland
Scotland	Scotland	Baleares	Baleares
Champagne-Ardenne 4.20.9	Champagne-Ardenne	Champagne-Ardenne	Champagne-Ardenne 4
Centre	Centre	Centre	Centre
Bourgogne	Bourgogne	Bourgogne	Bourgogne
Asturias	Asturias	Limousin	Limousin
Cantabria	cantabria	Calabria	Molise e Abruzzi
Pais Vasco	Pais Vasco	Madrid	Calabria
Aragon	Aragon	Galicia	Luxembourg
Cataluna	Cataluna	Asturias	Madrid
Limousin 4.20.10	Limousin	Cantabria	Galicia
Calabria	Calabria	Pais Vasco	Asturias
Madeira	Madeira	Aragon	cantabria
Madrid 4.20.18	Madrid	Castilla la mancha	Pais Vasco
Galicia	Galicia	Cataluna	Rioja
Castilla la mancha	Castilla la mancha	Pais Valenciano	Aragon
Pais Valenciano	Pais Valenciano	Andalusia	Castilla la mancha
Andalusia	Andalusia	Murcia	Cataluna
Murcia	Murcia	Madeira	Pais Valenciano
Lisboa	Lisboa	Lisboa	Andalusia
Molise e Abruzzi 4.20.13	Molise e Abruzzi	Molise e Abruzzi	Murcia
Luxembourg	Luxembourg	Luxembourg	Acores
Rioja 4.20.19	Rioja	Rioja	Madeira
Acores 4.20.20	Acores	Acores	Norte
Norte	Norte	Norte	Centro
Centro	Centro	Centro	Lisboa
Alentejo	Alentejo	Alentejo	Alentejo
Algarve	Algarve	Algarve	Algarve

The first number is referred to the larger cluster, the second is referred to the cut of the clustering tree, the third is referred to the cluster number.

TABLE IV

Subjective indicators: cluster related averages at the different aggregation levels (20-4)

Indicators	Clusters 1	2	3	4	Indicators	20 Clusters 1	2	3	4	5	6	7	8	9	10	11	12	13	14	15	16	17	18	19	20
M SOD	25.76	19.41	21.75	11.12	M SOD	38.01	10.01	18.53	23.39	40.94	15.44	10.22	13.40	12.77	3.36	14.82	11.25	12.94	10.00	32.92	29.73	42.74	15.70	0.00	8.22
ASOD	61.13	62.11	57.88	62.06	ASOD	54.36	73.96	67.07	62.99	54.70	62.83	64.41	61.95	67.03	62.83	66.54	53.47	73.50	80.00	50.84	57.27	48.37	50.67	85.71	60.26
AINSOD	10.08	15.16	14.97	20.45	AINSOD	5.67	14.13	10.61	10.41	4.16	16.36	21.46	17.08	15.62	27.20	15.68	28.99	10.78	10.00	11.12	10.05	7.41	26.31	14.29	21.01
MINSOD	3.04	3.33	5.40	6.37	MINSOD	1.96	1.90	3.79	3.21	0.20	5.37	3.91	7.57	4.57	6.60	2.96	6.28	2.78	0.00	5.12	2.95	1.48	7.32	0.00	10.51
COPERAI	20.54	25.53	48.13	27.23	COPERAI	22.12	8.59	19.41	38.98	30.25	20.20	47.62	45.31	14.82	14.02	15.08	21.39	42.86	10.00	44.10	68.63	38.08	26.17	71.43	41.42
CMEINF	60.80	65.91	45.49	65.52	CMEINF	55.60	70.47	64.26	51.93	54.05	63.80	49.09	43.65	76.89	82.31	75.68	69.69	19.05	80.00	49.97	30.98	59.20	70.79	28.57	55.85
CMESUP	18.66	8.56	6.37	7.25	CMESUP	22.28	20.94	16.33	9.09	15.70	16.00	3.29	11.04	8.29	3.68	9.24	8.92	38.10	10.00	5.93	0.39	2.73	3.04	0.00	2.73
NOREL	50.73	19.94	54.13	23.99	NOREL	42.97	66.82	40.66	25.09	62.68	59.68	73.71	52.61	44.35	6.14	20.31	7.91	5.36	0.00	51.50	33.39	27.84	27.33	28.57	3.98
REL	49.27	80.06	45.87	76.01	REL	57.03	33.18	59.34	74.91	37.32	40.32	26.29	47.39	55.65	93.86	79.69	92.09	94.64	100.00	48.50	66.61	72.16	72.67	71.43	96.02
MAXESG	64.82	51.46	45.17	30.40	MAXESG	69.89	72.35	60.09	54.49	60.32	60.86	49.28	34.48	35.57	26.66	52.03	43.92	41.67	60.00	54.96	37.42	40.29	34.34	33.33	13.79
NEUESG	19.20	18.11	23.34	18.81	NEUESG	14.34	21.20	23.51	21.25	31.59	16.71	32.46	27.06	23.07	17.53	17.02	15.35	16.86	10.00	15.95	20.41	18.06	17.08	16.67	16.39
MINESG	15.98	30.43	31.49	50.79	MINESG	15.77	6.45	16.40	24.27	8.09	22.44	18.26	38.45	41.36	55.82	30.95	34.73	41.48	30.00	29.09	42.16	41.65	48.58	50.00	69.82
ECOPES	37.64	33.77	43.73	45.05	ECOPES	40.40	46.90	32.68	37.20	33.73	36.19	32.00	41.05	39.04	37.85	36.91	33.59	60.58	0.00	45.75	64.43	20.26	51.57	14.29	49.78
ECONEU	19.92	18.40	18.31	20.88	ECONEU	13.15	36.72	21.61	26.14	8.00	25.90	18.13	27.49	22.63	24.38	17.01	12.84	27.78	10.00	12.52	11.50	10.64	12.75	42.86	20.20
ECOOTT	42.44	47.84	37.96	34.08	ECOOTT	46.45	16.38	45.71	36.66	58.26	37.91	49.87	31.46	38.33	37.77	46.08	53.57	11.65	90.00	41.74	24.07	69.11	35.68	42.86	30.02
FINPES	33.84	19.96	36.93	31.74	FINPES	34.23	47.38	31.83	22.42	24.98	33.29	32.66	30.15	31.26	26.60	18.17	19.95	37.29	20.00	40.94	50.08	19.52	30.57	14.29	38.50
FINNEU	36.78	48.09	29.49	40.64	FINNEU	35.66	33.86	43.60	50.04	37.57	33.14	31.39	44.07	43.09	26.52	49.85	43.31	48.61	70.00	18.96	19.04	34.67	38.37	85.71	36.16
FINOTT	29.39	31.95	33.58	27.62	FINOTT	30.11	18.76	24.57	27.54	37.45	33.57	35.95	25.78	25.65	46.88	31.98	36.74	14.10	10.00	40.09	30.88	45.80	31.06	0.00	25.35

TABLE IV

Continued

Objective and subjective indicators: cluster related averages at the different aggregation levels (20-4)

Indicators	Clusters 1	2	3	4	Indicators	20 Clusters 1	2	3	4	5	6	7	8	9	10	11	12	13	14	15	16	17	18	19	20
DEM	71.12	55.90	63.19	65.75	DEM	63.02	79.86	58.71	79.73	46.90	57.88	59.04	57.09	63.15	83.51	57.58	74.68	52.85	56.81	58.27	46.99	62.51	82.60	52.43	75.23
ECO	50.87	60.79	73.12	81.68	ECO	53.46	13.51	64.12	91.76	46.51	69.02	67.26	66.39	73.99	53.50	82.24	80.41	68.81	40.95	72.30	75.68	91.62	77.45	96.45	89.53
OCC	17.31	19.28	33.91	50.08	OCC	10.15	15.80	23.50	31.68	15.77	41.40	30.16	28.80	25.38	23.56	69.09	57.97	13.89	15.03	17.07	35.06	77.66	65.65	7.20	22.23
SEX	35.61	16.05	17.04	46.59	SEX	21.62	13.43	15.43	20.02	15.61	18.85	14.54	43.01	18.94	49.11	60.53	72.45	30.31	28.29	2.31	21.58	48.34	51.46	38.81	26.16
SAN	67.85	32.36	60.56	73.38	SAN	59.36	36.48	40.26	65.67	23.42	63.38	56.44	73.04	62.12	74.34	76.47	74.91	8.66	67.14	46.01	45.69	77.78	62.56	82.11	99.06
AGR	11.87	8.98	16.98	30.11	AGR	8.42	1.96	8.51	11.59	7.05	11.79	22.74	16.91	13.08	15.67	29.54	38.51	12.66	9.03	5.74	22.85	47.62	25.36	44.06	31.46
IND	37.07	63.18	46.84	54.78	IND	25.39	60.24	66.77	29.65	90.80	45.73	55.37	38.19	74.49	39.46	75.74	38.89	54.80	50.49	39.58	61.29	60.49	35.89	39.06	83.68
TER	52.83	32.17	50.74	57.26	TER	57.69	27.87	29.26	57.66	11.32	46.75	50.13	56.52	28.03	54.68	42.28	75.96	41.35	41.00	45.41	46.29	69.38	65.91	80.92	38.76
AUTO	30.80	48.54	48.34	57.63	AUTO	28.59	18.78	49.85	48.15	32.18	49.65	47.59	45.00	47.12	27.81	50.91	60.75	49.46	40.90	63.34	73.69	71.08	63.29	61.71	59.91
SUI	38.70	32.38	71.18	30.54	SUI	43.50	65.16	33.79	58.64	34.74	79.23	71.75	45.51	62.46	28.75	16.05	24.49	26.75	52.91	23.47	29.08	25.64	25.27	8.89	70.21
AMB	65.46	50.88	50.48	41.70	AMB	68.83	77.71	56.35	82.10	29.64	40.51	42.46	40.61	56.24	67.41	27.43	38.88	38.02	55.75	69.55	43.01	38.44	38.39	48.25	75.82
MSOD	20.56	31.62	12.98	13.17	MSOD	19.70	9.30	29.25	10.22	32.89	14.60	13.20	17.69	12.57	15.37	9.53	5.00	38.57	33.37	31.64	41.03	18.86	17.64	5.78	8.99
ASOD	66.22	55.01	64.36	60.39	ASOD	69.30	77.37	52.22	64.41	53.23	58.66	67.97	64.14	63.54	67.48	53.68	82.86	56.77	58.53	54.05	49.48	49.73	63.31	68.82	45.69
AINSOD	10.94	9.77	17.03	20.74	AINSOD	9.41	13.33	13.17	21.46	9.87	18.09	14.34	15.21	17.07	14.11	29.98	12.14	3.25	6.43	10.14	7.27	24.79	15.46	22.46	22.99
MINSOD	2.28	3.61	5.63	5.70	MINSOD	1.60	0.00	5.36	3.91	4.01	8.65	4.49	2.96	6.82	3.04	6.81	0.00	1.41	1.67	4.17	2.23	6.63	3.59	2.94	22.33
COPERAI	21.76	33.62	34.48	27.63	COPERAI	23.25	5.26	35.52	47.62	15.34	46.52	20.85	45.28	30.94	15.72	20.92	40.71	26.82	32.65	58.65	52.57	25.44	15.97	25.94	51.67
CMEINF	65.54	53.29	53.91	66.04	CMEINF	58.52	73.50	56.14	49.09	56.80	43.87	62.48	32.99	62.38	74.42	71.46	54.29	55.57	57.22	39.36	43.34	71.93	81.02	71.21	47.20
CMESUP	12.71	13.09	11.62	6.33	CMESUP	18.23	21.24	8.34	3.29	27.86	9.61	16.67	21.73	6.68	9.87	7.62	5.00	17.61	10.12	1.99	4.09	2.64	3.01	2.85	1.14
NOREL	28.86	48.24	56.68	19.39	NOREL	41.24	63.46	55.51	73.71	52.45	52.61	51.53	11.86	19.53	18.59	12.98	14.29	39.35	31.67	42.03	29.26	27.64	36.40	2.59	6.69
REL	71.14	51.76	43.32	80.61	REL	58.76	36.54	44.49	26.29	47.55	47.39	48.47	88.14	80.47	81.41	87.02	85.71	50.65	68.33	57.97	70.74	72.36	63.60	97.41	93.31
MAXESG	57.19	59.60	45.28	36.65	MAXESG	63.18	75.44	58.84	49.28	73.13	34.41	50.38	43.93	40.89	52.50	49.02	46.67	56.88	57.93	42.10	37.71	39.37	33.21	15.15	10.18
NEUESG	19.76	17.45	26.15	17.57	EUESG	21.03	19.30	18.99	32.46	13.02	25.22	23.87	19.61	22.19	17.39	15.55	13.33	16.15	22.94	18.28	22.55	14.37	20.01	15.85	17.27
MINESG	23.04	22.95	28.57	45.78	MINESG	15.78	5.26	22.18	18.26	13.85	40.38	25.75	36.46	36.91	30.11	35.43	40.00	16.97	19.13	39.62	39.75	46.26	46.77	69.01	72.55
ECOPES	34.93	42.32	36.99	41.84	ECOPES	37.61	50.35	38.85	32.00	35.65	44.05	34.76	54.55	42.36	35.58	41.47	7.14	41.98	29.21	60.30	18.84	46.77	37.55	46.46	46.92
ECONEU	17.50	15.68	26.75	19.16	ECONEU	15.31	35.79	15.22	18.13	18.85	25.71	31.34	25.94	25.72	15.03	15.18	26.43	10.58	26.42	11.55	15.96	14.16	15.64	20.49	22.99
ECOOTT	47.57	42.00	36.26	39.01	ECOOTT	47.07	13.86	45.93	49.87	45.50	30.24	33.90	19.51	31.92	49.39	43.35	66.43	47.44	44.36	28.15	65.20	39.07	46.80	33.05	30.09
FINPES	21.56	38.35	32.56	27.12	FINPES	28.60	50.35	38.86	32.66	32.12	31.60	33.12	32.91	28.46	19.11	24.45	17.14	34.11	15.71	49.56	21.59	24.95	23.15	31.85	44.09
FINNEU	48.88	28.34	39.43	42.31	FINNEU	45.93	35.79	22.70	31.39	33.79	43.23	40.67	46.74	38.01	50.12	38.64	77.86	35.53	50.85	18.58	40.47	41.53	41.85	37.17	33.36
FINOTT	29.56	33.31	28.01	30.57	FINOTT	25.47	13.86	38.44	35.95	34.10	25.17	26.21	20.35	33.54	30.77	36.91	5.00	30.36	33.43	31.86	37.94	33.52	35.01	30.99	22.55

TABLE V

Social well-being: cutting the clsutering tree at the different levels (20-16-12-4)

CLUSTER 20	CLUSTER 16	CLUSTER 8	CLUSTER 4
Schleswig-Holstein	Schleswig-Holstein	Schleswig-Holstein	Schleswig-Holstein
Niedersachsen	Niedersachsen	Niedersachsen	Niedersachsen
Hessen	Hessen	Hessen	Hessen
Limburg	Baden Wuerttemberg	Baden Wuerttemberg	Rheinland-Pfalz
Pais Vasco	Saarland	Saarland	Baden Wuerttemberg
Baden Wuerttemberg	Liguria	Picardie	Bayern
Saarland	Limburg	Provence-Alpes-Cot	Saarland
Liguria	cantabria	Liguria	Nord-pas de Calais
Cantabria	Pais Vasco	Limburg	Picardie
Aragon	Aragon	Madrid	Aquitaine
Rheinland-Pfalz	Rheinland-Pfalz	galicia	Midi-Pyrénéés
Bayern	Bayern	cantabria	Provence-Alpes-Cot
Nord-pas de Calais	Nord-pas de Calais	Pais Vasco	Emilia Romagna
Aquitaine	Aquitaine	Aragon	Lazio
Emilia Romagna	Emilia Romagna	cataluna	Piemonte+V. D'Aost
Lazio	Lazio	Pais Valenciano	Liguria
Piemonte+V. D'Aosta	Piemonte+V. D'Aost	Andalusia	Trentino
Friuli V.G.	Friuli V.G.	Murcia	Friuli V.G.
Toscana	Toscana	Rheinland-Pfalz	Toscana
Brabant (Wallon+Vlaams)	Brabant (Wallon+Vlaams)	Bayern	Limburg
Limburg	Limburg	Nord-pas de Calais	Brabant (Wallon+Vlaams)
Oost-Vlaanderen	Oost-Vlaanderen	Aquitaine	Antwerpen
West-Vlaanderen	West-Vlaanderen	Midi-Pyrénées	Limburg
LUSSEMBURGO	LUSSEMBURGO	Emilia Romagna	Oost-Vlaanderen
Castilla Leon	castilla leon	Lazio	West-Vlaanderen
Extremadura	extremadura	Piemonte+V. D'Aost	LUSSEMBURGO
Picardie	Picardie	Trentino	Madrid
Provence-Alpes-Cot	Provence-Alpes-Cot	Friuli V.G.	galicia
Madrid	Madrid	Toscana	Asturias
Galicia	galicia .	Brabant (Wallon+Vlaams)	cantabria
Cataluna	cataluna	Antwerpen	Pais Vasco
Pais Valenciano	Pais Valenciano	Limburg	Rioja
Andalusia	Andalusia	Oost-Vlaanderen	Aragon
Murcia	Murcia	West-Vlaanderen	castilla leon
Midi Pyrénées	Midi-Pyrénées	LUSSEMBURGO	extremadura
Trentino	Trentino	Asturias	cataluna
Antwerpen	Antwerpen	Rioja	Pais Valenciano
Asturias	Asturias	castilla leon	Andalusia
Rioja	Rioja	extremadura	Murcia
Franche-Compté	Franche-Compté	Franche-Compté	Franche-Compté
Namur	Molise e Abruzzi	Molise e Abruzzi	Limousin
Canarias	Luxembourg	Luxembourg	Lombardia
Castilla la mancha	Namur	Namur	Campania
Lisboa	Canarias	Canarias	Veneto
Alentejo	Castilla la mancha	Castilla la mancha	Umbria
Algarve	Acores	Acores	Marche
Abruzzi e Molise	Lisboa	Lisboa	Molise e Abruzzi
Luxembourg	Alentejo	Alentejo	Puglia
Acores	Algarve	Algarve	Basilicata
Limousin	Limousin	Limousin	Calabria
Calabria	Campania	Lombardia	Sicilia
Madeira	Calabria	Campania	Sardegna
Norte	Sicilia	Veneto	Luxembourg
Centro	Sardegna	Umbria	Namur
Campania	Madeira	Marche	Canarias
Sicilia	Norte	Puglia	Castilla la mancha
Sardegna	Centro	Basilicata	Acores
Lombardia	Lombardia	Calabria	Madeira
Veneto	Veneto	Sicilia	Norte
Umbria	Umbria	Sardegna	Centro
Marche	Marche	Madeira	Lisboa
Puglia	Puglia	Norte	Alentejo
Basilicata	Basilicata	Centro	Algarve

TABLE V

Continued

CLUSTER 20	CLUSTER 16	CLUSTER 8	CLUSTER 4
Hamburg	Hamburg	Hamburg	Hamburg
Basse-Normandie	Basse-Normandie	Bremen	Bremen
Pays de la Loire	Pays de la Loire	Nordrhein-Westfalen	Nordrhein-Westfalen
Bremen	Bremen	Ile de France	Berlin
Centre	Centre	Champagne-Ardenne	Brandeburg
Bourgogne	Bourgogne	Haute-Normandie	Macklenburg Vorpom
Alsace	Alsace	Centre	Sachsen
Hainaut	Hainaut	Basse-Normandie	Sachsen-Anhalt
Liege	Liege	Bourgogne	Thuringen
Nordrhein-Westfalen	Nordrhein-Westfalen	Lorraine	Ile de France
Champagne-Ardenne	Ile de France	Alsace	Champagne-Ardenne
Poitou-Charentes	Champagne-Ardenne	Pays de la Loire	Haute-Normandie
Auvergne	Haute-Normandie	Bretagne	Centre
Ile de France	Lorraine	Poitou-Charentes	Basse-Normandie
Haute-Normandie	Bretagne	Rhone-Alpes	Bourgogne
Lorraine	Poitou-Charentes	Auvergne	Lorraine
Bretagne	Rhone-Alpes	Languedoc-Roussill	Alsace
Rhone-Alpes	Auvergne	Bruxelles	Pays de la Loire
Languedoc-Roussill	Languedoc-Roussill	Hainaut	Bretagne
Bruxelles	Bruxelles	Liege	Poitou-Charentes
Berlin	Berlin	Berlin	Rhone-Alpes
Brandeburg	Brandeburg	Brandeburg	Auvergne
Macklenburg Vorpom	Macklenburg Vorpom	Macklenburg Vorpom	Languedoc-Roussill
Sachsen	Sachsen	Sachsen	Bruxelles
Sachsen-Anhalt	Sachsen-Anhalt	Sachsen-Anhalt	Hainaut
Thuringen	Thuringen	Thuringen	Liege

CLUSTER 20	CLUSTER 16	CLUSTER 8	CLUSTER 4
Groningen	Groningen	Groningen	Groningen
East Anglia	East Anglia	Friesland	Friesland
Balcares	Balcares	Dranthe	Dranthe
Friesland	Friesland	Overijssel	Overijssel
Dranthe	Dranthe	Gelderland	Gelderland
Overijssel	Overijssel	Flevoland	Flevoland
Gelderland	Gelderland	Noord-Brabant	Noord-Brabant
Flevoland	Flevoland	Utrecht	Utrecht
Noord-Brabant	Noord-Brabant	Noord-Holland	Noord-Holland
Utrecht	Utrecht	Zuid-Holland	Zuid-Holland
Noord-Holland	Noord-Holland	Zeeland	Zeeland
Zuid-Holland	Zuid-Holland	East Anglia	North
Zeeland	Zeeland	South East	Yorkshire Humber
South East	South East	South East	East Midlands
South West	South West	North West	East Anglia
North West	North West	NORTHERN IRELAND	South East
North	North	IRELAND	South West
Yorkshire Humber	Yorkshire Humber	DANMARK	West Midlands
East Midlands	East Midlands	Navarra	North West
West Midlands	West Midlands	Balcares	Wales
Wales	Wales	North	SCOTLAND
SCOTLAND	SCOTLAND	Yorkshire Humber	NORTHERN IRELAND
NORTHERN IRELAND	NORTHERN IRELAND	East Midlands	IRELAND
IRELAND	IRELAND	West Midlands	DANMARK
DANMARK	DANMARK	Wales	Navarra
Navarra	Navarra	SCOTLAND	Balcares

TABLE VI

Objective and subjective indicators: cutting the clustering tree at the different levels (20-16-8-4)

CLUSTERS 20		CLUSTERS 16	CLUSTERS 8	CLUSTERS 4 (larger clusters)		
Schleswig-Holstein	1.20.1*	Schleswig-Holstein	Schleswig-Holstein	Schleswig-Holstein	DE	1
Niedersachsen		Niedersachsen	Niedersachsen	Niedersachsen	DE	
Nordrhein-Westfalen		Nordrhein-Westfalen	Nordrhein-Westfalen	Nordrhein-Westfale	DE	
Hessen		Hessen	Hessen	Hessen	DE	
Rheinland-Pfalz		Rheinland-Pfalz	Rheinland-Pfalz	Rheinland-Pfalz	DE	
Baden Wuerttemberg		Baden Wuerttemberg	Baden Wuerttemberg	Baden-Wurttemberg	DE	
Bayern		Bayern	Bayern	Bayern	DE	
Saarland		Saarland	Saarland	Saarland	DE	
Antwerpen	1.20.14	Antwerpen	Antwerpen	Lombardia	IT	
Oost-Vlaanderen		Oost-Vlaanderen	Oost-Vlaanderen	Emilia Romagna	IT	
West-Vlaanderen		West-Vlaanderen	West-Vlaanderen	Lazio	IT	
LUSSEMBURGO		LUSSEMBURGO	LUSSEMBURGO	Piemonte+Valle D'Aost:	IT	
DANMARK		DANMARK	DANMARK	Liguria	IT	
Lombardia	1.20.10	Lombardia	Lombardia	Trentino	IT	
Emilia Romagna		Emilia Romagna	Emilia Romagna	Veneto	IT	
Lazio		Lazio	Lazio	Friuli V G	IT	
Piemonte+Valle D'Aosta		Piemonte+Valle D'Aosta	Piemonte+Valle D'Aosta	Toscana	IT	
Liguria		Liguria	Liguria	Umbria	IT	
Trentino		Trentino	Trentino	Marche	IT	
Veneto		Veneto	Veneto	Antwerpen	BE	
Friuli V G		Friuli V G	Friuli V G	Oost-Vlaanderen	BE	
Toscana		Toscana	Toscana	West-Vlaanderen	BE	
Umbria		Umbria	Umbria	LUSSEMBURGO	LU	
Marche		Marche	Marche	DANMARK	DK	
Hamburg	2.20.2	Hamburg	Hamburg	Hamburg	DE	2
Bremen		Bremen	Bremen	Bremen	DE	
Berlin	2.20.3	Berlin	Berlin	Berlin	DE	
Languedoc-Roussillon		Languedoc-Roussillon	Ile de France	Ile de France	FR	
Provence-Alpes-Cot		Provence-Alpes-Cot	Languedoc-Roussillon	Languedoc-Roussillon	FR	
Groningen		Groningen	Provence-Alpes-Cot	Provence-Alpes-Cote d'/	FR	
Zeeland		Zeeland	Groningen	Groningen	NL	
East Anglia		East Anglia	Friesland	Friesland	NL	
South-East		South-East	Drenthe	Drenthe	NL	
South-West		South-West	Overijssel	Overijssel	NL	
North-West		North-West	Gelderland	Gelderland	NL	
Baleares		NORTHERN IRELAND	Flevoland	Flevoland	NL	
NORTHERN IRELANI	2.20.16	IRELAND	Noord-Brabant	Noord-Brabant	NL	
IRELAND		Baleares	Limburg	Limburg	NL	
Ile de France	2.20.5	Ile de France	Utrecht	Utrecht	NL	
Flevoland		Flevoland	Noord-Holland	Noord-Holland	NL	
Utrecht		Utrecht	Zuid-Holland	Zuid-Holland	NL	
Noord-Holland		Noord-Holland	Zeeland	Zeeland	NL	
Zuid-Holland		Zuid-Holland	Bruxelles	Bruxelles	BE	
Bruxelles		Bruxelles	East Anglia	North	UK	
Friesland	2.20.13	Friesland	South-East	Yorkshire e Humber	UK	
Drenthe		Drenthe	South-West	East Midlands	UK	
Overijssel		Overijssel	North-West	East Anglia	UK	
Gelderland		Gelderland	NORTHERN IRELAND	South-East	UK	
Noord-Brabant		Noord-Brabant	IRELAND	South-West	UK	
Limburg		Limburg	Baleares	West Midlands	UK	
North	2.20.15	North	North	North-West	UK	
Yorkshire e Humber		Yorkshire e Humber	Yorkshire e Humber	Wales	UK	
East Midlands		East Midlands	East Midlands	Scotland	UK	
West Midlands		West Midlands	West Midlands	NORTHERN IRELANI	UK	
Wales		Wales	Wales	IRELAND	IE	
Scotland		Scotland	Scotland	Baleares	ES	

TABLE VI

Continued

CLUSTER 20		CLUSTER 16	CLUSTER 8	CLUSTERS 4 (larger clusters)		
Brandenburg	3.20.4	Brandenburg	Brandenburg	Brandenburg	DE	3
Mecklenburg-Vorpommern		Mecklenburg-Vorpommern	Mecklenburg-Vorpommern	Mecklenburg-Vorpomm	DE	
Sachsen		Sachsen	Sachsen	Sachsen	DE	
Sachsen-Anhalt		Sachsen-Anhalt	Sachsen-Anhalt	Sachsen-Anhalt	DE	
Thuringen		Thuringen	Thuringen	Thuringen	DE	
Nord-pas de Calais	3.20.6	Nord-pas de Calais	Nord-pas de Calais	Nord-pas de Calais	FR	
Picardie		Picardie	Champagne-Ardenne	Champagne-Ardenne	FR	
Haute-Normandie		Haute-Normandie	Picardie	Picardie	FR	
Basse-Normandie		Basse-Normandie	Haute-Normandie	Haute-Normandie	FR	
Lorraine		Lorraine	Centre	Centre	FR	
Hainaut		Hainaut	Basse-Normandie	Basse-Normandie	FR	
Liège		Liège	Bourgogne	Bourgogne	FR	
Champagne-Ardenne	3.20.7	Champagne-Ardenne	Lorraine	Lorraine	FR	
Centre		Centre	Alsace	Alsace	FR	
Bourgogne		Bourgogne	Pays de la Loire	Pays de la Loire	FR	
Alsace		Alsace	Bretagne	Bretagne	FR	
Pays de la Loire		Pays de la Loire	Poitou-Charentes	Poitou-Charentes	FR	
Bretagne		Bretagne	Aquitaine	Aquitaine	FR	
Poitou-Charentes		Poitou-Charentes	Midi-Pyrénées	Midi-Pyrénées	FR	
Aquitaine		Aquitaine	Rhone-Alpes	Rhone-Alpes	FR	
Midi-Pyrénées		Midi-Pyrénées	Auvergne	Auvergne	FR	
Rhone-Alpes		Rhone-Alpes	Hainaut	Hainaut	BE	
Auvergne		Auvergne	Liège	Liège	BE	

CLUSTER 20		CLUSTER 16	CLUSTER 8	CLUSTERS 4 (larger clusters)		
Franche-Compté	4.20.8	Franche-Compté	Franche-Compté	Franche-Compté	FR	4
Abruzzo e Molise		Abruzzo e Molise	Limousin	Limousin	FR	
Limburg		Limburg	Abruzzo e Molise	Campania	IT	
Luxembourg		Luxembourg	Brabant (Wallon+Vlaams)	Abruzzo e Molise	IT	
Limousin	4.20.9	Limousin	Limburg	Puglia	IT	
Brabant (Wallon+Vlaams)		Brabant (Wallon+Vlaams)	Luxembourg	Basilicata	IT	
Namur		Namur	Namur	Calabria	IT	
Lisboa		Lisboa	Acores	Sicilia	IT	
Alentejo	4.20.20	Alentejo	Madeira	Sardegna	IT	
Algarve		Algarve	Norte	Brabant (Wallon+Vlaam	BE	
Acores	4.20.19	Acores	Centro	Limburg	BE	
Madeira		Madeira	Lisboa	Luxembourg	BE	
Norte		Norte	Alentejo	Namur	BE	
Centro		Centro	Algarve	Madrid	ES	
Campania	4.20.11	Campania	Campania	Canarias	ES	
Puglia		Puglia	Puglia	Galicia	ES	
Calabria		Calabria	Basilicata	Asturias	ES	
Sicilia		Sicilia	Calabria	Cantabria	ES	
Sardegna		Sardegna	Sicilia	Pais Vasco	ES	
Madrid		Madrid	Sardegna	Navarra	ES	
Canarias		Canarias	Madrid	Rioja	ES	
Basilicata	4.20.12	Basilicata	Canarias	Aragon	ES	
Rioja		Rioja	Galicia	Castilla leon	ES	
Galicia	4.20.17	Galicia	Asturias	Castilla la mancha	ES	
Castilla la mancha		Asturias	Cantabria	Extremadura	ES	
Extremadura		Cantabria	Pais Vasco	Cataluna	ES	
Andalusia		Pais Vasco	Navarra	Pais Valenciano	ES	
Murcia		Navarra	Rioja	Andalusia	ES	
Asturias	4.20.18	Aragon	Aragon	Murcia	ES	
Cantabria		Castilla leon	Castilla leon	Acores	PT	
Pais Vasco		Castilla la mancha	Castilla la mancha	Madeira	PT	
Navarra		Extremadura	Extremadura	Norte	PT	
Aragon		Cataluna	Cataluna	Centro	PT	
Castilla leon		Pais Valenciano	Pais Valenciano	Lisboa	PT	
Cataluna		Andalusia	Andalusia	Alentejo	PT	
Pais Valenciano		Murcia	Murcia	Algarve	PT	

The first number is referred to the larger cluster, the second is referred to the cut of the clustering tree, the third is referred to the cluster number.

NOTES

[1] In the social sciences the geographical maps have been neglected as an analytic tool for a long time. The reason of this appears to lie largely in the common difficulties of using maps effectively and efficiently. Geographical Information System (GIS) is a computer technology for handling "geographic" data i.e. data where the detailed physical location is an essential element. GIS technology is a combination of digital mapping techniques and specialised data base management procedures. GIS are used to encode, store, maintain, retrieve, process, analyse and display data in their spatial context. GIS gives substantial advantages in data handling, analysis and presentation. The ability to link and display from different data sets (not necessarily with one identical geo-coding system) is both a powerful analytic tool and a way of presenting results with maximum impact. In this paper we considered the GIS for this ability to facilitate the statistical cluster analysis.

[2] Alongside this study C. Rampichini and S. Schifini D'Andrea (Social Indicators Research, Vol. 44, n. 1, 1998) analysed individual satisfaction between Italian regions. Moreover, work is now underway to develop a multilevel model for the analysis of life satisfaction among European regions (C. Rampichini and S. Schifini D'Andrea: 1998, Subjective, Objective and Contextual Components of Life Satisfaction in Europe, *Draft only*).

[3] For purposes of demonstration, in this paper, we have chosen a negative aspect of quality of life, that of "socio-economic unease."

[4] By "macro" we refer to a country-wide study, as opposed to "micro" which we use to refer to a study at the individual level.

[5] Eurostat data refer to 1994 and are found in the 1995–1996 and 1997 volumes (Cfr. Eurostat, Regions Series, Theme 1A).

[6] The regions of Eurostat are not exactly comparable with those of Eurobarometer, and thus, right from the phase of the singling out of territorial units there is already a lack of uniformity. For example, the Eurostat data show some countries without regional divisions (Luxembourg, Denmark, Ireland), Eurobarometer divides these same countries into regions (Luxembourg = 4; Denmark = 4; Ireland = 9). There are regions that Eurostat separate (for example, Italy: Piedmont and Val d'Aosta) which are grouped together by Eurobarometer; and in other cases, vice versa. There are countries in which there is Eurobarometer data but not Eurostat data (ex: Norway), and others in which there is Eurostat data but not Eurobarometer data (Finland, Sverige). We have excluded Greece due to the impossibility of isolating l'Attiki, with the city of Athens, which in Eurobarometer data is not reported as a separate region.

[7] Edited Eurostat data even have gaps at the level of single territorial units. For certain phenomena (e.g., for Holland: number of doctors; for the UK: number of hospital beds, cause of death) in the absence of regional data, data for the next level up was given. In particular, the UK is more problematic for purposes of comparison and thus the objective indicators often demonstrate a uniformity that most probably does not correspond to reality.

[8] This method is distinct from all other methods because it uses an analysis of variance approach to evaluate the distance between clusters. In short, this method attempts to minimize the Sum of Squares of any two (hypothetical) clusters that can be formed at each step. In general this method tends to create clusters of small size. We have noticed that when the similarity between observations is strong, analogous aggregations result even when other methods are used For example, here is the first cluster that is confirmed with Ward's method and with the complete tie method.

Hainaut	Liege		
Namur	Luxembourg		
Baden Wuerttemberg	Bayern		
Brandeburg	Macklenburg Vorpommern		
Sachsen	Sachsen-Anhalt	Thuringen	
Aragon	La Rioja		
Asturias	Pais Velenciano		
Cantabria	Castilla Leon		
Cataluna	Pais Vasco		
Champagne-Ardenne	Centre	Bourgogne	Pays de la Loire

[9] Clusters are indicated by three numbers in parentheses: the first is in reference to the larger cluster obtained at the level of 4 European divisions; the second to the level at which the tree is cut (in this case comprised of 20 parts); the third to the number of the particular cluster within the grouping under consideration.
[10] See note n. 7.
[11] See note n. 2.

REFERENCES

Diener, E. and E. Suh: 1997, 'Measuring quality of life: economic, social and subjective indicators', Social Indicators Research 40, pp. 189–216.
Diener, E., M. Diener and C. Diener: 1995, 'Factors predicting the subjective well-being of Nations', Journal of Personality and Social Psychology 69, pp. 851–864.
Diener, E., E. Suh and L. Shao: 1995, 'Nationals differences in reported subjective well-being: why do they occur?', Social Indicators Research 34, pp. 7–32.
Diener, E.: 1995, 'A value based index for measuring national quality of life', Social Indicators Research 36, pp. 107–127.
European Commission: 1994, Eurobarometer 42 (Bruxelles).
Eurostat: 1995, 1996, 1997, Regions Statistical Yearbook (Luxembourg).
Inglehart, R. and J. R. Rabier: 1984, 'Du bonheur sentiment personel et norme culturelle', Futuribles 81, pp. 3–27.

Rampichini, C. and S. Schifini D'Andrea: 1998, 'A hierarchical ordinal probit model for the analysis of life satisfaction in Italy', Social Indicators Research 44, pp. 41–69.

Department of Statistics "G. Parenti"
University of Florence
Italy
E-mails: alex@ds.unifi.it; schifini@ds.unifi.it

JEROEN BOELHOUWER

SOCIAL INDICATORS AND LIVING CONDITIONS IN THE NETHERLANDS

ABSTRACT. The Dutch Social en Cultural Planning Office (SCP) monitors social changes and social services, evaluates social policies, gives information about expected developments in the future and gives recommendations for further policy. Key issues are the assessment of economic, demographic and social changes and the influence of these factors on the social and living conditions of the population. The SCP uses social and economic indicators to examine these developments. Besides researching specific themes (such as social exclusion, the consequences of long-term unemployment, the social position of the elderly and use, costs and productivity of social services) the SCP has developed an overall monitoring tool for the living conditions: the living conditions index (LCI). Nowadays the index is composed of indicators which reflect conditions in eight areas: housing, health, consumer durables, leisure activity, sport activity, social participation, mobility and holiday. In the future, the SCP will attempt to develop a conceptual model that will link the living conditions index to other social indices like livability (housing and level of services), poverty and socioeconomic deprivation.

1. THE DUTCH SOCIAL AND CULTURAL PLANNING OFFICE

In the Netherlands there are four planning offices, which form a network from which government can draw during the process of setting out a policy. They are: the Netherlands Bureau for Economic Policy Analysis (CPB), the National Physical Planning Agency (RPD), the National Institute of Public Health and the Environment (RIVM) and the Social and Cultural Planning Office (SCP). Besides these planning offices there is a provider of official statistics: Statistics Netherlands (CBS).

As the names indicate, each of the planning agencies is concerned with a different aspect of society: economy, town and country planning, health and the environment, and social and cultural affairs. Together they cover almost all areas of government.

Social Indicators Research **60:** 89–113, 2002.

Speaking of planning can, in this context, be misleading. The planning offices do not make a blueprint for the future society. They analyse developments, evaluate policy and make recommendations for improving that policy. From these starting points, however, they tend to look into the future and make suggestions for upcoming policies.

The Social and Cultural Planning Office was established by Royal Decree in 1973. In the Royal Decree the official definition of the task is threefold:

- to carry out research designed to produce a coherent picture of the state of social and cultural welfare in the Netherlands and likely developments in this area;
- to contribute to the appropriate selection of policy objectives and to provide an assessment of the advantages and disadvantages of the various means of achieving those ends;
- to seek information on the way in which interdepartmental policy on social and cultural welfare is implemented with a view to assessing its implementation.

The SCP is an inter-ministerial institute which conducts independent research on social and cultural developments and advises the policy-makers. The SCP considers all areas of government policy, as far as social aspects are involved. It concentrates on the fields of health, welfare, social security, labour market and education and especially on the intersections between these different social fields.

The government is the principal user of the SCP products. Ministers, the parliament and civil servants are the primary target groups of the SCP. A second category are the regional and local authorities. They too need information about social trends and governmental social policies as a frame of reference for their own social policies. The bureau reports frequently on local and regional developments. The publications are also used often for scientific purposes by universities and researchers. Another category of consumers are the management and professionals of the service-sector, subsidized by government, like schools, hospitals and theatres. The SCP frequently publishes about issues that are relevant to them.

Each report gets more or less extensive press coverage, by which the general public (and the target groups mentioned above) get to know about the findings and results of SCP-research. Scientific aspects of SCP research are highlighted in national and international journals.

2. SOCIAL INDICATORS AND THE SCP

For over a century now, statistics and indicators are being used to express characteristics of societies. The beginning of the social indicators movement can be set in 1966, when Bauer was asked by NASA to explore the social effects of their space program. This has stimulated other organizations to develop similar studies. Perhaps the most influential of them was the "Social Indicator Development Program" of the Organisation for Economic Co-operation and Development (OECD). This Program began in 1970 and lead to a list of social indicators in 1982, followed by a "compendium" in 1986 (called "Living Conditions in OECD Countries"). Currently many countries, and even some regions within them, have come up with a bundled form of social statistics, titled "Social Indicators" or "The quality of life in ...." In the Netherlands this publication is called the "Social and Cultural Report," product of the SCP.

This is the most important, and most voluminous, publication of the SCP and is filled with analyses based on empirical data, official statistics and policy papers. It is published every two years and deals with various aspects of Dutch society, such as: demographic developments; economy, the welfare state, work and social security; values and norms in society; public administration; emancipation; health and health care; housing; education; crime and justice; leisure, media and culture; and (social) participation. The central theme of the 1998 Report was: "Twenty-five years of social change."

When the first copy of the Social and Cultural Report 1998 was handed to the Prime Minister, he said: "The Social and Cultural Report has developed into a reliable, critical and abundant source of information for politics, policy, the field, science and journalism. That was what the government intended at the foundation and it still is the most important assignment."

Social and Cultural Report 1998
25 years of social change in the Netherlands

Demographic Developments, Emancipation and Values and Norms in Society
* Parenthood is being postponed.
* Most mothers with small children have returned to work, but emancipation stops at the one-and-a-half income household.
* First and foremost, the Dutch want safety.

The Multi-ethnic Society
* The proportion of ethnic minorities in Dutch society has increased sixfold in one-quarter of a century to nearly 10% of the population and is still growing fast.
* The ethnic minorities are strongly over represented among the underprivileged groups of society. However, as more and more members of these groups achieve social success, the minorities exhibit increasing social diversity.
* As the ethnic minorities grow in number, the Netherlands is also becoming more diverse in a cultural respect, which however does not make the Netherlands a *multi cultural* society.

Economy and the Welfare State, Work and Social Security
* Between 1977 and 1995 inequality in income showed a substantial rise. In 1977, the purchasing power of a household on benefit was 93% of the average purchasing power of all households; by 1995 this figure had dropped to 79%.
* In 1997, a majority of the population felt most social security schemes to be inadequate, while this was still a minority four years ago.

Political Diversity, Public Administration, Participation
* The electorate has become more flexible: voters are less inclined to consistently vote for one single party.
* Turnout for elections has further decreased, but at the same time the involvement of the general public in organizations for a 'good cause' has shown a strong increase.

Health and Health Care
* In 1998 there is more "illness" among the population than 25 years ago. Aging, early detection and an increased alertness to health problems are responsible for this.
* More and more people seek help for psychological problems.

Housing
* Renting is less and less popular.
* The urban housing stock has difficulty in competing on the housing market.

Education
* The educational expansion went hand in hand with less inequality in education.
* Young people with limited capacities and a vocational orientation have more and more difficulty as requirements continue to rise.

Crime and Justice
* Between 1970 and 1994, registered crime nearly quadrupled. This brought crime in the Netherlands to the same level as in other Western countries.
* Thanks to societal developments, new problems are presenting themselves, such as fraud on the stock exchange and crime on the electronic superhighway.

Leisure Time, the Media and Culture
* Partners in two-income households spend more time on duties and obligations (child care, work and studying) and have a total of 14 hours less in free time than partners in a traditional household with a single breadwinner.
* Less free time is spent at home.

The SCP mainly has two types of products. The Social and Cultural Report is part of the *first one:* the periodical publications. Another important, periodical, publication is the Social and Cultural Outlook which is published yearly.[2] The purpose of the Social and Cultural Outlook is to describe briefly (several aspects of the) living conditions of the Dutch population and to analyse current developments in important areas of government policy. Recurring issues are: the public opinion on government and politics, the living conditions of the Dutch population, and the public, subsidised, sector. Besides, every year a topical subject is examined, like residents of deprived neighbourhoods, (feelings of) insecurity, and the lower end of the labour market. See for the headlines of the Social and Cultural Outlook 1998 Appendix A.

Besides the Social and Cultural Report and the Social and Cultural Outlook other periodical publications deal with special categories of the population. The bureau reports regularly on the elderly, the youth, the mentally and physically handicapped people, women and ethnic minorities. See for last years publications

Appendix B. The *second category* of products are the research-results on specific issues, like poverty, car use and living without a job (for some examples, see Appendix B). In addition, the director and his staff participate in advisory bodies and governmental co-ordinating committees.

Most of the SCP publications deal with several different aspects of the living conditions. The SCP has also developed an overall monitoring instrument for the living conditions: the so called living conditions index.

3. THE SCP'S LIVING CONDITIONS INDEX

After a dip in the attention paid to social indicators, the interest in social issues gradually revived. Not only for specific areas, but also for a measuring instrument that integrates various areas. An international example is the "Human Development Index" of the United Nations Development Programme (UNDP), which integrates indicators in three areas: health, education and income, and compares various countries on the HDI. In the Netherlands too, governmental policy in the past years shifted from attention for different areas to a more integrative approach. Examples are the so-called "major cities policy" (with special attention for the specific, and diverse, problems of the four major cities in the Netherlands) and the growing attention for livability (in the major cities as well as in the rural areas). Policy on improving the quality of life does nowadays not only aims at the struggle against unemployment, but also at improving the living conditions, safety and social and societal participation.

3.1. *Basic Considerations*

Riding the crest of the internationally emerging social indicators movement, the Social and Cultural Planning Office in 1974 initiated a survey on well-being. The intended result was an index for the social side of the Netherlands. More specifically, the study focussed on the dispersion and concentrations of well-being.[3] The aims assigned by the SCP to the study were fivefold: to depict social and cultural conditions as a single entity; to evaluate this entity in terms of positive and negative; to create a time series for observing changes; to monitor developments in the separate indicators over time; and to situate the description of social and cultural conditions in a broader context of background information. It was not the primary aim to publicize absolute figures each year. After all, it means very little to announce that, for example, "well-being was 5.9 in 1980." The primary aim was to identify trends.

The first step in developing the index was to determine which areas were to be included in the umbrella notion of well-being. The fact that one task of the SCP is to make policy recommendations to the government was an important starting-point. That's why clusters were selected that were capable of being influenced by government policy. The actual indicators, as well as the variables comprising these indicators, were then defined within each cluster.

A number of requirements were set for the indicators. First, they were to be focussed on *"output."* The number of dwellings actually built was less important for this purpose than peoples housing conditions, and the number of doctors was not as important as the state of health of individuals. Second, the indicators were to be *general in nature*, applicable to the entire population rather than to specific groups. Third, they were to measure *objective* characteristics of living conditions, in order to avoid personal preferences and individual interpretations of concepts. Fourth, it was to be clear, at least implicitly, whether they had a *positive or a negative effect* on well-being. Finally they had to be measured at an individual level. This makes it possible not only to monitor developments at the national level, but also to break down well-being for different groups in society.

Until 1993 the term used was "the index on well-being." However, the term "well-being" is often associated with subjective feelings of happiness. Since the index in question was designed to create an objectified picture, the SCP now prefers the term "living conditions index."

3.2. *Some Changes over Time*

Nowadays the index is composed of indicators which reflect conditions in eight areas: housing, health, leisure activity, sport activity, social participation, mobility, vacation and consumer durables. Taken together, the indicators provide an objectified description of living conditions.

But there has never been a cut-and-dried formula for the contents of the SCP index. What variables, indicators and clusters should be included or omitted has always been the subject of debate. They have changed over time, for instance because of outdated parts or because of new trends and fields of importance, indicated by policymakers. However, the SCP tried to take great care for preserving the comparability of the data over time. This enabled us to monitor how the different factors influencing living conditions interrelate and change over time.

Table I contains a summary of indicators that were used in the living conditions index between 1974 and 1997.

Onc of the greatest merits of the living conditions index has been the time series of twenty years until 1993. Unfortunately this series could not be continued because of changes data collecting by Statistics Netherlands. It changed the surveying design as well as the questions, the order in which they are asked, and the methods of selecting and contacting respondents. Statistics Netherlands now integrates a number of surveys, among which the living conditions survey, into what is called the "permanent study of living conditions" (POLS).

These alterations logically caused a break in the trend registered so far. On the other hand, this has provided us with an opportunity to carry out a thorough revision of the LCI. Only a single break in the trend will then occur, and a new time series can be started. So from 1997 on new data is collected biannually, using new questions and modified survey methods in a new design.[4]

One of the reasons to revise the LCI was that some parts of it had grown out of date. Items that were important 20 years ago are not necessarily so any longer. A consumer article then considered a luxury may now be commonplace, or even antiquated. Furthermore, due to technological progress there are now articles available that did not exist, or were not available to the general public, in 1974. So slide projectors have made way for personal computers and CD players.

Another reason for the revision was that policy nowadays deals with aspects of life that affect living conditions, not all of which could be covered adequately by the LCI. Examples are social participation, residential environment and public safety.

TABLE I

Indicators used in the Living Conditions Index in the Course of its History

	1974	1977	1980	1983	1986	1988/89	1990–1993	1997
Housing								
Type of ownership	x	x	x	x	x	x	x	x
Type of building	x	x	x	x	x	x	x	x
Structural condition	x	x	x	x	x	x		
Desire to relocate				x	x			
Central heating		x						
Number of rooms				x				x
Area of living room								x
Scary spot in the neighbourhood								x
Year of construction								x
Health								
Number of long-term illnesses	x	x	x					
Number of psychosomatic symptoms	x	x	x	x	x	x	x	x
Stayed home sick in past 3 months	x	x	x					
Number of 8 serious illnesses				x	x	x	x	x
Number of other illnesses				x	x	x	x	x
Feeling of being ill		x						
Hospitalized in past year				x				
Purchasing power/consumer durables								
Nousehold income	x	x	x	x				
Number of consumer durables	x	x	x	x	x			
Number of household appliances					x		x	x
Number of hobby articles					x	x	x	x
Leisure activities								
Number of leisure activities	x	x	x					
Number of hobbies				x	x	x	x	x
Number of non-domestic entertainment activities				x	x	x	x	x

TABLE I

Continued

	1974	1977	1980	1983	1986	1988/89	1990–1993	1997
Organizational membership				x	x	x	x	x
Mobility								
Car ownership	x	x	x	x	x	x	x	x
Season ticket railway								x
Social participation								
Active contribution to activities of organization								x
Contact with neighbourhood residents		x						
Volunteer work				x	x	x	x	x
Social isolation (scale)	x	x	x					x
Sport activity								
Dport participation	x	x	x	x	x	x	x	
Number of times sporting a week								x
Number of sports								x
Vacation								
Vacation in past year					x	x	x	x
Vacation to a foreign country								x
Number of vacation articles					x	x	x	x
Miscellaneous								
Educational attainment level	x	x	x	x	x			
Paid employment				x	x			

We also used the opportunity to broaden and deepen several clusters, such as whether the vacation was in the Netherlands or abroad, and with greater numbers of sports and leisure activities specified in the survey.

Throughout the years we also made some adjustments in the arrangement of the clusters and indicators. In 1980 the SCP decided to split the former indicators "number of leisure activities" and "number of consumer durables" into three new ones each (see Table I). The reason to do this was that the former clusters appeared to be too broad to get a good picture of differences between groups.

In 1997 the cluster "leisure activities" was split into two new ones. One of them now contains indicators which not necessarily lead to social contacts: organizational membership; number of hobbies; and number of non-domestic entertainment activities. The other cluster ("social participation") contains indicators of which can be expected that they contribute to having social contacts (see Table I). The splitting up has to do with the greater attention social participation nowadays draws.

We also included a separate cluster "sport activity." Sport activities were formerly added to the cluster of "leisure activities." The reason for creating a new cluster is that sport participation has effect on leisure activities as well as on health and social participation.

3.3. *Living Conditions and Resources*

As you may have noticed, the index itself contains no indicators for education, income or payed employment since 1989. This change was motivated by theoretical considerations. Until 1989 the LCI contained indicators which can be seen as "output" or "realised opportunities," like the type of housing and the activities someone participates in. On the other hand the index contained a number of elements which contribute to realising the opportunities: level of education, income and payed employment. According to us these elements could better be seen as *resources* which enhance people's opportunities to achieve certain living conditions.

We now use these resources to describe the backgrounds of living conditions and have removed them from the index.[5] When describing these backgrounds we posit a causal relation: the more resources a person has, the more likely he or she is to enjoy better living conditions.

In this way the living conditions index reflects the degree to which people realise their opportunities. This makes it possible to consider whether government policy is needed to improve the conditions so that more people can realise their opportunities.

This modification, and the theoretical considerations that motivated it, now raise the question of what to do with health. From the view that resources create the preconditions for achieving certain living conditions, there is something to be said for classifying the health cluster under the resources. One might argue that good health is a prerequisite for good living conditions as defined by the index. On the other hand, one could also regard peoples state of health as an *outcome* of government measures or other factors that make for optimal living conditions. For this reason we have decided so far to retain health as part of the index proper.

3.4. *Living Conditions and Subjective Indicators*

The index contains furthermore no individual judgements. For this the most important argument is that we analyse living conditions in terms of *policy-relevant indicators.* Our purpose is to furnish the government with concrete handles for achieving a desired result. Identifying the exact sources and determinants of happiness, if at all possible, would be so complicated that research on subjective feelings would yield little information relevant to policy-making. Because of their obvious relationship, however, we regularly examine the relationships between the living conditions index, satisfactions, subjective health and general happiness (see Table II).

As can be seen in the table: the connection between happiness and the overall living conditions index is stronger than that between happiness and the separate indicators of the index.

3.5. *Constructing One Single Index*

A well-known problem is how to integrate the different indicators and clusters into one single index. There are a lot of different alternatives to cope with this problem. One of them is following the trends in a relative simple way, as used by Zapf and his colleagues from the university of Mannheim. They developed a linear additive model with ordinal scaling to compare different periods in time using +, – and =. One of the difficulties using this method is that a series of +, –, +, – between 1960 and 1970 can mask a rise from, let's say, 5 to 8 in the same period (5, 4, 9, 8). Another possible disadvantage of this method is that it gives every indicator an equal weight. Another approach is the one which takes as starting point a minimum package of needs (goods and services). The extent to

TABLE II

Correlation between (Indicators of) the Living Conditions, Happiness and Subjective Health, 1997 (Pearsons Correlation Coefficients)

	Living conditions	Happiness[a]	Subjective health[b]
Happiness	0.33	1.00	
Subjective health	0.40	0.31	1.00
Type of dwelling	0.20	0.10	0.08
Area of living room	0.40	0.12	0.14
Number of rooms	0.37	0.11	0.11
Type of ownership	0.44	0.15	0.15
scary environment	0.18	0.05	0.10
Year the dwelling was build	0.21	0.08	0.06
Diversity of hobby activities	0.31	0.13	0.11
Diversity of non-domestic entertainment activities	0.68	0.20	0.28
Organizational membership	0.45	0.09	0.12
Active contribution to an association or club	0.46	0.10	0.10
Volunteer work	0.23	0.08	0.05
Social isolation	0.51	0.29	0.20
Number of times a week sporting	0.51	0.13	0.19
Number of different sports	0.66	0.19	0.26
Recent vacation	0.60	0.21	0.19
Vacation abroad	0.53	0.16	0.17
Number of vacation articles	0.33	0.11	0.12
Car ownership	0.53	0.17	0.15
Ownership of a public transport season ticket	0.08	0.02 (n.s.)	0.04
Number of household appliances	0.44	0.15	0.12
Number of hobby articles	0.63	0.19	0.23

TABLE II

Continued

	Living conditions	Happiness[a]	Subjective health[b]
Score on a psychosomatic symptoms scale	0.34	–0.25	–0.49
Number of 9 serious illnesses	–0.19	–0.08	–0.31
Number of other illnesses	–0.34	–0.13	–0.47

[a]"To what degree do you consider yourself a happy person?" 1 = unhappy; 2 = not that happy; 3 = not happy and not unhappy; 4 = happy; 5 = very happy.
[b]"How is, in general, your health?" 1 = bad; 2 = sometimes good and sometimes bad; 3 = so so; 4 = good; 5 = very good.
n.s.: not significant.
Source: CBS (POLS, 1997); calculations by SCP.

which these needs are met can then be measured as a percentage of this minimum package. The index is then a aggregated figure of these percentages. In a similar way Johnston developed a quality-of-life index based on yearly changes in 21 objective indicators of "social concern." He gave greater weight to a declining development than to a rising one.[6] These examples mainly use objective, or objectified, indicators: what do people have or should have (according to a set of standards). Sometimes they use perceived satisfactions as a supplement. This approach differs from that of researchers who take happiness and satisfactions as a starting point.

Because of the lack of external criteria for weighting the indicators, the SCP chose for a rather pragmatic than fundamental solution. The starting point was the common dimension of the chosen indicators, which all contribute positively or negatively to the living conditions. Moreover, a single indicator which correlates better with the others should have a greater weight. Another starting point was that it had to be an *individually based* index, since we not only wanted to follow developments for the Netherlands as a whole, but for different groups in society as well.

In this way the SCP living conditions index is constructed, statistically, from the above mentioned clusters. The way in which this is done has slightly changed over time. In the beginning we used factor analysis to construct the index. We now use nonlinear canonical correlation analysis (OVERALS) to do so. This procedure enables us to cluster the indicators not only theoretically, but in the analysis as well. Besides that, the procedure can be used to weigh the indicators. OVERALS also has the advantage that variables do not have to be measured at the interval level (which is an assumption of PCA). Another advantage is that the *categories* of the indicators receive weights besides the indicators themselves, thus enabling us to compare the categories too.[7]

Table III contains an overview of the component loadings of the separate indicators which are the basis for the living conditions index in 1997.[8] Conceptually, the component loadings may be thought of as analogous to the factor loadings given in factor analysis (SPSS, 1990). The important indicators are: number of non-domestic entertainment activities; number of hobby articles and number of sports. On the other hand, possession of a season ticket for the railway; type of building and a scary spot in the neighbourhood do not contribute very much to the living conditions index.

3.6. *Controversial Indicators*

There has been some controversy about the role of car ownership in the index. People with cars score higher on living conditions than those without, and some observers asked whether that was rightly the case, in view of the growing awareness of the environment and of vehicle pollution. Although the pollutive nature of cars obviously cannot be denied, having a car does give many people a sense of freedom, of being able to come and go as they please. This is presumed to have a favourable effect on their living conditions. In view of the arguments on both sides, it has now been decided to include possession of a public transport season ticket alongside car ownership, since the former can engender a similar sense of freedom.

We planned to include a cluster on safety in the living conditions index, for two reasons: meeting the growing political interest on this subject and adding more information on the residential environment. The indicators chosen for this cluster had to do with falling victim to some offences, like bike or car theft, pick pockets and maltreatment. However, we could not include such a cluster. There appeared to be

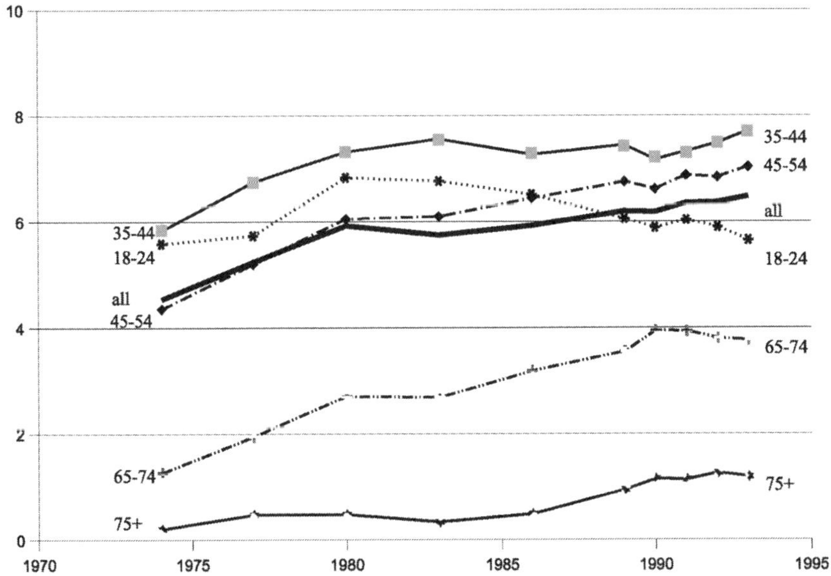

Figure 1. Living conditions in the Netherlands from 1974 to 1993, for all and for age groups.

no relation between the chosen indicators and the other indicators that form the LCI.[9] The conclusion had to be that there is no structural relationship between living conditions as a whole and falling prey to offences: it is more likely that this comes by accident and can happen to anybody anywhere.

Still, the index has not yet reached its final composition (if it ever will). In the nearby future we shall examine, for example, whether limitations due to lasting illnesses, disorders or handicap can be included in the LCI.

4. DEVELOPMENTS OF THE LIVING CONDITIONS BETWEEN 1974 AND 1997

The development of the living conditions in the Netherlands is shown in Figure 1. It shows that between 1974 and 1993 living conditions improved. As a consequence of the 1980 (oil) crisis, there was a dip in 1983. Nevertheless, in 1986 the living conditions had already reached the same level as before the crisis. The overall improvement in living conditions can be attributed primarily to a growing number of home owners and the greater number of house-

TABLE III

Component Loadings of the Indicators and the Influence of the Eight Clusters on the Living Conditions Index 1997 (Regression, bèta-Coefficients)

Indicators	Component loadings	Leisure activities	Sport durables	Consumer participation	Vacation	Social	Housing	Mobility	Health
Season ticket railway	0.08							x	
Type of building	0.17						x		
Scary spot in neighbourhood	0.17						x		
Number of 8 serious illnesses	–0.19								x
Volunteer work	0.23					x			
Year of construction	0.25						x		
Number of hobbies	0.30	x							
Number of other illnesses	–0.33								x
Number of rooms	0.33						x		
Number of vacation articles	0.34				x				
Score on health scale	–0.34								x
Area of living room	0.36						x		
Type of ownership	0.41						x		

TABLE III

Continued

Indicators	Component loadings	Leisure activities	Sport durables	Consumer participation	Vacation	Social	Housing	Mobility	Health
Number of household appliances	0.44			x					
Organizational membership	0.46	x							
Active contribution to activities	0.46					x			
Social isolation	0.50					x			
Number of times sporting	0.52		x						
Car ownership	0.53							x	
Vacation in foreign country	0.53				x				
Vacation last year	0.60				x				
Number of hobby articles	0.63			x					
Number of sports	0.67		x						
Number of non-domestic entertainment activities	0.69	x							

Source: CBS; POLS 1997 (calculations by SCP).

hold appliances. In addition, car ownership increased and more people were joining organizations and engaging in sports. As said, collection of the data ceased in 1993 and was not continued until 1997. There has not yet been enough time to thoroughly examine the breakings in the trend, so (for the time being) the trends can not be continued.

The SCP not only monitors the living conditions for the Dutch population as a whole, but for various groups as well. Breaking down the index for various groups reveals that not all people have benefited from the greater prosperity to the same extent. Although the living conditions of most groups have improved, the pace of improvement is not equal (see Figure 1). Moreover, the youngest age-group (18–24 years old) was confronted with declining living conditions since 1980. The reasons for this drop were diverse: their scores on most indicators declined.[10] Besides, some groups have consistently endured rather poor living conditions between 1974 and 1993. These are the older people, the single-person households, and the city-dwellers. In addition, groups with low levels of education or low incomes (from social benefit, especially from the state old-age or widows and orphans schemes) have made below-average gains.

Table IV shows the living conditions in 1997 for several groups.[11] We have taken into account some demographic characteristics, as well as some of the resources. Unfortunately, not all data are available yet (like income and source of income). As a substitution, we constructed a variable reflecting the most important daily activity in combination with having (or not having) a paid job.

The Table IV shows that the following groups are in relative poor living conditions:

* persons aged 75 years or older;
* one person households and one parent households;
* unemployed people (especially if the most important daily activity is being a housewife/-man);
* people with low education.

The best living conditions are experienced by students, particularly if they have a paid job besides their study. The main reasons for their good living conditions are the relative great number of entertainment activities and the relative large number of social contacts they have.

TABLE IV

Influence of Some Background Characteristics on the Living Conditions in 1997 (Analysis of Variance ANOVA)

	Not corrected	èta	corrected	bèta
Entire population	100		100	
Age				
18–24 years	105		101	
25–34 years	104		101	
35–44 years	105		102	
45–54 years	102		101	
55–64 years	97		100	
65–74 years	91		99	
75 years or older	76		87	
		0.51		0.24
Type of household				
1 person household	91		94	
1-parent family	90		92	
(married) couple with a child (<18 years)	105		102	
(married) couple without children	99		101	
3 adult or more, including a (married) couple	104		103	
Other	103		102	
		0.34		0.21
Most important daily activity[a]				
Paid work	105		102	
Working student	110		107	
Non-working student	104		103	
Working housewife/-man	105		102	
Non-working housewife/-man	91		96	
Volunteer work	100		102	
Other	88		93	
		0.49		0.25

TABLE IV

Continued

	Not corrected	èta	corrected	bèta
Completed educational level				
Primary school	87		91	
Lower vocational education	97		97	
Lower secondary education	102		102	
Higher secondary/vocational education	104		102	
High education, university	109		107	
		0.49		0.36
Explained variance				48%

[a]Within the category volunteer work no distinction has been made between working and non-working, because the majority of volunteers does not work.
NB: everything above 1 hour is counted as "working." It turned out that there was no difference in scores for people working more and people working less than 12 hours a week.
Source: CBS (POLS, 1997); calculations by SCP.

5. THE FUTURE: A MODEL-BASED APPROACH

At this moment we work at a conceptual model with which we can link the living conditions to other SCP-research, like indices of livability (housing and level of services) and socioeconomic deprivation (see Figure 2). In this model we shall examine relations with satisfactions and happiness as well. The purpose of this new study is to find out in what way such social areas are interrelated and to what extent personal or neighbourhood characteristics influence them. The need for such a model comes forth from the growing attention for social indicators, and especially the growing need for integrated information, in the Netherlands.

The first step, to be taken within the upcoming months, is to study more thoroughly the relationship between the living conditions of individuals and their residential environment. Currently policymakers in the Netherlands are very interested in figures about socially deprived neighbourhoods and districts.

Two recent studies of the Social and Cultural Planning Office to this matter, reveal that:

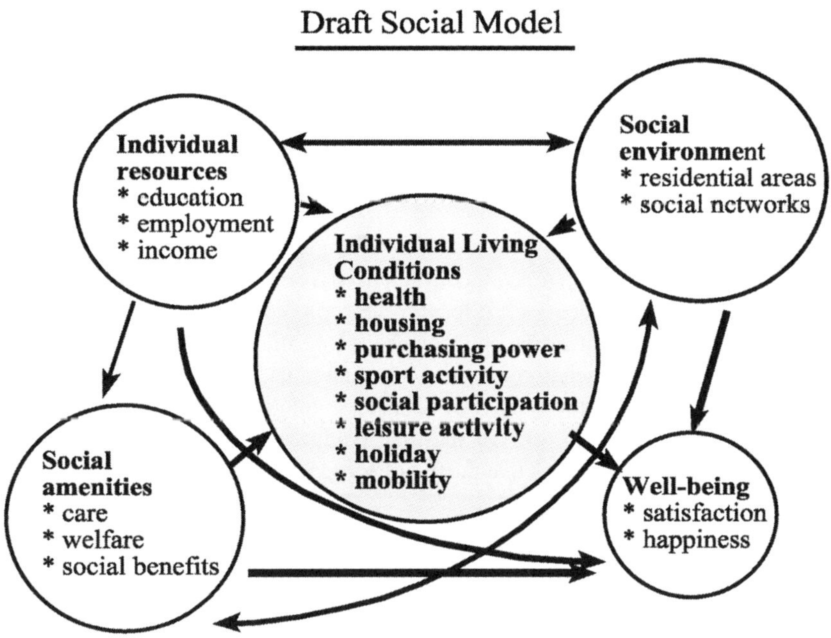

Figure 2. The future of the living conditions index in a conceptual social model.

* The social status of many urban neighbourhoods has dropped, while rural neighbourhoods have seen their status rise;
* Decline in the status of a neighbourhood is accompanied by general deterioration: the area becomes unsafe;
* Most poor rural areas are in the north of the country. However: they generally have lower concentrations of poor people than poor areas of the major cities.

These studies, however, concentrated on separate aspects: one on social status, the other on poverty. The aim of the model, as said, is to integrate these aspects with the living conditions index to confront individual and environmental characteristics.

APPENDIX A: HEADLINES OF THE SOCIAL AND CULTURAL OUTLOOK 1998

Public opinion and the government

People in the Netherlands have a growing optimism about the Dutch economy. A big majority gives government a pass on socio-economic policies. However: maintaining order and care for the elderly people are unsatisfactory. Almost two-third of the population find the differences in incomes too big and find the benefits for the elderly (the old age pensions) too low.

Europe

The vast majority of the population thinks positively about the European Union.

Drugs inconvenience

8% of the population is inconvenienced by drugs in the neighbourhood on a regular basis; 14% is sometimes inconvenienced. Half of the population in those neighbourhoods has fallen victim to an offence, which is twice as much as in neighbourhoods without drugs convenience. More than 40% of the population of drugs-convenience neighbourhoods feel unsafe. These percentages are much higher in the four major cities. Nevertheless: tolerance for the use of soft drugs is growing (though 40% of the total population and the majority of the people aged 50 or more, think that the use of soft drugs has to be punished severe).

Living conditions

The living conditions of the Dutch in the long term are still rising. However, also in 1997 people aged 75 or more; single parent households; and one person households, are confronted with worse living conditions.

Education

The educational level of the Dutch population keeps rising. The average number of years of education has risen to almost 12 years. School dropout gradual reduces.

Work and income

Between 1994 and 1997 the working population has grown with almost 500.000 people. Unemployment decreases: however somewhat more than 1.000.000 are searching for a job. Income inequality, which had grown at the end of the 1980's, is declining.

High-risk groups and local social policies

Based on education, work and income a number of high-risk groups has been appointed. To a great extent they live in the deprived areas of the major cities. They include: 55.000 youngsters (ethnic minorities are over represented); 188.000 long standing unemployed (ethnic minorities are over represented); 266.000 children of households with minimum incomes; 190.000 elderly and handicapped people with low income and a great need for care; 25.000 homeless; between 185.000 and 320.000 alcohol addicts; and between 34.000 and 54.000 problematic hard drugs users.

APPENDIX B: A SELECTION OF THE SCP-PUBLICATIONS IN 1997

Last years SCP-publications that deal with special categories of the population:

* "Youth report 1997": This study focuses on a specific group: young people with problems.
* "Report on the Disabled 1997": The focus areas are education, employment, income, residential situation, take-up of care and use of leisure time.
* "Report on Minorities 1997": This publication examines the school attendance, educational attainment and school careers of ethnic minority pupils. It also assesses their employment prospects.
* "Social atlas of the woman: part 4: changes in the primary living situation": This report discusses the respective positions of, and relationships between, men and women households and on the labour market.

Examples of other SCP-reports:

* "From high to low; from low to high": This study explains how social status of residential areas is determined and how it can change in the course of time.
* "Poverty Monitor 1998" (in cooperation with Statistics Netherlands): presents a complete and up-to-date picture of poverty in the Netherlands.
* "Life without a job": This study explores the impact of not working on the individual.
* "Survey of demand for housing and care for the elderly": This report concerns the possible increase in the number of elderly people requiring help and the consequences for the uptake of housing and care facilities for the elderly.
* "Social and individual determinants of car use": The SCP has developed a model to investigate which factors influence behaviour that is relevant for the environment.

NOTES

[1] An English translation of the 1996 Report (with special attention to the big cities) is available. An English translation of a popular version of the Social and Cultural Report 1998 and a translations of the 2000 Report (The Netherlands in a European Perspective) are available as well.
[2] From the year 2000 on, the Social and Cultural Outlook is replaced by a new bi-annual report called: The Social Side of the Netherlands.
[3] Well-being was defined as "the totality of all aspects that can be considered beneficial to people's living conditions," see Mootz & Konings-van der Snoek, 1990.
[4] It should be noticed that the survey for the living conditions index is only held among persons living on their own (and their household). This implies that

people (temporarily) living in institutes or without a permanent address are not questioned, by which they are no part of the sample.

[5] The removal of the so-called resources from the LCI did, however, not affect the main structure of the index. Without these indicators, the remaining ones correlated in the same way as they did before. See the Social and Cultural Report 1988.

[6] These examples are based on Horn, 1993.

[7] OVERALS looks first at the influence of the separate indicators within one cluster. Then every cluster is equally weighted in the combined index; irrespective of the number of indicator included in a cluster. This also is an advantage to previous used techniques.

[8] Component loadings are projections of the quantified variables in the object space (when there are no missing data, the component loadings are equivalent to the Pearson's correlation, between the quantified variable and the object scores).

[9] There is one exception: we found a, small, positive relation between number of non-domestic entertainment activities and bike-theft. Besides, there are some relations between falling victim and categories of background indicators. For example: men fall more victim to threats and maltreatment than women; people who do lots of different sports fall more prey to pick pockets; and in general younger people (18–24 years old) and people living in flats fall more victim to all kinds of crimes.

[10] A possible explanation for the declining living conditions of people aged 18–24 are changes in their scholarships into the so-called "pace-scholarship." As a result of this, students had less spare time to spent at activities and paid work.

[11] As you will notice we also changed the way we present the index. In the beginning the factor-scores were re-calculated into a scale which ranged, approximately, from 0 till 10. The current index is set at 100 for 1997 for the whole Dutch population.

REFERENCES

Andrews, F. M. (ed.): 1986, Research on Quality of Life (Institute for Social Research, Ann Arbor, MI).

Bauer, R. A. (ed.): 1966, Social Indicators (MIT Press, Cambridge, MA).

Campbell, A.: 1981, The Sense of Well-Being in America (McGraw-Hill, New York).

Diener, E. and E. Suh: 1997, 'Measuring quality of life: economic, social, and subjective indicators', Social Indicators Research 40, pp. 189–216.

Horn, R. V.: 1993, Statistical Indicators for the Economic Sciences (Cambridge University Press, Cambridge).

Mootz, M. and M. Konings-van der Snoek: 1997, De mate van welzijn: verdeling en concentraties van welzijnsaspecten 1974–1989 (Social and Cultural Planning Office / VUGA, Rijswijk/The Hague).

Noll, H.: 1998, Social Indicators and Social Reporting: the International Experience (http://www.ccsd.ca/noll1.html and http://www.ccsd.ca/noll2.html).
Nussbaum, M. C. and A. Sen (eds.): 1993, The Quality of Life (Oxford University Press, New York).
Organisation for Economic Co-operation and Development: 1973, List of Social Concerns. Common to Nost OECD Countries (OECD, Paris).
Roes, Th.: 1998, 'Linking social monitoring and policy-making. Experiences of the Dutch Social and Cultural Planning Office', in W. Hang et al. (eds.), Statistics as a Public Service (Swiss Federal Statistical Office, Bern).
Social and Cultural Planning Office: 1996, various editions, Sociale en culturele verkenningen (Social and Cultural Planning Office / VUGA, Rijswijk / The Hague).
Social and Cultural Planning Office: 1996, Social and Cultural Report 1996 (Social and Cultural Planning Office / VUGA, Rijswijk / The Hague).
SPSS: 1990, SPSS Categories (SPSS, USA).
United Nations Development Programme: 1998, Human Development 1998 (Oxford University Press, New York / Oxford).
Veenhoven, R.: 1996, 'Developments in satisfaction-research', Social Indicators Research 37, pp. 1–46.
Vogel, J.: 1995, The Social Indicator Tradition. Paper presented at Eurostat meeting 20, 21 February 1995.

Social and Cultural Planning Office
P.O. Box 16164
2500 BD The Hague
The Netherlands
E-mail: j.boelhouwer@scp.nl

E. SCOTT HUEBNER and RICH GILMAN

AN INTRODUCTION TO THE MULTIDIMENSIONAL STUDENTS' LIFE SATISFACTION SCALE

ABSTRACT. QOL researchers have primarily focused their attention on adults. The purpose of this presentation is to describe the rationale, development, and psychometric properties of a multidimensional life satisfaction scale appropriate for children and youth, the Multidimensional Students' Life Satisfaction Scale (MSLSS: Huebner, 1994; Huebner et al., 1998). This multidimensional self-report scale was designed for use with students from third through the twelfth grades. The current version of the MSLSS includes 40 items intended to assess satisfaction with five specific domains (School, Self, Family, Friends, and Living Environment). The presentation will summarize a series of recent studies assessing its reliability, factor structure, and convergent and discriminant validity. Additionally, the potential usefulness of children's life satisfaction scales for research and clinical applications were discussed.

INTRODUCTION

The impetus for the construction of the Multidimensional Students' Life Satisfaction Scale (MSLSS) was the increased interest in the promotion of positive psychological well-being in children and adults. In contrast to models that infer well-being from the absence of psychopathological symptoms, psychologists, such as Seligman (1998) have argued for the need to nurture a science and practice of psychology based on the presence of positive psychological indicators. Similarly, Cowen (1991) has recommended that psychological well-being should be defined using criteria such as "a basic satisfaction with onesself and one's existence . . . or life satisfaction" (p. 404).

Life satisfaction has been defined as a "global evaluation by the person of his or her life" (Pavot et al., 1991: p. 150). Although hundreds of studies of life satisfaction of adults have been conducted (see Diener, 1984; 1994), life satisfaction in childhood has only recently become the focus of empirical work. Recent investiga-

Social Indicators Research **60:** 115–122, 2002.

tions have demonstrated the importance of the life satisfaction construct in understanding the psychological well-being of children and adolescents. For example, life satisfaction reports have been differentiated from other well-being constructs such as self-esteem (Huebner et al., in press; Terry and Huebner, 1995), depression (Lewinsohn et al., 1991), and positive and negative affect (Huebner, 1991c; Huebner and Dew, 1996).

Systematic research efforts have been hampered by the lack of validated instruments for children and adolescents (Bender, 1997; Huebner, 1997). Children's life satisfaction scales have been limited to unidimensional measures of global or general life satisfaction, which yield only a single overall score (e.g., Perceived Life Satisfaction Scale: Adelman et al., 1989; Students' Life Satisfaction Scale: Huebner, 1991a, b).

The MSLSS was designed to provide a multidimensional profile of children's life satisfaction judgments. Such differentiated assessment are expected to provide more focused research and clinical applications. For example, students who indicate relatively high levels of dissatisfaction with their family experiences should require different clinical interventions than students who indicate greatest dissatisfaction with their school experiences. Such differentiated subjective indicators may also yield interesting findings when used in combination with the traditional objective indicators (e.g., divorce rates, family income levels, per pupil school expenditures) often used to assess the quality of life of children and youth.

Specifically, the MSLSS was thus designed to (a) provide a pofile of children's satisfaction with important specific domains (e.g., family, school, friends) in their lives; (b) assess their general or overall life satisfaction; (c) demonstrate acceptable psychometric properties (e.g., subscale reliability); (d) reveal a replicable factor structure demonstrating the meaningfulness of the five dimensions; and (e) be used with effectively with children across a wide range of ages (grades 3–12) and ability levels (e.g., gifted children, children with mild mental disabilities).

CHARACTERISTICS OF THE MSLSS

Item Selection

In the initial test development, several authors developed 14 items to represent each of the five specific domains of family, friends, school, living environment, and self. The specific life satisfaction domains were selected on the basis of a literature review, pilot interviews with school age students, student essays, and previous research (e.g., Huebner, 1991). The items were written to be easy to read and comprehend, thus being potentially useful across a wide range of age and ability levels. The results of subsequent item and factor analyses yielded a 40-item final version of the scale. The items and scoring procedures can be found in Huebner (1994).

The 40-item final version of the MSLSS may be administered to children and adolescents in groups as well as individually. The children are asked to complete the demographic information at the top of the scale first. The instructions for the scale (including a sample item) are provided prior to the MSLSS items. With younger children (grades 3–5) and children with learning difficulties (e.g., learning disabilities, mental disabilities), it is recommended that researchers read aloud the directions and encourage students to ask questions as necessary. The readability of the scale is estimated at the 1.5 grade level, therefore most students require little assistance in responding to the questions.

Normative Data

To date, the MSLSS has been administered to four samples of students in South Carolina. These samples have included 312 students in grades 3–8 (Huebner, 1994), 413 students in grades 3–5 (Huebner, 1994), 291 students in grades 6–8 (Huebner et al., 1998), and 321 students in grades 9–12 (Gilman et al., 1998). Greenspoon and Saklofske (1997) have also reported on a sample of Canadian students. Validation studies in Spain (Cassas, personal communication and Korea (Park, personal communication) are also underway. A modified version of the MSLSS, which separated the Friends domain into same-sex and opposite-sex relations scales, has also been studied with 266 high school students in South Carolina (Dew, 1996).

Mean scores for all domains and the total score were all above the midpoint in the South Carolina and Canadian samples, indicating positive levels of life satisfaction. Such findings are consistent with studies of adults (Diener, 1984, 1994) and other studies of children using different measures (e.g., Huebner et al., 2000).

Reliability

The MSLSS has consistently yielded acceptable internal consistency coefficients across the four American samples and the Canadian sample. Alpha coefficients for the MSLSS total score ranged from 0.90 to 0.92, suggesting high overall reliability. These coefficients have been noted to compare favorably to those reported for adult life satisfaction scales (Bender, 1997). Further, the internal consistency estimates for the five domains are acceptable for research purposes. Alphas ranged from 0.79 to 0.85 for the Family domain, 0.81 to 0.85 for the Friends domain, 0.83 to 0.85 for the School domain, 0.72 to 0.84 for the Self domain, amd 0.79 to 0.83 for the Living Environment domain.

Test-retest coefficients have also been reported (Dew, 1996; Huebner et al., 1998) for two- and four-week time frames, falling mostly in the 0.70–0.90 range. These data provide some preliminary support for the stability of the scale.

Validity

The results of exploratory factor analyses have supported the dimensionality of the MSLSS in American (Huebner, 1994) and Canadian samples (Greenspoon and Saklofske, 1997). Confirmatory factor analyses, conducted on samples of children in grades 6–8 (Huebner et al., 1998) and grades 9–12 (Gilman et al., 1998) have provided further support for the multidimensional hierarchical model, consisting of a general life satisfaction higher-order factor at the apex of the hierarchy along with five specific domains below.

Convergent and discrminant validity have also been demonstrated through predicted correlations with other self-report well-being indexes (Greenspoon and Saklofske, 1997; Huebner, 1994; Gilman et al., 1998; Huebner et al., 1998), parent reports (Dew, 1996), teacher reports (Greenspoon and Saklofske, 1997), and social desirability scales (Huebner et al., 1998). For example, the MSLSS

School domain correlated 0.68 with the Quality of School Life Scale (Epstein and McPartland, 1977), the MSLSS friends domain correlated 0.56 with the Loneliness and Social Dissatisfaction Scale (Asher et al., 1984), the Family domain correlated 0.61 with the Parent scale from the Behavioral Assessment Scale for Children (Reynolds and Kamphaus, 1992), and the MSLSS Self domain correlated 0.62 with the General Self-Esteem scale of the Self-Description Questionnaire-I (Marsh, 1990). It should be noted that a suitable criterion measure for the Living Environment domain has yet to be identified, however.

Findings of relationships with demographic variables (e.g., age, gender, race) were also consistent with expectations (e.g., see Huebner, 1994; Huebner et al., 1998).

DISCUSSION

The initial research findings provide support for the use of the MSLSS for research purposes with students in grades 3–12. Given that the item content and response options incorporate both positive and negative indicators of subjective well-being, the MSLSS may operate as a global and domain-specific "affectometer" (Kamman et al., 1984), allowing sensitivity to changes across the spectrum of well-being (e.g. from "mild" to "moderate" life satisfaction). The MSLSS may thus serve as a useful measure of subjective quality of life in studies of various group comparisons (e.g., school, city, nation), whenever the perspective of the child is to be considered. Various researchers (e.g., Frisch et al., 1992; Huebner et al., 1998) have speculated on possible clinical applications of life satisfaction measures, such as the MSLSS, as well.

Additional research is clearly needed, however. First, more representative samples must be employed to assess the generalizability of the current findings. National US samples that include children and adolescents from other parts of the US and different ethnic backgrounds (e.g., Hispanic, Asian Americans, etc.) are crucial. Also, normative data for child clinical populations (e.g., behavior disordered, mentally handicapped) should be illuminating. For example, Ash and Huebner (1998) have reported on unique aspects of MSLSS reports with gifted middle school students.

Finally, cross-national investigations should be conducted to assess the replicability of the satisfaction dimensions in other countries.

Second, additional studies of the stability of MSLSS scores are needed. Longer time frames (e.g., 6 months, one year) would provide greater clarity with respect to the meaning of the construct with children. Studies of the sensitivity of the scale to life changes (e.g., school or neighborhood changes, psychotherapeutic interventions) are imperative for demonstrating the usefulness of the MSLSS as an outcome measure for applied and research purposes.

Third, additional validation studies should be undertaken, particularly with respect to possible clinical applications. For example, predictive validity studies (e.g., determining the ability of the MSLSS to predict important clinical outcomes, such as depression or changes in peer relationships) would be valuable.

Finally, further studies investigating the relationship between life satisfaction and the affective domain are particularly important for children and adolescents. Given the greater intensity and variability of affect in youth (Larson et al., 1980), the nature of the association between affect and life satisfaction judgments may be different than that for adults.

In summary, preliminary studies with the MSLSS suggest its usefulness, particularly as a research tool. Nevertheless, much additional research remains to be done to clarify the nature and boundaries of this construct with children and youth.

REFERENCES

Adelman, H. S., T. Taylor and P. Nelson: 1989, 'Minors' dissatisfaction with their life circumstances', Child Psychiatry and Human Development 20, pp. 135–147.

Ash, C. and E. S. Huebner: 1998, 'Life satisfaction reports of gifted middle school children', School Psychology Quarterly 13, pp. 310–321.

Asher, S. R., S. Hymel and P. D. Renshaw: 1984, 'Loneliness in children', Child Development 55, pp. 1456–1464.

Bender, T.: 1997, 'Assessment of subjective well-being in children and adolescents', in G. Phye (ed.), Handbook of Classroom Assessment: Learning, Achievement, and Adjustment (Academic Press, San Diego), pp. 199–225.

Cowen, E.: 1991, 'In pursuit of wellness', American Psychologist 46, pp. 404–408.

Dew, T.: 1996, The Development and Validation of a Life Satisfaction Scale for Adolescents. Unpublished doctoral dissertation, University of South Carolina.

Dew, T. & E. S. Huebner: 1994, 'Adolescents' perceived quality of life: an exploratory investigation', Journal of School Psychology 32, pp. 185–199.

Diener, E.: 1984, 'Subjective well-being', Psychological Bulletin 95, pp. 542–575.

Diener, E.: 1994, 'Assessing subjective well-being: progress and opportunities', Social Indicators Research 31, pp. 103–159.

Epstein, J. & J. M. McPartland: 1977, The Quality of School Life Scale (Riverside, Riverside, CA).

Frisch, M., J. Cornell, M. Villanueva and P. J. Retzlaff: 1992, 'Clinical validation of the Quality of Life Inventory: a measure of life satisfaction for use in treatment planning and outcome assessment', Psychological Assessment 4, pp. 92–101.

Gilman, R., E. S. Huebner and J. Laughlin: 1998, Validation of the Multidimensional Students' Life Satisfaction Scale. Manuscript submitted for publication.

Greenspoon, P. and D. H. Saklofske: 1997, 'Validation of the Multidimensional Students' Life Satisfaction Scale with Canadian children', Journal of Psychoeducational Assessment 15, pp. 138–155.

Huebner, E. S.: 1991a, 'Initial development of the Students' Life Satisfaction Scale', School Psychology International 12, pp. 231–240.

Huebner, E. S.: 1991b, 'Correlates of life satisfaction in children', School Psychology Quarterly 6, pp. 103–111.

Huebner, E. S.: 1991c, 'Further validation of the Students' Life Satisfaction Scale: the independence of satisfaction and affect ratings', Journal of Psychoeducational Assessment 9, pp. 363–368.

Huebner, E. S.: 1994, 'Preliminary development and validation of a multidimensional life satisfaction scale for children', Psychological Assessment 6, pp. 149–158.

Huebner, E. S. and G. Alderman: 1993, 'Convergent and discriminant validation of a children's life satisfaction scale: its relationshipto self- and teacher-reported psychological problems and school functioning', Social Indicators Research 30, pp. 71–82.

Huebner, E. S., W. Drane and R. Valois: 2000, 'Levels and demographic correlates of adolescent life safisfaction reports', School Psychology International 21, pp. 281–292.

Huebner, E. S., J. Laughlin, C. Ash and R. Gilman: 1998, 'Further validation of the Multidimensional Students' Life Satisfaction Scale', Journal of Psychoeducational Assessment 16, pp. 110–134.

Kamman, R., M. Ferry and P. Herbison: 1984, 'The analysis and measurement of happiness as a sense of well-being', Social Indicators Research 15, pp. 91–115.

Larson, R., M. Csikszentmihalyi and R. Graef: 1980, 'Mood variability and psychosocial adjustment of adolescents', Journal of Youth and Adolescence 9, pp. 469–490.

Lewinsohn, P., J. Redner and J. Seeley: 1991, 'The relationship between life satisfaction and psychosocial variables: new perspectives', in F. Strack, M. Argyle and N. Schwartz (eds.), Subjective Well-being (Plenum Press, New York), pp. 193–212.
Marsh, H.: 1990, Self-Description Questionnaire Mmanual (University of Western Sydney, Campbelltown NSW Australia).
Pavot, W., E. Diener, C. R. Colvin and E. Sandvik: 1991, 'Further validation of the Satisfaction with Life Scale: evidence of cross-method convergence of well-being measures', Journal of Personality Assessment 49, pp. 149–161.
Reynold, C.R. and R. Kamphaus: 1992, Behavior Assessment System for Children (BASC) (American Guidance Services, Circle Pines, MN).
Seligman, M.: 1998, 'What is the good life?', American Psychological Association Monitor 30(1), p. 2.
Terry, T. and E. S. Huebner: 1995, 'The relationship between self-concept and life satisfaction in children', Social Indicators Research 35, pp. 39–52.

University of South Carolina
Columbia, South Carolina
USA
E-mail: Huebner@sc.edu

E. Scott Huebner

Georgia State University
Atlanta, Georgia
USA

Rich Gilman

MAHAR MANGAHAS and LINDA LUZ GUERRERO

SELF-SUSTAINED QUALITY OF LIFE MONITORING: THE PHILIPPINE SOCIAL WEATHER REPORTS[1]

ABSTRACT. In the Philippines, measurement of social indicators covering Quality of Life and other social concerns has been institutionalized by means of a unique Social Weather Reporting system. The Social Weather Reports are based on a series of national surveys operated on a self-sustaining, syndicate-cum-omnibus basis by a private research institute which operates as an "enterprising non-profit." The surveys began on a semestral basis in 1986 and have been run quarterly since 1992. Among their regular topics are self-rated poverty, QOL gaining/losing and optimism/pessimism, victimization by common crimes, satisfaction with the performance of government institutions and officials, public opinion on contemporaneous critical issues, and electoral prospects. Since the topics all deal with public issues, subscribers to the Social Weather Reports are mostly from the public sector, plus some corporate and diplomatic institutions. Access of non-subscribers to the survey findings is on a delayed basis; all surveys are archived for public use. The most important factors behind the success of the Social Weather Reports have been their consistent focus on indicators of democracy and governance and their record in predicting the outcomes of the 1992, 1995, and 1998 national elections in the Philippines.

HISTORICAL DEVELOPMENT OF PHILIPPINE SOCIAL INDICATORS

In the Philippines, the social indicators movement dates from the Social Indicators Project of the Development Academy of the Philippines,[2] which drew up a set of indicators for representing national well-being, including not only some existing indicators but also some experimental ones which it tested in a provincial pilot survey (Mangahas, 1976, 1977). Inasmuch as the project was undertaken during the authoritarian regime (1972–1986) of Ferdinand Marcos, the most noteworthy among its innovations were self-rated poverty and some subjective indicators of political well-being.

Social indicators do not grow on trees, as though waiting to be harvested, but are deliberately constructed by institutions. In due

Social Indicators Research **60:** 123–144, 2002.

time, the DAP advanced from its previous conceptual work to the practical demonstration of new social indicators based on social surveys, in what was called the Social Weather Stations or SWS project. The term "social weather stations" stems from the idea that social indicators, somewhat like meteorological indicators, might be regularly collected from "observation posts" of social progress (cf. Ghai, Hopkins and McGranahan, 1989). In 1981–1983, DAP conducted several such surveys in Metro Manila, and one national survey, but ultimately the book which would have published the findings (Mangahas, Miranda and Paqueo, 1984) was suppressed, notwithstanding the DAP charter's guarantee of academic freedom.

The possibility of generating social indicators privately, rather than by the government, was established in the final phase of the Marcos era, when a civic group, the Bishops'-Businessmen's Conference on Human Development or BBC, took the initiative to conduct and publicly report two surveys on political and social conditions of the time. The BBC required these surveys to be nationwide (n = 2,000), despite the large cost, lest anything smaller be dismissed as case studies in biased locations. One survey was funded by businessmen, and the other was joined, with sponsor's consent, with an Asia Foundation-supported poll about the legal profession.

The highly favorable public reception to the mix of opinion poll data – showing public disapproval of Marcos's legislation by decree and detention of persons by fiat (BBC, 1985) – and subjective social indicators provided by these private surveys encouraged the 1985 incorporation of the private non-stock, non-profit institute Social Weather Stations or SWS, named after the DAP project, for the purpose of generating survey data for social advocacy.

SWS is a creature of the social indicators movement. It understands that a nation has a multiplicity of social concerns – pointedly including a critical concern for good governance under democratic conditions – and that achievements along any social concern should be both equitable and sustainable (Mangahas, 1994). SWS defines its mission as generating new survey data along key social concerns for the three purposes of:

Education: So eyes may see social conditions.
Conscientization: So hearts may feel social problems.
Analysis: So minds may understand their solutions.

Two general values underlying the SWS mission are (a) a discomfort with the social status quo, and (b) a preference for democracy as a system. In relatively young democracies such as the Philippines there is a high public demand for quality-of-life monitoring when blended with opinion polling (cf. recent South African experience, per Møller, 1997). An SWS survey shows that Filipino appreciation of opinion polls is no less than that of Americans (Guerrero and Mangahas, 1997). As a highly influential type of social survey, opinion polling has great potential as a source of support for Quality of Life (QOL) monitoring done in tandem.

This paper describes how the QOL in the Philippines is tracked by a Social Weather Reporting system which is not only well-accepted by influentials, but also financially sustainable. Key to SWS's success is a credibility earned by undertaking reliable surveys on controversial issues with integrity, and in particular by consistently making accurate election predictions and "exit polls"[3] (Posadas and Sandoval, 1992; Guerrero and Ramirez, 1998; Mangahas, May 1998; Laquian and Laquian, 1998). Politicians at the helm of many SWS client-agencies have become eager for their latest survey ratings, knowing the strong correlation with chances of winning a national election (Mangahas, March 1998). The phrase "social weather" is so popular that SWS is trademarking it.

After the May 11, 1998 presidential election, 37% of Filipino adults in the nation – 52% in Metro Manila – knew of the SWS election surveys. Among those aware of the surveys, 33% called them Very Credible, 53% called them Somewhat Credible, 10% were Undecided if they were credible or not, 3% said they were Somewhat Not Credible, and only 0.6% said they were Not At All Credible, giving the SWS election surveys an excellent Net Credibility Rating of + 83 (i.e., credible minus not credible).[4]

MONITORING QOL IN THE SOCIAL WEATHER REPORTS

SWS aims for its survey data to be socially relevant, simple to understand, and up-to-date. The accuracy of SWS surveys in elections – one of the very few social matters having an independent population count with which to compare a sample count – has helped immensely to convince skeptics of the technical quality of the quality-of-life surveys, in the same way that George Gallup's election track record promoted his bread-and-butter market research.

A Social Weather Report covers a wide array of social concerns, such as economic well-being, public safety, the quality of governance, and so forth, as well as readings of public opinion on contemporary issues. The Report's value-added increases in proportion to its ability to fill gaps in official statistics[5] (Mangahas, 1991). The attached charts – on poverty, gainers/losers and optimists/pessimists with respect to QOL,[6] victimization by common crimes, satisfaction with the performance of the President, and satisfaction with government performance along selected issues – show some of the QOL indicators regularly tracked in the Reports.

For any topic, whether economic, political or social, the state of equity is conveniently depicted by means of a simple classification system from consumer research as practiced in the Philippines. The Marketing and Opinion Research Society of the Philippines has guidelines, pertaining to dwelling appearance and amenities, which enable survey interviewers to judge respondents as Class A (rich), Class B (upper class), Class C (middle), Class D (mass), or Class E (very poor). The pertinence of socioeconomic class as a powerful discriminating variable is illustrated in Chart 3.[7]

Social Weather Reports should be issued at intervals as short as possible, to show that they are up-to-date. The sampling procedures draw from market research practices, inasmuch as these were developed in order to deliver results on time.[8] SWS is partial to subjective indicators of well-being mainly because they are respondent-friendly and thus easy to generate from surveys.

For instance, using the self-rating approach, SWS measured the incidence of poverty semestrally over 1986–1990, and quarterly from 1991 to the present, producing a national time-series of 43 data points from mid-1983 to the 4th quarter of 1998. On the other hand, using the orthodox comparison of income to a poverty line, the government tracks poverty only once every three years, thus far producing data only for the five points of 1985, 1988, 1991, 1994, and 1997, the last point being no longer applicable at present since it fails to account for the current Asian economic crisis. The practical distinction between income-defined-poverty and self-rated poverty is not that one is objective and the other subjective, but that income is so complicated that surveying it is too expensive to do even on an annual basis. Yet only if tracked quarterly can poverty data compete for public attention with the quarterly-estimated Gross National Product, which is merely growth-oriented.

Competition for public attention demands, furthermore, that social indicators be national in scope, and thus based on nationally-representative surveys. The need for wide geographical scope and for frequent updating puts a heavy financial responsibility on a private institution carrying out a social indicators monitoring program on a sustained basis. Thus, for reasons of economy, the SWS sample sizes were reduced in 1987 from the former 2 000 (error margin of 2.2% in estimating national percentages) to 1 200 (2.9% error margin). The periodicity of the Social Weather Reports was increased gradually, in line with financial capability. During 1988–1991 the semestral national surveys were interpersed with extra rounds limited to Metro Manila, and starting 1992 the national surveys became quarterly.

FINANCIAL SUSTAINABILITY

SWS can be called *an enterprising non-profit*, using the terminology of a recent article in the *Harvard Business Review* (Dees, 1998). Like any a non-profit institution with a social mission, it needs financial means to sustain its mission. As advantages, it has no stockholders and thus pays out no dividends, and has corporate-income-tax-free status under Philippine law. Like many non-profits, SWS started off with only enough financial capital to pay for printed letterhead, with mainly volunteer labor, and with in-kind donations. Out-of-pocket survey expenses in the early years came from philanthropic sources, namely Ford Foundation for four national surveys jointly done by SWS with Ateneo de Manila University in 1986–1987, and the Philippine economic planning agency, NEDA, for another set of four rounds in 1988–1989.

In order to be sustainable, an enterprising non-profit must generate enough revenue from some part of its operations in order to meet regular costs. In the common case that its ultimate constituents are disadvantaged groups of society with little purchasing power themselves, it usually targets a market of third-party payers with a vested interest in the welfare of those groups (Dees, 1998). This market has included, in addition to government and international agencies, a handful of corporate enterprises who realize that they are affected by changes in the social environment. Since enterprising non-profits should take care that "the tail of market profits does not wag the dog of the social mission," in the case of SWS the survey agenda is driven primarily by the public-sector market and only marginally by the private corporate market.

SWS's approach for achieving financial sustainability involves: (a) charging annual subscription fees to clients, mainly government agencies, for the privilege of advance information from a common data set available in Social Weather Report or SWR surveys, (b) accepting commissioned questions as rider-items in the regular SWR survey, operating as an omnibus, and (c) accepting business-like contracts for social, political or economic surveys in areas of its expertise. SWS seeks to earn market-scale surpluses from such operations in order to cross-subsidize its main mission activities. As a private, self-sustainable system of monitoring a nation's quality-of-life, the quarterly Social Weather Reports are, to our knowledge, unique in the world.

The Social Weather Report subscription system

SWS got weaned early from foundation funding, unlike its initial partner, the Jesuit-run Ateneo University, which did its own social surveys for five more years (1988–1992) before eventually succumbing to foundation-fatigue. The first Social Weather Report subscriber was the Department of Agriculture, which signed up in 1988 and renewed annually for about five years. The Department of Agrarian Reform and the Department of Labor and Employment which signed up next, have remained SWS subscribers up to the present.

President Fidel V. Ramos (July 1992–June 1998), whose narrow election victory was accurately predicted by SWS, took a Social Weather Report subscription through the National Security Council at the start of his term, and then regularly invited SWS to present the main Report to his cabinet each quarter; President Joseph E. Estrada (July 1998–) has continued the practice. Many cabinet members followed President Ramos's lead, adding to the SWS subscriber list the portfolios of health, education, defense, foreign affairs, interior/police, justice, tourism, transportation and communications, natural resources and environment, economic planning, finance, budget, internal revenue, housing, and social welfare. As the Office of the Vice-President (who headed an anti-crime commission at the time), the Senate, the House of Representatives, and the Supreme Court came in, all three branches of government became subscribers of the Social Weather Report. A few private companies, government corporations, and individual politicians make up the balance.

SWS maintains quarterly liaison with its subscribers so that it can design questions corresponding to their current interests, for inclusion in the next survey round of the Social Weather Report. The number of items has grown so large that a survey "round" now typically requires two, and sometimes three, questionnaires simultaneously implemented on separate national samples, each generating its own dataset. SWS differentiates its service to each subscriber, after dealing briefly with the material of common interest, by focusing each presentation on the subscriber's special concern. It is reasonable to interpret a renewal of the annual subscription as evidence that the user has found it to be worth the price, presently set at ₱320 000 (about US$8 000) for four quarterly Social Weather Reports.

To keep the subscription system viable, data from one quarter's Social Weather Report, copyrighted by SWS, are not supposed to be published in the mass media until rendered "obsolete" by the arrival of data for the succeeding quarter. SWR data have been frequently cited by subscribers in public statements, such as the President's State of the Nation Address. A special book prepared by De La Salle University and the Fletcher School for Law and Diplomacy for the 1996 APEC summit meeting in the Philippines included an "SWS survey tour" of the country (Mangahas, 1996).

The omnibus survey system

To help make the survey vehicle for a Social Weather Report financially viable, it also serves as an omnibus for research sponsors amenable to the common sample size, geographic scope, type of respondent, and project schedule. This omnibus, for public issues, has advantages similar to those currently used for research on business issues (cf. Davis, 1986). For the use of its omnibus, SWS charges no entry fee, but either a price per questionnaire item (less if closed-ended than if open-ended), or else a total fee negotiated on the basis of the interview time required for the client's survey module.

The SWS national omnibus is quite suitable for politicians aspiring to run for positions of President, Vice-President, or Senator,[9] all of which are elected by the nation at large. The standard survey divides the country into at least four major areas, Metro Manila, the rest of Luzon (sometimes further divided into North Luzon and South Luzon), Visayas, and Mindanao, each with n = 300 for a sampling error margin of 6% per area. Sponsors need not use every geographic area; for example, the omnibus was cost-effective for a metropolitan agency interested in data about traffic-reduction schemes in Metro Manila specifically.

Omnibus sponsors may commission as little as one item to as many as twenty items per survey. For instance, many politicians, officials, and even private personalities commission only a single item, namely their public name recognition. Those with electoral ambitions may commission a few more items on what makes them popular, as well as unpopular. On the other hand, the omnibus has also carried much more detailed survey modules to test the effectivity of information campaigns for government programs on housing and on overseas employment.

Omnibus sponsors can obtain tabulations of their items not only by common socio-demographic variables, but also by the survey's QOL indicators and other items, which SWS is at liberty to share with them. If necessary, they may have a documented survey data diskette, including both commissioned items and correlates, aside from hard copy of the marginals crosstabulated by location, locale, gender, age, and socio-economic class.

The running of the omnibus surveys at regular intervals enables users to track time-trends. For instance, over 1994–1997, USAID/ Manila wanted to determine whether its activities were contributing to its strategic objectives, measured by qualitative indicators on democracy, natural resource management, population, health, and economic growth. A 1996–1998 project is using non-traditional performance indicators to assess the Social Security System's impact on families and to learn about Filipino perceptions and sentiments about the social security program. Since the Social Weather Report surveys cover social, economic, and political issues under the broad theme of *quality of life*, the implementation of a questionnaire combining syndicated or common items with omnibus or commissioned-items on different public issues has not been a problem.

Dedicated surveys

SWS has undertaken a number of special surveys,[10] many of which involve QOL indicators for specific sectors. These applications of social indicators also help to generate funds to sustain the Social Weather Reports. In 1988–1989, SWS studied the socio-economic impact of the Upper Pampanga River Integrated Irrigation System on the farmers of Nueva Ecija province. SWS was tasked in 1989–1993 to design indicators of rural well-being, particularly for agrarian reform beneficiaries. In 1996–1998 it did two national surveys of the characteristics, attitudes, needs, aspirations and problems of the Filipino youth. SWS did five surveys for the Quezon City government during 1993–1997, to study the city's quality of life, and the impact of existing and proposed city government programs (Sandoval, 1998).

SWS has been trusted by the government to survey public opinion on controversial issues. In 1993, an SWS survey established that residents of a village in Zambales province were opposed to the building of a coal-fired power plant in their area, but also had so much trust in the President that he visited them personally, and was able to change their minds about the project. On the other hand, in the same year, the government shelved its plan to operate a casino in Cagayan de Oro City, following an SWS survey showing majority opposition to it.

Some studies have combined riders on the national omnibus with dedicated surveys. In 1993–1994, SWS combined a large rider with a survey of 300 metropolitan firms to study how Medicare program coverage could be expanded. Using data collected over 1985–1996,[11] SWS studied the state of the legal profession and the judiciary by joining omnibus-riders, face-to-face sample surveys of lawyers in key cities, and mail surveys of about 1 000 judges throughout the country (Mangahas, La Viña, Rood, Casambre and Arroyo, 1996).

KEEPING TO THE SOCIAL INDICATORS MISSION

Aside from the publications[12] expected of academic institutions, SWS is actively involved in promoting social science knowledge through *data dissemination* and *training*. Such activities, which are not expected to be financially self-sustaining, serve to show that "the tail of market profits does not wag the tail of the social mission," despite success of SWS as an enterprising non-profit.

SWS is the only private Philippine survey institution which permanently archives all of its data for public use; its by-laws inhibit it from conducting purely proprietary surveys. By November 1998, the SWS Survey Data Bank included 165 Philippine surveys, encompassing 177 167 interviews, on 20 866 survey questions, not counting standard backgrounders. Of these 165 surveys, 75 are Social Weather Surveys, 68 of them being national in scope. In addition, the Data Bank has over 150 datasets from foreign surveys, many directly comparable with the SWS surveys. SWS has established its academic credentials internationally by representing the Philippines in the International Social Survey Programme since 1991, the World Values Survey in 1995/1996, and the Comparative Study of Electoral Systems in 1994/1998, all major cross-country survey networks.

For researchers' convenience, SWS has organized two electronic databases for a *System for Easy Access to the Archives of Social Weather Stations*, or *SEARCH-SWS*. One database allows access to the results of Social Weather Report surveys since 1986, crosstabulated by location and socio-economic class, and the other contains question wordings of items used in the Social Weather Report surveys, following the original survey instruments. SWS is directly promoting the use of its survey data among social science departments of major universities, and has newly established a modest Student Paper Research Prize to encourage the use of the surveys in theses and dissertations.

To help educate the public on the value of social surveys in a democratic setting, SWS is regularly involved in training on prin-

TABLE I

SWS data bank of Philippine surveys (as of 5 November 1998)

	Data sets*	Respondents	Items**	Data Bits
1984	1	2,000	19	38,000
1985	2	10,163	146	686,400
1986	2	3,200	260	411,200
1987	4	4,100	371	352,800
1988	3	1,800	367	244,200
1989	4	3,200	656	475,100
1990	11	11,946	1,209	1,661,200
1991	11	14,235	1,868	2,366,400
1992	17	18,397	1,594	2,310,900
1993	16	10,898	2,245	1,817,100
1994	10	9,420	1,639	1,760,100
1995	19	16,051	2,100	2,007,800
1996	23	19,866	3,011	2,764,600
1997	19	20,750	2,810	3,251,600
1998	23	31,141	2,571	2,934,100
TOTAL	165	177,167	20,866	23,081,500

*National surveys (96 datasets) and special area surveys (69 datasets).
**Excludes standard background variables.

ciples of social surveys, quality-of-life indicators, and opinion polls. It has organized training programs and seminars for staff of the Bureau of Agricultural Statistics, the Bureau of Internal Revenue, and a number of local governments and academic institutions. It conducted special seminars for media companies on precision-journalism in 1995, short before the senatorial elections. SWS has also provided training on social surveying and opinion polling to eleven research institutes located in several provinces and cities.

CONCLUDING REMARKS

In his "Where Do We Stand in the Mid-1990s?," Kenneth Land (1996) observed that social indicators work has switched from a *technocratic* model to an *enlightenment* model. The technocratic model aims for data to promote technical solutions for social problems. The enlightenment model seeks to place QOL issues on the political agenda by supplying data for public debate through the mass media – which according to Vogel (1997, p. 104) is actually "the original purpose of social indicators: to send signals to governments, business, other organizations and the general public." These call to mind the deliberate order in the SWS mission statement: generate data first to stimulate the eye, next to influence the heart, finally to guide the mind.

SWS believes that the path towards effective social indicators is as much institutional as it is technical. There is considerable room for private institutions in the generation of social statistics for public use (Guerrero and Mangahas, 1989). These institutions should develop indicators that are *meaningful, understandable, credible, frequent*, and *sustainable*.

Meaningfulness stems from keeping critical concerns on the agenda, in particular, remembering to include governance and political wellbeing Understandability requires developing a public communication program. Credibility comes from following academic practices of transparency and passing the litmus test of predicting how citizens will vote. The frequency of social indicators should match, at least, that of the orthodox economic growth indicators. An enterprising non-profit can attain sustainability by exploiting the cost-effectivity of the omnibus approach in surveying and by actively engaging in survey research contract work, especially where quality-of-life indicators play a role.

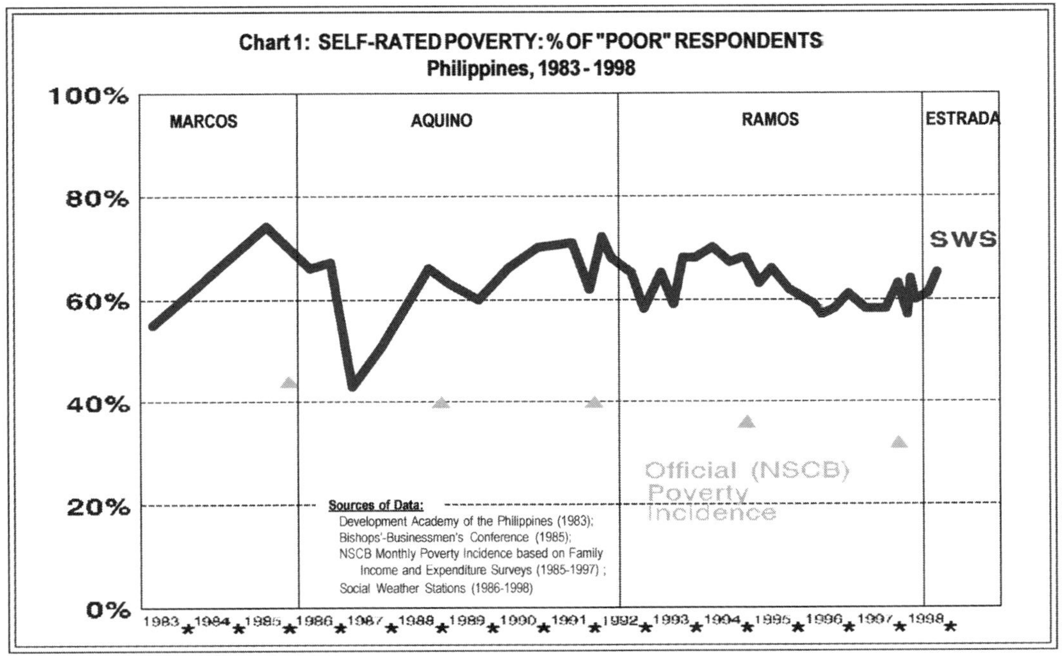

Chart 1. Self-rated poverty: % of "poor" respondents (Philippines, 1983–1998).

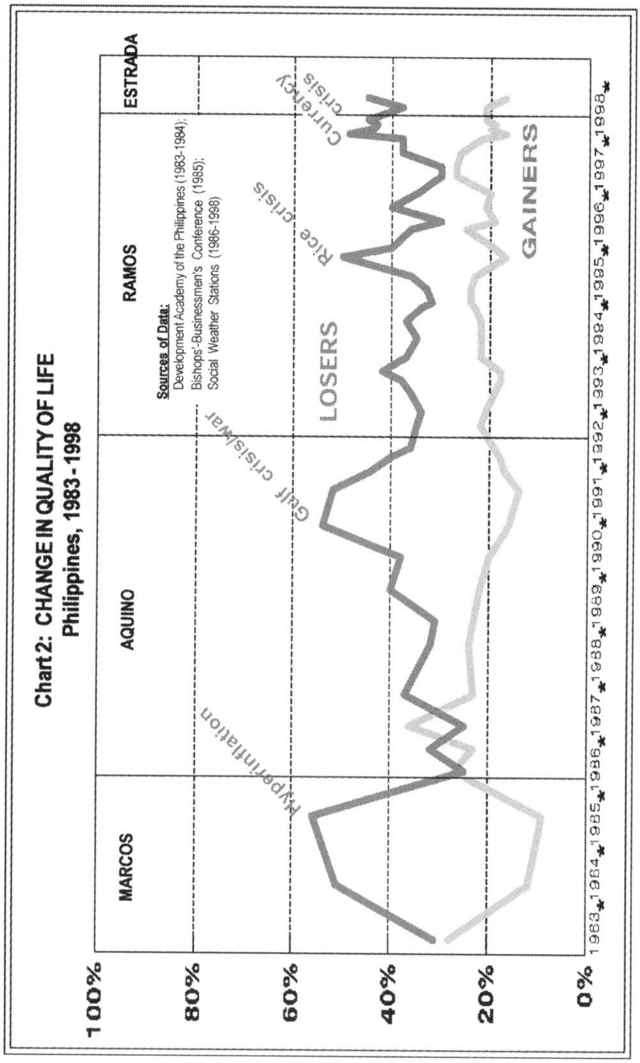

Chart 2. Change in quality of life (Philippines, 1983–1998).

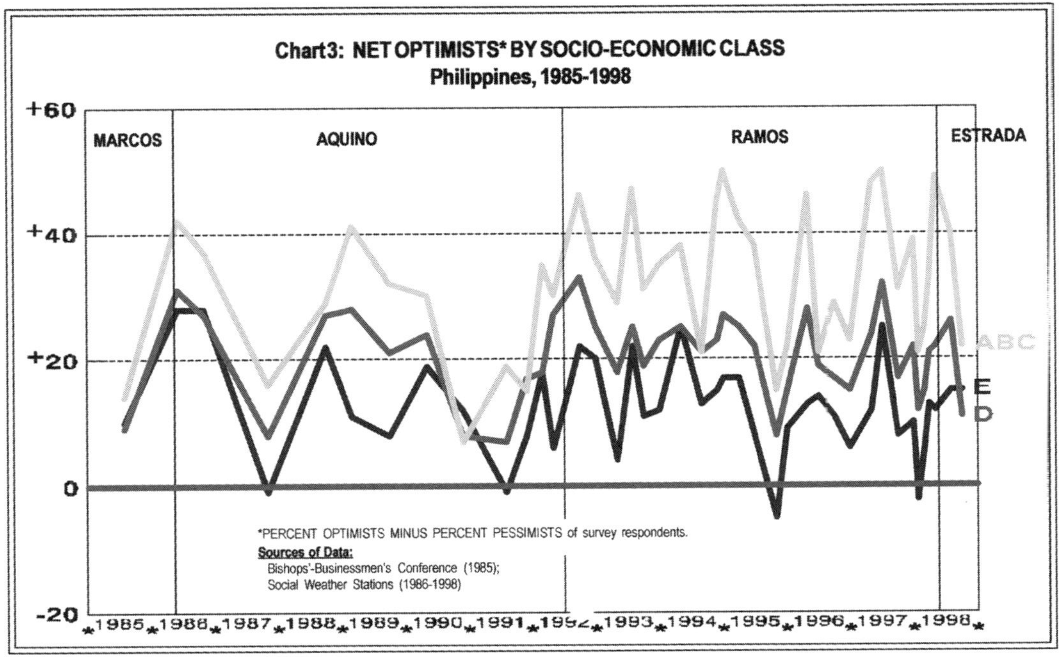

Chart 3. Net optimists* by socio-economic class (Philippines, 1985–1998).

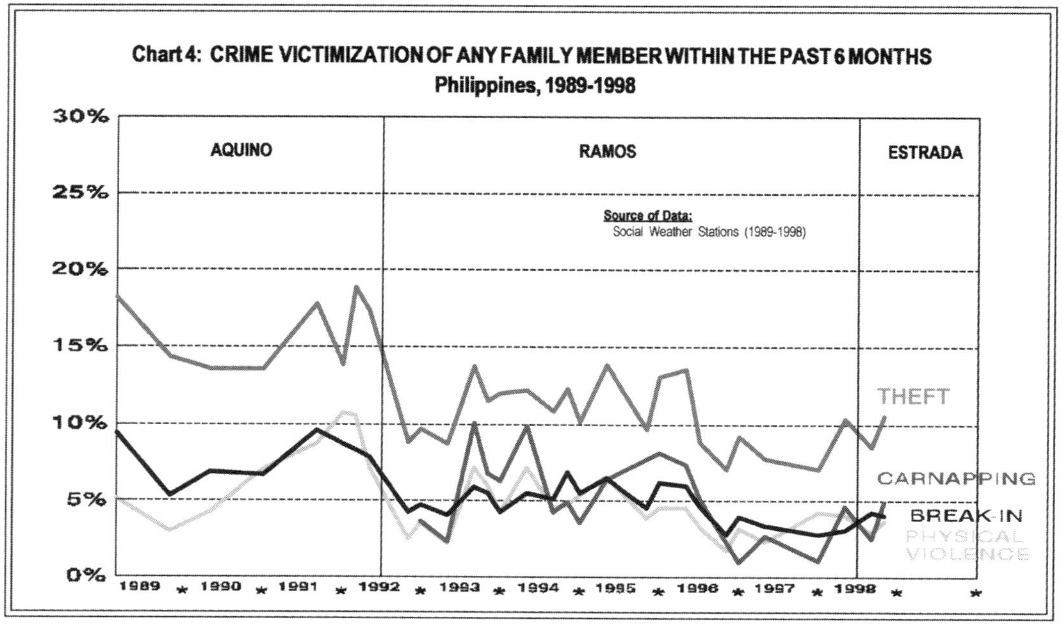

Chart 4. Crime victimization of any family member within the past 6 months (Philippines, 1989–1998).

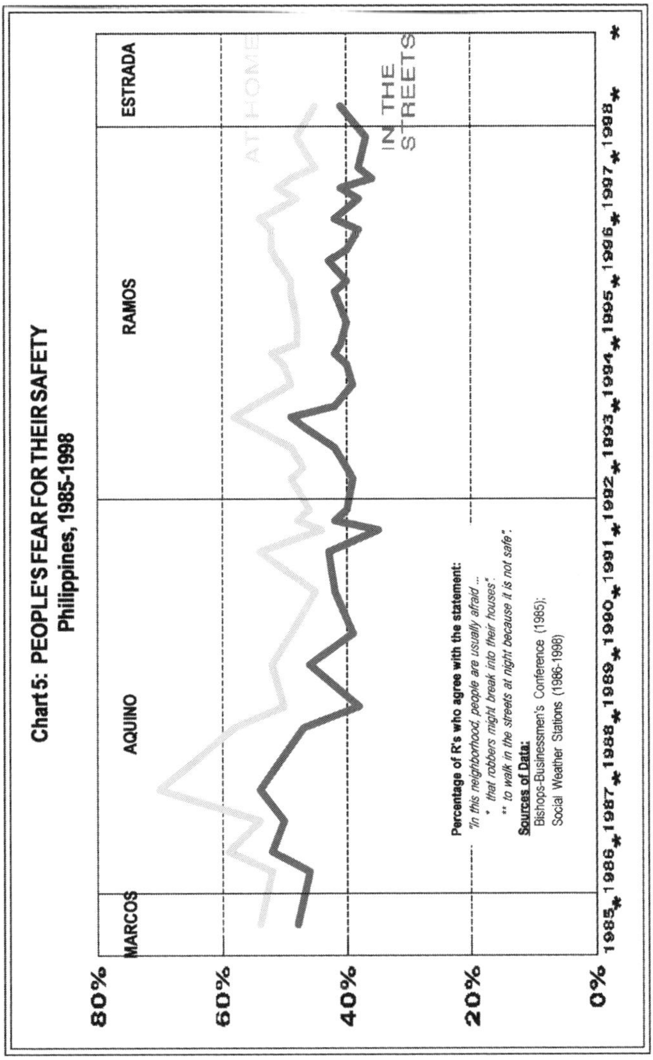

Chart 5. People's fear for their safety (Philippines, 1985–1998).

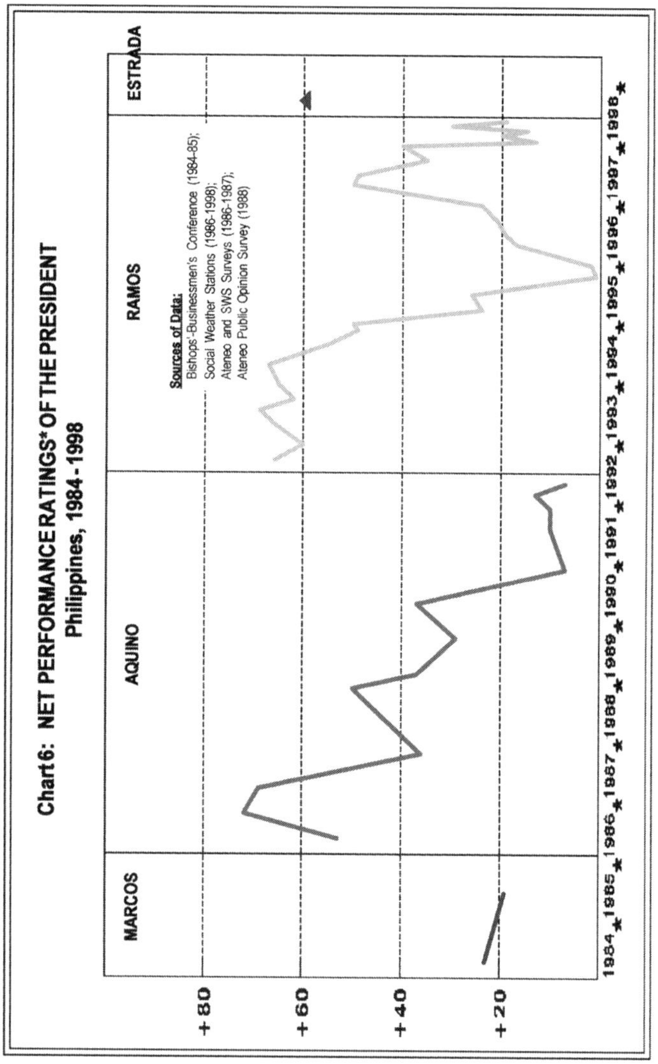

Chart 6. Net performance ratings* of the president (Philippines, 1984–1998).

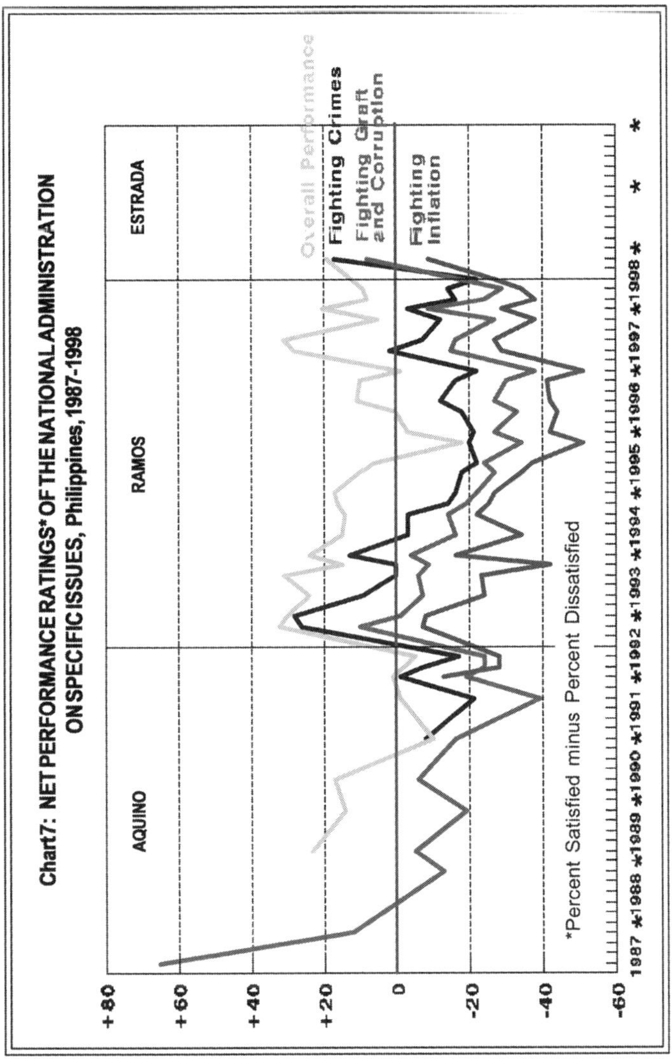

Chart 7. Net performance ratings* of the national administration on specific issues (Philippines, 1987–1998).

NOTES

[1] Presented as an Invited Paper at the Second Annual Conference of the International Society for Quality-of-Life Studies, Williamsburg, Virginia, USA, December 3–6, 1998; a revised version of "Social Weather Reporting in the Philippines," paper presented at the 14th World Congress of Sociology, Working Group 6 (Social Indicators), July 26–August 1, 1998, Montreal, Canada.
[2] The DAP is a state institution mainly concerned with training the upper ranks of the bureaucracy.
[3] Strictly speaking, the SWS "exit polls" of 1992, 1995, and 1998 were done in the dwellings of the sample of respondents on voting day, after they had already voted; to have the interviewers literally waiting outside polling places to accost voters as they leave was deemed too hazardous on account of the tendency of political partisans to mill around polling places.
[4] Based on the Social Weather Survey of June 27 to July 14, 1998, with a national sample size of 1,200.
[5] On the other hand, SWS gives low priority to the issues of indexation and of cross-country comparability. Indexation is a way of coping with a surplus of data; but the social indicators problem is one of data deficits rather than surpluses. Any requirement that a social indicator be internationally comparable before adopting it stultifies a country's initiatives to develop its own indicators.
[6] The gainers/losers indicator comes from the survey question, "Is your quality of life now better than, the same as, or worse than it was 12 months ago?" The optimists/pessimists indicator is from the question, "Do you expect your quality of life 12 months from now to get better than, stay the same as, or get worse than it is now?" Replies of "no change" are not charted.
[7] In this case, classes A, B, and C were grouped together since the survey sample size did not warrant separating them.
[8] SWS has always used probability sampling rather than quota-sampling, however.
[9] The term for all of these positions is six years. There are 24 Senate seats, 12 of which are vacated every 3 years. The Vice-President and Senators may be reelected once, but the President may not be reelected.
[10] Fieldstaff, data encoders and tabulators are provided by TRENDS-MBL, a respected market research company regularly subcontracted by SWS over the past 13 years.
[11] The openness of the SWS Survey Data Bank enables new projects to build on all earlier SWS surveys related to a research topic, whether or not commissioned by the same sponsor.
[12] SWS publishes monographs and Occasional Papers by SWS Fellows, and twice-monthly Social Weather Bulletins on specific survey topics, including tables, charts and the original survey questions. For general information, see the SWS webpage at http://www.sws.org.ph.

REFERENCES

Bishops'-Businessmen's Conference for Human Development: 1985, The BBC Nationwide Socio-Political Opinion Surveys of 1984 and 1985 (Manila).

Richard Davies: 1986, 'Omnibus surveys', in Robert Worcester and John Downham (eds.), Consumer Market Research Handbook (McGraw-Hill Book Company for the European Society for Opinion and Marketing Research, London, Third Edition).

Gregory Dees, J.: 1998, 'Enterprising nonprofits', Harvard Business Review (January–February), pp. 55–67.

Ghai, D., M. Hopkins and D. McGranahan: 1989, 'Some reflections on human and social indicators', in K. Haq and U. Kirdar (eds.), Development for People: Goals and Strategies for the Year 2000 (North South Roundtable, Islamabad and UNDP Development Study Programme, New York).

Linda Luz B. Guerrero and Mahar Mangahas: 1989, A Survey of Private Sector Statistics for Social, Economic and Political Analysis (paper for the 5th National Convention on Statistics, sponsored by the Philippine Statistical Association and the National Statistical Coordination Board, Manila, December 5).

Linda Luz B. Guerrero and Mahar Mangahas: 1977, 'Polling about polls in the Philippines', Social Weather Bulletin, 97(May), pp. 9–10.

Linda Luz B. Guerrero and Ophelia Ramirez: 1998, The 1992 and 1995 Philippine Exit Polls (Social Weather Stations Occasional Paper, Quezon City, March).

Kenneth C. Land: 1996, 'Social indicators and the quality-of-life: where do we stand in the mid-1990s?', SINET 45(February), pp. 5–8.

Aprodicio Laquian and Eleanor Laquian: 1998, Joseph Ejercito 'Erap' Estrada: The Centennial President (Institute of Asian Research, University of British Columbia, Vancouver, and College of Public Administration, University of the Philippines, Quezon City).

Mahar Mangahas (ed.): 1976, Measuring Philippine Development (Development Academy of the Philippines, Metro Manila).

Mahar Mangahas: 1977, 'The Philippine social indicators project', Social Indicators Research 4, pp. 67–96.

Mahar Mangahas: 1991, 'Monitoring the economic and social weather in the Philippines', in Kenneth J. Arrow (ed.), Issues in Contemporary Economics, Volume 1: Markets and Welfare (Macmillan for the International Economic Association, London).

Mahar Mangahas: 1994, The Philippine Social Climate: From the SWS Surveys (Anvil Publishing, Metro Manila).

Mahar Mangahas: 1996, 'A survey tour of the Philippines', in W. Scott Thompson and Wilfredo V. Villacorta (eds.), The Philippine Road to NIChood (De La Salle University and Social Weather Stations, Manila).

Mahar Mangahas: 1998, The SWS Pre-Election Surveys of 1992 and 1995 (Social Weather Stations Occasional Paper, Quezon City, March).

Mahar Mangahas: 1998, 'How the SWS exit poll was done, basic results of the SWS exit poll, and comparing SWS exit poll and namfrel tallies', Columns in the Manila Standard of May 15, May 18, and May 22 respectively.

Mahar Mangahas, Felipe B. Miranda and Vicente B. Paqueo: 1982, Measuring the Quality of Life: A 1982 Social Weather Report (Development Academy of the Philippines Press, Makati, Metro Manila, publication suppressed; ISBN 971-152-000-1).

Mahar Mangahas, Antonio G. M. La Viña, Steven Rood, Athena Lydia Casambre and Dennis M. Arroyo: 1996, Monitoring the State of the Judiciary and the Legal Profession (Social Weather Stations, Quezon City).

Valerie Møller: 1997, 'South Africa's emergent "Social Indicators Movement"', Social Indicators Research 41, pp. 1–14.

Conchita L. Posadas and Gerardo A. Sandoval: 1992, 'How did SWS fare in predicting the May 11, 1992 election results?', Social Weather Bulletin 92(June), p. 12.

Gerardo A. Sandoval: 1998, Surveys in Quezon City, Philippines, 1993–1997 (paper presented at the World Association for Public Opinion Research Regional Conference on Opinion Research and Democracy, Manila, January 30–31).

Joachim Vogel: 1997, 'The future direction of social indicator research', Social Indicators Research 42, pp. 103–116.

Social Weather Stations

SECTION II

POLICY, FINANCE, MARKETING, AND BUSINESS

BONNIE BRAUN, PATRICIA D. OLSON and JEAN W. BAUER

WELFARE TO WELL-BEING TRANSITION

ABSTRACT. Welfare to well-being leads to better quality of life for families and communities. Around the world, societies are experimenting and shifting policies that address welfare to well-being for families and communities. In the U.S., the greatest shift in several decades has occurred with the welfare reform policies. These shifts have placed at issue the extent to which individuals and families and governments contribute to self-sufficiency and sustainability of their members and the collective whole in society. The paper addresses: a framework for thinking about sustaining well-being in the context of making transitions from welfare for the few to well-being for the many; a research illustration of focus group findings on the meaning of self-sufficiency for families who are currently receiving one type of welfare (food stamps); and the opportunities emerging in the context of the interaction of the family and society at the community, state, national and global level that allows for a wholistic response to issues around well-being and quality of life studies.

INTRODUCTION

Welfare and Well-Being

Supporting the poor with public dollars is a policy decision practiced by many countries. Willingness to use public assistance to support people varies over time. As the 20th century ends, many countries are rethinking their public assistance policies.

In the United States, welfare policies were put in place during the Great Depression beginning with the Social Security Act. Aid to Dependent Children (ADC) legislation subsidizing widows with children but without incomes began in the 1930s. ADC evolved in to Aid to Families with Dependent Children (AFDC), called welfare by most. In addition to AFDC, the U.S. put into place numerous public assistance programs aimed not only at income assistance but food, housing, energy, health and child welfare. The intent of these

Social Indicators Research **60:** 147–154, 2002.

federal programs was to support families until they could become economically self-sufficient (Braun et al., 1995).

However, by the 1980s, "welfare had become a longer term support to families than originally intended." The welfare roles were growing and the ability to sustain the cost was in question. Thus, Congress passes the "Family Support Act" which provided income for work performed with the intention of moving single mothers off public assistance.

As the 1990s arrived, most citizens, politicians and direct beneficiaries were agreeing that the "system" wasn't working. They disagreed on alternative policy. The drivers for reform were primarily the need to reduce the federal deficit, the intent to shift the responsibility for the programs and some of the funding from the federal to states and localities, and the desire to emphasize person responsibility and self-sufficiency. The Personal Responsibility and Work Opportunity Reconciliation Act of 1996 changed over sixty years of social policy and created the Temporary Assistance to Needy Families (TANF). With these "welfare reform" changes and the related Agricultural Appropriations Act of 1997, a window of opportunity opened for focusing on the well-being of children, youth, and families – the fundamental unit of a community and the economy (Braun and Bauer, 1998a).

With the transition occurring as a result of federal and state welfare reform, the opportunity arises to shift from welfare for the few to well-being for the many and from short term self-sufficiency to long term sustainability. It also shifts the focus from a questionable level of living for a few to a proposed desired quality of life for all. This shift raises the question of what might be the outcome of welfare reform if viewed from a well-being framework.

The Family and Consumer Sciences profession frequently uses the concept of "well-being" as an expression of a state of life for humans, individually and collectively. Zimmerman (1992) argues that well-being should be a key component of any public policy affecting families. While scholars debate the origins and applications of the concept, it seems to be one that the general public, policy makers, researchers, educators and practitioners can use as a starting point for discussing the human condition. Well-being is defined as the condition of health, happiness, and freedom from wants. It is a

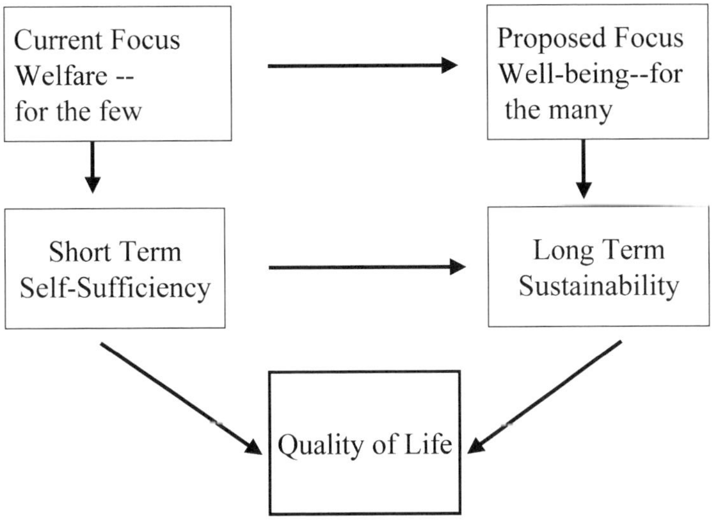

Figure 1. Welfare to well-being transitional framework.

state of being in which basic needs are met and for that state to be sustainable, it is one that maintains a sense of future well-being as well as current well-being.

Systems for Welfare and Well-being

A systems perspective is needed to understand what is happening between welfare and well-being, self-sufficiency and sustainability and how this all leads to a change in the quality of life for families. Families affect each other and the overall quality of society. There is reciprocity between families and society at the community, state, national and global level. The goals of policymakers would be enhanced if we could find ways to sustain families and communities to sustain society locally and around the world (Braun and Bauer, 1998b). A systems approach allows a look at arenas for action toward quality of life that move from the individual to the global society (Bronfenbrenner, 1979; Bulbolz and Songtag, 1993).

Contrasts Between Welfare and Well-being

Welfare discussions tend to focus on the past (of what was) and the present (of what is). Well-being, while having a past and present component, focuses on the future. The concept of self-sufficiency is a cornerstone of welfare; the concept of sustainability of well-being.

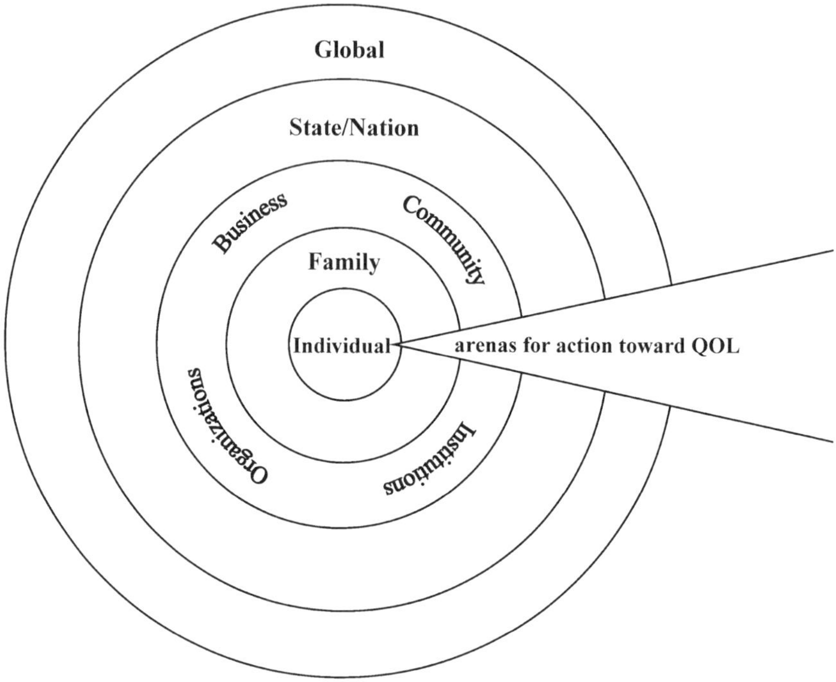

Figure 2. An ecological view of arenas for actions towards the quality of life.

What do the terms self-sufficiency and sustainability mean and what is their relationship to each other? Although policymakers rhetorically have expressed their concern for increasing self-sufficiency among the poor, little attention has been given to defining self-sufficiency or considered how it is best achieved (Sandfort and Hill, 1996). The American Heritage Dictionary (1998) defines self-sufficient as the ability to provide for oneself without help of others. Sufficient is defined as an adequate means to live in modest comfort.

In the field of economics, self-sufficiency is usually an objective measure using income-to-needs comparison (above or below the poverty line). All income coming into the household is counted, including earned income and transfer payments such as Temporary Assistance to Needy Families (TANF) and Food Stamps. Self-sufficiency is often defined dichotomously. In contrast sociology and social work use a broader definition to self-sufficiency and often utilizes many subjective measures. Lie and Morney (1992) indicated that self-sufficiency is a continuum rather than a state of "is or is not." The variable has components of resources and money, psychological, and skills. They used three arenas of current functioning to measure self-sufficiency. These were the individual arena (self-esteem, social adjustment, educational attainment, career goals, alcohol use, substance abuse), relational arena (parenting knowledge and skills, money management, household management skills), and the environmental arena (housing, transportation, childcare, and social isolation).

Historically, the concept of sustainability has been studied by anthropologists and applied agricultural economists in determining the survival of developing countries. Hansen (1994) in a study of sustainability and self-sufficiency found that there is a broad disagreement in defining sustainability. In a study of sustainability he states that three main approaches are the production of enough food, preservation and stewardship of natural resources and preservation of social units and cultural values. The American Heritage Dictionary (1998) defines it as the ability to keep in existence or maintain.

If self-sufficiency is the ability to provide for oneself in an adequate and modest comfort and sustainability is the ability to maintain and preserve social units and cultural values, then both of these contribute to quality of life. It is interesting to note that the policies do not support these broader definitions, but use the word for welfare policy. This means there is a need for further research for a better understanding of the welfare concepts and well-being concepts as used in public policy.

Researching Measures of Well-being for Public Policy

Various indicators of well-being can be collected from multiple sources and perspective and used to determine the past, current and desired state of well-being for children, youths, families, communities and even society. The indicators can be used to monitor change and measure the impacts of the change on the well-being of the system. In order to measure consistently, and increase the understanding of self-sufficiency and not dependence, the U.S. Congress requested that a yearly report on the welfare dependence and well-being of families be made (USDHHS, 1996). To monitor effects of policies on families requires agreement on indicators of well-being and the methods of tracking changes in the indicators. A year after the initial "Indicators of Welfare Dependence and Well-Being" was released, numerous government and private sector individuals and groups are organizing their resources to do the needed research. In Minnesota a team used focus groups to learn how families were coping with welfare reform, to assess the extent to which the family was being affected and what they were thinking and doing as a result of many changes in their lives.

In Minnesota, focus groups were conducted over two years with both rural and urban mothers who lived with at least one child under nine years old and who were either participating or were eligible to participate in the federal Food Stamp program (a welfare program). The 88 mothers ranged in age from 17 to 51 and had an average of 2 children per household. Forty percent of the households included a wage-earning individual. Twenty three percent of the mothers were either living with a spouse or partner and the rest were living as a single parent with their children (Magistad et al., 1998). The findings indicate that families raising children on Food Stamps are often very resourceful and skilled at making their limited resources last longer to meet their basic needs. The are skilled at stretching their resources so that housing, food, health care, transportation and other basic needs are met. However, in many families simply there are not enough resources to make ends meet and be self-sufficient. Therefore, family alone was not enough for these mothers. They turned to the community for support for their daily lives. Welfare reform in the U.S. affected policy towards the resources at the community and societal level. Thus it is important to move from welfare to well-being and focus on well-being and sustainability that adds to the quality of life for all.

Responses to Issues around Well-being and Quality of Life

Opportunities for all us emerge in the context of the interaction of the family and at the community, state, national and global level that allows us to look at the policies for well-being. The arenas for action are at every level. This paper used only the one example for research for the family and community level.

CLOSING

In closing, the intent of this paper was to serve as a stimulus for scholars, educators, practitioners, policy makers, agency and organization personnel and citizens to examine concepts embedded in "welfare" and in "well-being." The common definitions vary and so the challenge is to discuss and find ways to monitor and measure what is happening in families at the community, state, national, and global levels. The impact of welfare reform will change a wide range of people and institutions in the years to come and to shift the focus from short term self-sufficiency, to the long term, sustainable well-being of individuals, families, and society and improve the quality of life for families and society.

ACKNOWLEDGEMENTS

The paper was supported by Minnesota Agricultural Experiment Station Project (MIN 52-055) and the College of Human Ecology, Office of Outreach, University of Minnesota. The researchers wish to thank all the parents receiving Food Stamps who were part of the focus groups discussed in the paper. All correspondence should be directed to Dr. Bauer at Family Social Science Department, 275 McNeal Hall, 1985 Buford Avenue, St. Paul, MN 55108. She can be reached at jbauer@umn.edu or at (612)-625-1763.

REFERENCES

Braun B. and J. Bauer: 1998a, 'Welfare reform: an opportunity to engage universities in community and economic development', Journal of Public Service and Outreach 3(1), pp. 33–37.

Braun, B. and J. Bauer: 1998b, 'From welfare to well-being: a framework for dialogue and action', in M. I. Henry, D. I. Mitstifer and F. M. Smith (eds.), Toward a Theory of Family Well-being II, pp. 71–76.

Braun, B., K. Craig, J. Bauer and C. J. Peck: 1996, 'Welfare reform issues, implications and public policy', in I. Leech (ed.), Consumer Interests Annual 42 (American Council on Consumer Interests, Columbia MO), pp. 365–371.

Braun, B., K. Craig, J. Henton, T. Knipp and M. Naddaff: 1995, Welfare Reform: Justice for Children and Families (National Association of State Universities and Land-Grant Colleges, Special Task Force on Welfare Reform, Board on Human Sciences, Washington DC).

Bronfenbrenner, U.: 1979, The Ecology of Human Development: Experiments by Nature and Design (Harvard University Press, Cambridge, MA).
Bubolz, M. M. and M. S. Sontag: 1993, 'Human ecology theory', in P. Boss, W. Doherty, R. LaRossa, W. Schumm and S. Steinmetz (eds.), Sourcebook of Family Theories and Methods (Plenum Press, New York), pp. 419–448.
Hansen, A.: 1994, 'The illusion of local sustainability and self-sufficiency: famine in a border area of Northwestern Zambia', Society of Applied Anthropology 53, pp. 11–20.
Henry, M. I., D. I. Mitstifer and F. M. Smith: 1998, Toward a Theory of Family Well-being II (Kappa Omicron Nu Honor Society, East Lansing, MI).
Lie, G. and R. M. Morney: 1992, 'A controlled evaluation of comprehensive social services provided to teenage mothers receiving AFDC', Research on Social Work Practice 2, pp. 429–447.
Magistad, B. M., J. W. Bauer, M. S. Frazer and M. S. Stum: 1998, Families on Food Stamps: Perspectives about Making Ends Meet. Final report MIN 52-055. Working paper, Family Social Science Department, University of Minnesota, St. Paul MN.
Pickett J. P. et al.: 1998, The American Heritage Dictionary of the English Language (The Learning Company, electronic division 1998 Learning Company Properties, Inc., San Jose, CA).
Sandfort, J. R. and M. S. Hill: 1996, 'Assisting young, unmarried mothers to become self-sufficient: the effect of different types of early economic support', Journal of Marriage and the Family 58, pp. 311–326.
United States Department of Health and Human Services: 1997, Indicators of Welfare Dependence. Annual Report to Congress (USDHHS, Washington DC).
Zimmerman, S.: 1992, Family Policies and Family Well-being (Sage Publications, Inc., Newbury Park, CA).

Family Studies Department
University of Maryland
College Park, Maryland
USA

Bonnie Braun

College of Human Ecology
University of Minnesota – Twin Cities
St. Paul, Minnesota
USA

Patricia D. Olson

Family Social Science Department
University of Minnesota – Twin Cities
St. Paul, Minnesota
USA

Jean W. Bauer

ESTHER M. MADDUX

A BEHAVIORAL MODEL TO OPTIMIZE FINANCIAL QUALITY OF LIFE

ABSTRACT. The purpose is to present a behavioral model to enable individuals to change self-defeating behavior patterns to reduce financial stress and optimize financial quality of life. Strategies for reducing financial stress include identifying and naming the source of financial stress as well as identifying behavioral and financial strategies to reshape behavior to create an optimal quality of life. The paper discusses how behavior patterns are learned, how emotional distortions evolve, and how emotional distortions can be dissolved.

Optimal financial quality of life means being able to arrange money to do the things one wants to do. When individuals and families are unable to manage their money effectively, money problems can result.

Money problems can cause fights and increase tension in a relationship. The Consumer Credit Counseling Service of Atlanta conducted a recent survey of people who came to the organization for debt or budget counseling. Sixty percent of married respondents reported fighting about money with their spouse. Nineteen percent said financial problems negatively affected their relationships with their parents. Thirteen percent said the same was true for friends. Over ninety-three percent reported that financial problems increased the amount of stress in their lives (CCCS Atlanta, 1998).

Financial stress can originate from external and internal sources. **External sources** are circumstances that create financial stress that one may not be able to control. Circumstantial problems include job cutback or loss, income reduction due to death, disability from accident, illness, or divorce. **Internal sources** are self-defeating spending behavior patterns that can be changed. Internal factors may include lack of financial management knowledge or skills, and unwise spending decisions that lead to impulsive or compulsive behaviors. Self-defeating behavior patterns can be changed to attain a more optimal quality of life.

Social Indicators Research **60:** 155–177, 2002.

Illustration 1
The Behavioral Chain of Reaction

Event ⇨ Thoughts/beliefs/assumptions ⇨ Feelings ⇨ Decision ⇨ Action ⇨ Consequence

1. An **event** occurs.
2. One has personal **thoughts, beliefs, or assumptions** about the event.
3. **Feelings** result from emotional responses to thoughts, beliefs, or assumptions about the event.
4. One **decides** how to act in response to the feelings.
5. One **acts** on the decision.
6. There is a **consequence** or result of the action.

The purpose of this paper is to present a behavioral model to enable individuals to change self-defeating behavior patterns to reduce financial stress and optimize their financial quality of life. Strategies for reducing financial stress include:

1. Identify and name the source of financial stress;
2. Identify behavioral and financial strategies to reduce financial stress to create an optimal quality of life.

IDENTIFY AND NAME THE SOURCE OF FINANCIAL STRESS

Financial management is managing one's self with respect to the way he or she spends money. "One's self" is one's individual personality which influences all aspects of daily living including spending habits. One's **personality** is the total qualities and traits, including character or behavior, of the individual (Berube, 1985).

Behavior is what one does. It is the way one acts, reacts, functions or performs (Morris, 1971). Behavior is how one responds to events that happen to him or her in life. Events that invoke a behavioral response can be an internal drive or an external stimulus. When an event occurs, one has personal thoughts, beliefs or assumptions about the event. There is a chain reaction between the events in one's world, beliefs about those events, and resulting feelings, decisions, actions and consequences. Illustration 1 illustrates the components of the behavioral chain of reaction.

Behavior patterns don't just happen. They are learned through the shaping of brain cells. At birth, the natural self is moldable and adaptable to external influences. Each individual is born with

Illustration 2

PERSONALITY
AT BIRTH
⇓
NATURAL SELF
Natural Feelings and Natural Behaviors
The Potential For What One Can Be

a **prototype pattern** of what his or her life can potentially be. That potential includes **instincts**, natural actions or behaviors, and **intuition**, natural feelings. One's potential for what one can be is his or her **natural self**, the pure and authentic self (Campbell, 1971). See Illustration 2.

How Behavior Patterns Are Learned?

Behavior patterns are created after birth as a result of stimuli coming into the brain from the environment in which a child exists. The human brain functions to sense, process, perceive, store, and act on information from outside and inside the body solely to promote survival (Perry, 1995). The brain can change its architecture to further develop, reshape, weaken or remain the same to cope with experience. This functional architecture is the source of habits, thoughts, consciousness, memory, and mind. "The brain develops and organizes as a reflection of developmental experience, organizing in response to the pattern, intensity, and nature of sensory and perceptual experience" (FL Starting Points Initiative, 1998).

The brain has four parts: the brainstem, the cerebellum, the limbic system, and the cortex. The brainstem controls blood pressure, heart rate, and body temperature. The cerebellum controls automatic movements and balance such as appetite and sleep. The limbic system regulates emotions. The cortex regulates thought and the senses and can activate behavioral responses to an emotional trigger (FL Starting Points Initiative, 1998).

The limbic system is the portion of the brain that processes emotional matters. It activates the fight or flight response system. It is powerful enough to override rational thought and innate response patterns. Some emotional reactions and emotional memories can bypass the reasoning and logic center of the brain, the cortex. The limbic system can trigger an emotional response before the cortical centers have fully understood what is happening. The power of emotions can disrupt thinking and decision-making (FL Starting Points Initiative, 1998).

A child learns patterns through the senses which can eventually lead to a successful quality of life or a not so successful quality of life. From about age 4 to 10, there is enormous brain activity that is influencing behavior patterns. Brain cells are vigorously learning which behaviors to keep and which to discard (FL Starting Points Initiative, 1998).

The brain's ability to adapt is maximal during the first 10 to 12 years of life and reduces significantly by the early teenage years. Thereafter, the brain still changes in response to it's environment, but not to the same degree. As one gets older, it is not as easy for one to learn new things. If the brain does not receive appropriate stimulation within a developmentally prescribed time, it may never completely develop it's mental and emotional potential (FL Starting Points Initiative, 1998). Any deprivation of optimal developmental experiences result in primitive, immature behavioral reactivity (Perry, 1995).

Behavior has pattern and shape that evolves from childhood and develops in a highly predictable manner (Ilg, 1981). One behaves as one learns to behave. Behaviors are learned by associating experiences with rewards. Parents need to affirm that a child is of great value simply because he or she exists. Parents must somehow be both tolerant and intolerant, accepting and demanding, strict and flexible. (Peck, 1983). It is the task of parents to assist their children to achieve their own independence and separateness so individuality can emerge (Kerr, 1988). The degree to which one's individual identity develops is known as differentiation. **Differentiation** is the emergence of one's individual identity as opposed to being enmeshed within one's family unit. **Enmeshment** is the entanglement of the individual identity within the family unit's identity.

In healthy personal interactions, there is giving of respect from the worthy to the worthy. Each individual regards and honors the value or worth of self and others. Fully developed communication patterns allow each family member to feel loved, cared for,

Illustration 3

Characteristics of Troubled and Nurturing Families

Characteristics of Troubled Families	Characteristics of Nurturing Families
Enmeshed individual self-identity is entangled with family identity Self-image -based on anxiety, neediness of others, emotionally distorted perceptions of others -individual identity is not respected -if parent withholds affection or attention, child may not receive validation of value and importance -lack of validation prevents child from developing emotional skills to face and bear conflict effectively Pressured -pressured to seek acceptance and approval Emotional -emotionality/subjectivity has strong influence on family relationships Reactive -functions in reaction to what others expect	-Well-differentiated -One's own self-identity is allowed to emerge -Low-degree of emotionality or pressure for togetherness -Individual is respected/affirmed -Individual is permitted to develop personal autonomy to grow, think, feel, and act for self -Each family member feels loved, cared for, trusted and respected -Individuals express needs and get them met -Individual views parents, siblings, others as people with roles in his or her life as well as distinct/separate individuals -Beliefs, values, convictions are consistent -Individual is part of family, yet an individual within it. -Self-worth is high -Communication is direct, clear, specific, accurate, and honest -Rules are flexible, appropriate, and subject to change -Linking to society is open and hopeful

trusted, and respected. Effective communication patterns empower individual family members to express their needs and get them met.

In a well-differentiated family, there is a low degree of emotionality, or pressure for togetherness. A child is permitted to develop personal autonomy, to grow, think, feel, and act for self. The child can view parents, siblings, and others as people with roles in his or her life, as well as distinct and separate individuals. Self-image is not formed based on the anxieties and neediness of others, nor the emotionally distorted perceptions of others. The child is not pressured to seek acceptance and approval. Beliefs, values, and convictions are consistent. The child is a part of the family, yet an individual within it (Kerr, 1988).

Satir (1972) suggests that each family can be placed somewhere along a scale from very nurturing to very troubled. Satir characterizes vital and nurturing families as follows: "Self-worth is high. Communication is direct, clear, specific, accurate, and honest. Rules are flexible, human, appropriate, and subject to change. The linking to society is open and hopeful." See Illustration 3.

In a poorly-differentiated family, emotionality and subjectivity have a strong influence on family relationships. A child functions in reaction to what others expect (Kerr, 1988; Scherhorn, 1990). The child's individual identity is not respected. If parents withhold affection and attention, the child may not receive **validation** of value and importance. This lack of validation prevents the child from developing the emotional skills to face and bear conflict effectively (Scherhorn, 1990). The patterns learned in childhood continue into adulthood.

There are four **stages of human maturity**: infancy, childhood, adolescence, and adulthood. Certain physical, intellectual, mental, and emotional characteristics are associated with each level of human maturity (May, 1992). When emotional development does not keep pace with physical and intellectual development, the intellectually and physically mature adult behaves based on primitive, immature emotional responses. Immature emotional responses hinders one from maximizing his or her full potential because he or she is not accessing his or her natural self.

How does the natural self get repressed? When one is born, other people naturally become a part of the child's life. The child enters a world he or she did not create where there are rules he or she didn't make (Hoffman, 1979; Pittman, 1987). Those people influence the child's actions by the way they interact with him or her. Those interactions can be effective and healthy or they can be ineffective and unhealthy. The child learns by observing and responding to the stimuli in his or her environment. If one is respected and affirmed as a child in his or her family of origin, he or she enters adulthood with a strong sense of self. **Repression** of the natural self occurs if others dominate and successfully impose their wills on the child with little or no regard for his or her feelings or needs. In an unhealthy parent/child relationship, the parent sacrifices the child's self to preserve the parent's self-image of perfection. The child becomes a scapegoat. The parent unconsciously blames the child and holds the child responsible for the parent's emotional developmental deficiencies.

Children are told to honor father and mother so they do. Because parents are the child's primary frame of reference, the child learns to operate under the illusion that his or her family's situation is the ideal situation of how life should be. Unfortunately, one sometimes arrives in adulthood without realizing that his or her mommy and daddy were not perfect and did not always teach him or her the best skills to live life. The survival skills one learned to keep mommy or daddy satisfied aren't always skills that yield successful results in other environments. Children learn to define their needs and acquire their own methods for getting their needs met.

When one is not allowed the freedom to appropriately express his or her natural feelings, especially anger and hurt, those feelings are repressed (Bradshaw, 1992). Repression occurs when one learns that in order to please the will of the other person, he or she has to adapt to what others need or want. A child learns to imitate his or her parents to please them. If one is rewarded for pleasing others and punished if he or she does not, he or she learns to give in to the demands of others. Consequently the child represses his or her natural self to please others (Campbell, 1971; Peck, 1983).

When **repression** of the natural self takes place, the thought or feeling being repressed does not quietly disappear. The thought or feeling is tucked away out of awareness into the person's unconscious. Tucking away these thoughts and feelings from conscious awareness into the unconscious requires an energy force that always remains present.

This tucked away or repressed energy force is known as an **emotional distortion** or autonomous (troublesome) complex. An emotional distortion is a psychic formation that remains subliminal (tucked away) until it receives a charge of energy sufficient to carry it over the threshold into conscious awareness. Its association with consciousness does not mean that it is absorbed into the mind, only that it is perceived. It is not subject to conscious control and can be neither inhibited nor voluntarily reproduced. Therein lies the autonomy of the complex. It appears and disappears in accordance with its own inherent tendencies, independently of the conscious will (Campbell, 1971). See Illustration 4.

The troublesome complex can create a feeling of imbalance that leads to a sense of emptiness and chaos. When emotional feelings are overwhelmingly painful or unpleasant, and not dealt with directly and appropriately, defense mechanism behaviors form that express themselves as inappropriate adaptations. Inappropriate adaptations for dealing with unexpressed feelings or unmet needs may be exhibited as external experiences such as physical illness, withdrawal and stopping talking, explosive outbursts, verbal aggression, or escapist behaviors.

Illustration 4

PERSONALITY AT BIRTH

⇓

NATURAL SELF

Natural Feelings and Natural Behaviors
The Potential For What One Can Be

Event occurs

Ineffective reaction to major life experience - one reacts to please others
Causes emotional distortion of natural self

/ ↓ \

Outer Self ← ← ↓ → → **Inner Self**

(Awareness/Conscious) (Unawareness/Unconscious)

↓ ↓

Result: Behavior pleases other person (maybe)

Natural feelings repressed

↓

Emotional Distortion with a negative energy charge is formed

Escapist behaviors are substitutes that are enacted rather than acknowledging and dealing with true feelings. Bradshaw (1988) describes these escapist behaviors as **abortive adaptations**. Abortive adaptations may include alcoholism, drug addiction, spouse/child abuse, affairs, religion, excessive work patterns, gambling, eating disorders, sexual addiction, compulsive shopping, and compulsive clutter. Some people exhibit more than one addiction such as gambling and alcoholism or alcoholism and eating disorders (Krych, 1989). Escapist behaviors do not permanently satisfy longings for approval, love, value, and validation (Lieberman, 1988).

Langrehr (1991) cites examples of ineffective financial behavior as excessive use of money to maintain power or control over others, to buy love or belonging, or to hoard money due to fear. There are three classifications of spending behavior: planned, impulsive and compulsive/addictive. **Planned spending** is thought-out, controlled spending (Rook, 1987). **Impulsive spending** is acting without deliberation (unplanned spending) (Waddell, 1989). Impulsive buying is making a purchase in response to a sudden, unexpected urge to buy something (Gardner, 1988). In a study of the effects of impulse purchases, the urgency to substitute shopping for dealing with unmet needs resulted in feelings of anxiousness and guilt, not power.

O'Guinn (1989) classifies impulsive spending as acute behavior and compulsive spending as chronic. Another difference is the severity of the consequences (O'Guinn, 1989). **Compulsive spending** can be a mechanism to cope with stress, escape demands, or overcome unpleasant situations. d'Astous (1990) suggests that perhaps all consumers can be positioned along a generalized urge to buy continuum. Those in the upper extreme can be called compulsive or addictive spenders.

Bradshaw (1990) also classifies compulsive spending as an addiction. With shopping addiction, "it's not the stuff we want; it's the activity of buying the stuff that is symbolically representative of what we don't have." Scherhorn (1990) suggests that addictive spending is an ineffective reaction to a major life experience with which one is unable to cope. This experience triggers very clear, strong feelings that can serve as a red flag to pay attention to those feelings.

According to Faber (1989), compulsive behavior is chronic buying. The consumer is unable to stop or moderate the behavior. Compulsive buying *may* produce short-term positive feelings, but ultimately disrupts life and produces negative consequences.

Faber (1988) describes compulsive behavior as:

1. physical and/or psychological dependence on the substance or activity;
2. occasional loss of control regarding the behavior and subsequent interference with normal life functioning;
3. presence of a drive, impulse, or urge to engage in the behavior;
4. denial of the harmful, consequences of continuing the behavior; and
5. repeated failure in efforts to control or modify the behavior.

Compared to other consumers, compulsive buyers have a lower level of self esteem, scored higher on a general test of obsessive-compulsiveness, have a higher propensity for materialism, are significantly more envious, have a higher fantasy level, and a much higher debt load. There was no significant difference on possessiveness. The primary motivation behind compulsive consumption

Illustration 5
Feelings Before and After Compulsive Shopping

Feelings Before ⇒	Compulsive Shopping Experience ⇒	Feelings After
Abandoned		Accepted
Anxious or nervous		Assertive, powerful
Awareness of shortcomings		Attractive
Depressed		Control
Despair at being deserted		Important, respected
Disappointed, hurt		Relaxed, calmer
Frustrated		Safe and secure
Isolation		Self-confident
Harassed		Loved, appreciated
Lack of concern by others		
Left out, ignored		
Lonely, empty, bored		
Loss of precious things		
Misunderstood		
Need to punish self		
Need to punish or get even		
Pain and suffering		
Powerless		
Reversal of fortune; once proud now humiliated		
Shame and loss of honor		
Stressful or tense		
Unattractive		
Unimportant, worthless		
Unloved, unappreciated		

Source: Waddell, 1989.

is not the desire to own the purchased items, but the psychological benefit derived from the buying process itself (Faber, 1988, 1989). Compulsive consumers seem to get very little pleasure out of the things they buy. Consequences of compulsive buying include extreme levels of debt, anxiety and frustration, subjective sense of loss of control, and domestic dissensions (O'Guinn, 1989).

Waddell (1989) defines compulsive behavior as "an irresistible impulse to perform an irrational act." Occasionally spending money spontaneously or impulsively is human nature, and sometimes buying something to cheer oneself is healthy. Even an occasional excess is acceptable. But spending becomes harmful when it is chronic or compulsive and is not controlled.

Waddell (1989) suggests "identity issues" often are at the root of compulsive spending behavior. Feelings of low self-esteem and insecurity may develop when parents have exceptionally high expectations of a child or create an environment so the child feels inferior or inadequate. If a child suffers severe emotional deprivation, a method of coping may be to acquire things to feel good, accepted, or powerful. Illustration 5 identifies feelings Waddell has associated with before and after compulsive shopping experiences.

When one suppresses the natural self, the repressed feelings do not go away. The repressed feelings leave conscious awareness and become tucked away or suppressed in the unconscious. The unexpressed feelings are harbored inside in the unconscious and accumulate overtime.

Over time, the natural self rebels against the suppression by others and seeks acknowledgment. The natural self will seek this acknowledgment in either appropriate or inappropriate ways. Inappropriate or **self-defeating behaviors** occur when patterns, actions, and feelings are not in agreement with one's natural self. Self-defeating behaviors occur when what one wants is not consistent with what one does. The perceived conflict between what one wants and what one does leads to internal imbalance with one's emotions which is experienced as dissatisfaction. This feeling of dissatisfaction is an indicator that one has emotional potential yet to be developed.

If one learned in childhood to successfully negotiate for his or her natural self and act on true feelings, compromise and collaboration with one's self and others can occur. However, if the natural self was suppressed, one may not have developed appropriate skills to acknowledge his or her natural self to know what one does want. The result is that inappropriate adaptations will be used to bring about a feeling of balance in times when authentic needs are not being acknowledged and met.

How Emotional Distortions Evolve

When a child is born, he or she is born as his or her natural self. Other people influence the child's actions by the way they interact with him or her. If interactions are positive, respectful, and affirming, the individual will develop a strong sense of self-identity. With a strong sense of self, healthy personal interactions allow one to respect the worth of others and of self. When one has a strong, positive self-identity, one does what is consistent with one's wants. One consistently behaves in a manner appropriate to true feelings including situations that have been historically emotionally stressful.

If interactions are negative and ineffective, repression of the instinctual, natural self occurs. As the child molds itself in response to those about him or her, the child's personality[1] separates into an outer self that is designed to please others and an inner self that contains the natural self that was tucked away as well as the potential for what one can be. The **outer self** is sometimes referred to as the conscious. The **inner self** is sometimes called the unconscious.

James A. Hall, M.D., psychiatrist and Jungian analyst, in his book, *The Jungian Experience, Analysis and Individuation*, has further defined the structural elements of the personality. Dr. Hall defines the **archetypal self** as the regulating center of the personality or psyche as a whole, the conscious and the unconscious. It contains the potential that each individual has the capacity to be. The archetypal self is like a thermostat connected to a heating/air conditioning system in one's home. The thermostat senses the temperature of the environment and responds by adjusting the flow of hot or cool air. The archetypal self senses the tone of emotional interaction and responds accordingly.

Dr. Hall describes other components of the personality which are archetypes, complexes, ego, persona, shadow, and anima/animus. An **archetype** is a structuring pattern of the mind. It is a pattern of response to experiences. A psychological **complex** is a normal building block of the mind. It is a group of related images having a common emotional tone. It is formed as a residue of emotion acting within an archetypal organizing field.

The **outer self** or conscious self consists of those things of which one is aware, the ten percent of information one knows about one's self. It is the way one perceives himself or herself as well as the social mask one puts on for others. It is the multiple roles one plays in relation to other people (Brehoney, 1996). The conscious self is composed of two parts, the ego and the persona.

The **ego** is a psychological complex of behaviors and emotions which influences how one perceives one's self as well as how one interacts and relates to others. The ego adapts to it's environment. The ego decides what is acceptable and worthy of consciousness. It decides what is unacceptable and separated or dissociated into the unconscious. The ego may manifest itself in one of three states:

1. **Ego-image** – the self that one creates as one adapts to one's environment. Those who are less mature in emotional development often operate on illusions. An **illusion** is a false perception or belief (Berube, 1985);

2. **Affect-ego** – an emotional situation in which the ego experiences a strong, negative feeling tone associated with a troublesome complex indicating one's natural self has been strongly violated;
3. **Authentic ego** – one's true and natural self.

The **persona** is the bridge to outer relationships. It is the conscious self that we use to relate to others. It is the set of behavior patterns we have adapted to relate to others.

The **inner self** or unconscious self includes those things that are out of our awareness. It is made up of about 90% of what we know about ourselves.

The unconscious is composed of the shadow and the animus. The **shadow** is a psychological complex of behaviors and emotions which influences how we relate to our inner self including our feelings, attitudes, and desires. The unconscious contains:

- Those things which one knows but is not thinking of at the moment.
- Those things of which one was once conscious but has forgotten.
- Everything perceived by the senses, but is not noted by the conscious mind (Brehoney, 1996).

The shadow contains non-acceptable, repressed personal material from the past. It often contains unrecognized positive qualities that are needed for further individuation.

The unconscious also contains the patterns one has absorbed from one's family history. Family legacies are those things that one has taken in from family interactions in one's family of origin as well as behaviors passed down from previous generations. Family legacies include behavior patterns, healthy and unhealthy, that are learned and carried forward from one generation to another.

The unconscious is everything which, involuntarily, and without paying attention to it, one feels, thinks, remembers, wants, and does. It is all the future things which are taking shape in one and will sometime come to consciousness (Brehoney, 1996).

The **animus** is the bridge to inner relationships. It is how we relate to our inner self – our feelings, attitudes, and desires. It is the set of behavior patterns we have adapted to relate to our inner self. The ideal self is aware of true feelings, attitudes, and desires. A

Illustration 6

Characteristics of Outer and Inner Self

Outer Self (Conscious)	**Inner Self (Unconscious)**
Those things of which we are aware; 10% of what we know about our self	Those things out of awareness; 90% of what we know about self
Ego: -Complex of behavior and emotions which influences how one perceives one's self as well as how one relates to others -Decides what is acceptable and worthy of consciousness as well as what is unacceptable and separated or dissociated into consciousness -Ego manifests itself in three ways: 1. Ego image: the outer self one creates as one adapts to one's environment; often based on illusions, which are false perceptions or beliefs 2. Affect image: ego with a strong feeling tone associated with a troublesome complex indicating natural self has been strongly violated 3. Authentic ego: one's true and natural self	**Shadow:** Complex of behaviors and emotions which influence how we relate to our inner self Contains -Those things we know but aren't thinking of at moment -Those things of which one was conscious but has forgotten -Everything perceived by senses; but not noted by conscious mind -Contains non-acceptable repressed personal material from the past -Contains unrecognized positive qualities needed for further individuation - the potential for what we can be Family patterns of behavior that have been passed from one generation to another
Persona: Bridge to outer relationships The set of behavior patterns we have adapted to relate to others	**Animus:** Bridge to inner relationship The set of behavior patterns we have adapted to relate to inner self - our feelings, attitudes, and desires. Healthy - aware of true feelings, attitudes, desires Unhealthy - project feelings, attitudes, desires to others

less developed emotional self projects feelings, attitudes, and desires to others. **Projection** is a defense mechanism in the unconscious by which one's own feelings, attitudes, or desires are attributed to someone else (Berube, 1985). The weaknesses or strengths an individual sees in others is the inward reflection of an individual's inner state of being. If one is weak in a characteristic within one's self, one seeks a special relationship with another who is perceived to have strength in the weak characteristic. If one is excessively critical of another, that criticism is often a reflection of a weakness within the giver of the criticism. See Illustrations 6 and 7.

We learn to **adapt** by developing coping skills to survive in our environment. At birth, we emerge from an archetypal world and construct a personal world for ourselves out of whatever materials we are given by fate and circumstance (Hall, 1986). One's level of emotional strength influences how successful one is in all aspects of life – financial, physical, spiritual, social, family, and career. Emotional conflict within one's self prevents one from reaching his or her full potential and thus achieving an optimal quality of life.

ILLUSTRATION 7

AT BIRTH
NATURAL SELF

Imposition of other's will suppresses natural self of child
Parents sacrifice child to preserve own self-image of perfection

/ \

Conscious ⇔ **Unconscious**

Ego
Persona

Shadow
Animus

Repress natural self to please others
When the natural self is separated into the conscious and unconscious, sense of self-identity ranges from mild to severely weak
Operate under illusions, which is false perceptions or beliefs
Develop emotional distortions manifested as abortive adaptations
Practice self-defeating behaviors
Act out of fear

\ /

Correction: alter behaviors to arrive at healthy level of emotional maturity and healthy interpersonal interaction

Natural Self

Behave consistently based on true feelings, including situations which have been historically particularly stressful
What you do is consistent with what you want
Respect worth of self and others
At peace

How Emotional Distortions Dissolve

To achieve optimal quality of financial life one must be able to transcend inner personal conflict and transform behavior into healthy patterns that lead to wise spending decisions. To examine and transcend personal inner conflict, one needs a safe environment to:

1. explore self-defeating behavior patterns that hinder normal functioning.
2. dissolve troublesome complexes that cause abnormal behavior,
3. transcend self-defeating behavior patterns, and
4. transform them into life-enhancing behavior patterns.

Life-enhancing behavior patterns are healthy, positive, mature, and rational responses to life events. Life-enhancing behaviors allow one to consistently behave based on true feelings including situations that have been historically particularly stressful (Hall, 1986).

Self-defeating behavior patterns exist when what one does makes one unhappy. What one does is not consistent with what one wants. Troublesome complexes are present when one feels all is not right with his or her life. Often the **presenting symptom** that signals dissatisfaction with one's life is an abortive attempt to find the right path. The **underlying reason** for the abnormal behavior and personal discomfort is a troublesome complex that needs to be diagnosed, analyzed, and dissolved.

How does a troublesome complex take shape? When a person interacts with others, the ego decides what is acceptable and worthy of persona and ego or unacceptable and dissociated into the **shadow**. If another person forces his will on one, one's ego responds to the real or perceived dominant stimulus of the other person's strong will. The ego decides that the acceptable response by the persona is to respond out of fear to what the dominant person demands. One's own needs are suppressed into the shadow of one's unconscious to please the other person. The dissociated part of the self forms an abnormal behavior pattern with an energy charge that has a negative emotional tone. The more times the same pattern is repeated the stronger the emotional tone becomes. This is known as an **emotional distortion or troublesome complex**. When an event pushes one over the edge and activates the troublesome complex, the anxiety from awakening the repressed material alters the ego-image so the emotional tone of the complex takes over. The personality of the complex replaces the usual ego-image. The ego undergoes a marked change and takes on a very different personality known as the affect image (Hall, 1986). The strong negative feeling tone of the affect image indicates the natural self has been strongly violated.

When all is not right with one's life, uncovering the source of one's inner conflict can relieve personal discomfort. Dr. James Hall, M.D. (1986) suggests that one examine clues given off by pressure from the unconscious to find relief. If one consistently behaves based on one's true feelings or one's natural self, then one experiences an ideal level of psychological health and may be defined as individuated. However if one experiences great discomfort and the sensation that all is not right with one's life, then the unconscious may be excessively activated. The amount of pressure from the unconscious is an indicator for understanding one's level of individuation and the need for a change in the way one lives his or her life. If repressed feelings in the unconscious put excessive pressure on the conscious; disorders can result, ranging from mild anxiety through neurosis to severe mental illness (Hall, 1986).

The development of a positive self-identity can be achieved by examining one's behaviors, identifying self-defeating behavior patterns that need to be changed, and then making the changes. This can be achieved through personal study and self discovery, through sessions with a supportive psychotherapist, or perhaps more extreme external support, medication and hospitalization. Neglecting to deal with serious unconscious conflict can lead to physical illness (Hall, 1986). Closely and honestly examining personal behaviors can lead to insight that can decrease the uncomfortable pressure from the unconscious.

Dr. Hall (1986) suggests that there are several stages of movement through the individuation process that can lead to diminishing a troublesome complex:

1. Establish personal boundaries by learning to identify and name feelings associated with events when one is treated with disrespect, and specify goals that can move one toward reducing the discomfort.
2. Recognize and break down image ego and affect ego.
   a. Identify behaviors based on illusions which are false perceptions or beliefs
   b. Identify behavior patterns associated with troublesome complexes. Recognize feeling, identify the inner need that is not being met, then give yourself what you need.
3. Identify unwanted characteristics in the shadow and reshape them into positive characteristics you desire. The unwanted characteristic in one's shadow can be usually noted in another person of the same sex that irrationally one doesn't like. Identify the disturbing characteristic in the other person and develop a strategy to build that weakness into a strength.
4. Integrate animus. The animus can be detected when a person is unconscious of the actual conflicts that disturb him or her and project the cause onto the partner. The animus can also be

detected when another person does not live up to our expectations. In these situations, one's own complex has usually been unconsciously projected onto the other person. Become aware of true feelings, attitudes, and desires by examining the characteristics that you have projected onto others or in the behaviors of others that disturb you.

5. Synthesize and integrate insights into everyday life (Hall, 1986).

Resistance to personal growth indicates a self-image crisis. The barrier to successful personal growth is fear of rejection, the fear of one's own internal self-rejection. Fear is a learned emotion that is a response to attacks from others when they try to impose their will on us. Fear arises when what you want conflicts with what you do. Fear causes the separation of the natural self into the inner self and outer self that one abortively adapts to please others.

Upon honest self-examination, one discovers that he or she has been more highly influenced by unconscious assumptions and motivations than often realized. These unconscious processes are often a defense mechanism attempting to protect the ego image from perceived threats. Attention to one's unconscious is necessary. The attention required diminishes as self-integration increases (Hall, 1986). Self-integration is the process of accessing the natural self by dissolving the feeling of emptiness and chaos that was created when the natural self was separated into the outer self and inner self.

The goal of individuation is to understand the meaning of an activated, troublesome complex, to examine the complex, understand the history of the complex, analyze the complex, dissolve the complex, and be compassionate to one's self through out the process. Dissolving a possessive complex can be achieved by experiencing an active troublesome complex in a safe situation (Hall, 1986).

Individuation can occur when one finds safe environments to practice reshaping abnormal behavior patterns that impair normal functioning, dissolve troublesome complexes to be able to transcend self-defeating behavior patterns, and transform them into life-enhancing behavior patterns (Hall, 1986).

Individuation is a process, not a goal, that actualizes one's innate potentialities. Influencing one's own psychological processes is like learning another language. Learning the new language requires attending to the emotional tone and content associated with a troublesome complex. It requires conscious reflection on the emotional charge the troublesome complex carries and how it influences one's behavior. It requires courage and perceptiveness to transcend the troublesome complex and transform behavior into a meaningful life (Hall, 1986).

The stages in the process of individuation or learning the new language are as follows:

1. **Stuck/unchanged** – old feelings are unchanged.
2. **Transition** – old identity is loosened and cannot be reinstated. Bring unconscious material into conscious examination. Contents of the shadow are simply aspects of oneself that could have been lodged in the ego or the persona, but were relegated to the shadow because they were unacceptable to the ego.
3. **Luminality** – sense of insecurity that accompanies significant psychological transformation of basic identity patterns.
4. **Regressive restoration** – move backward to an earlier personality organization that is inadequate to the present growth potential, but is secure in a sense because it is completely known.
5. **Transcendence** – go beyond, transcend, the tension caused by the separation of the natural self into the conscious and the unconscious. During transcendence, there can be fluctuation in feelings, sometimes old feelings are unchanged; sometimes feelings are free from conflict. The troublesome complex must be dealt with repeatedly as long as it is a primary focus of feeling or affect. It needs to be dealt with as long as it carries an emotional charge.
6. **Clearly transcended** – much more difficult to regress to old behavior patterns.
7. **Transformation/growth** – a complete perceptual change (Hall, 1986).

Individuation means integrating dissociated unconscious material back into your awareness where it naturally belongs. The goal of individuation is to consistently behave based on true feelings including situations that have been historically stressful and painful. Individuation means being able to live with passion and depth in whatever situation one encounters (Hall, 1986).

Illustration 8

Behavioral Strategies to Achieve Financial Security

PERSONAL CHARACTERISTICS	SELF-DEFEATING BEHAVIORS	LIFE-ENHANCING BEHAVIORS
1. Needs awareness	Lack of awareness of unsatisfied/unmet needs	Be aware and identify unmet/unsatisfied needs Give self what is needed
2. Self-identity - the value we attach to our personal identity	Weak self-identity Stay stuck in place or regress	Develop strong sense of self Recognize need to change Identify self-defeating behaviors Change self-defeating behaviors
3. Self-control	Inadequate acknowledgment of personal power	Use personal power effectively Modulate and control one's action in age-appropriate ways Build and demonstrate inner control
4. Responsibility	Act irresponsibly Blame others	Accept responsibility for personal behavior
5. Self-direction	No direction No financial goals Not clear about values No spending priorities Confused between needs/wants Indecisive/reactive Impulsive Compulsive Narrow-minded, closed thinking Uninformed Exclusive	Set goals to achieve financial self-sufficiency Set financial goals Identify and clarify values Set spending priorities Distinguish between needs and wants Have a financial and spending plan Be proactive in decision-making; Make conscious, planned decisions Be open-minded; explore alternatives Include others when appropriate Build assets Think net income when making decisions Develop financial skills
6. Self-reliance	Dependence	Be independent and financially self-reliant
7. Safety and security	Fear View mistake or criticism as character attack	Overcome fear to achieve financial security Distinguish between real and imagined fear View mistakes as an opportunity to grow and as a signal for looking for different perhaps better ways to do things View criticism as information; focus on appropriate behavior not on worth as an individual
8. Facts	False assumptions	Check out and act on facts
9. Expectations	Unreasonable, unrealistic expectations	Be reasonable & realistic in expectations
10. Respect	Lack of respect for self and others Aggressive/nonassertive	Be respectful of self and others Be assertive
11. Positive thoughts and affirmations	Think negatively and put self down	Think positively and affirm successes
12. Feeling (Type, level of intensity)	Ignore/deny feelings	Acknowledge feelings Recognize, listen to, interpret the behavior connected with the feeling Express needs appropriately
13. Informed/aware of alternatives	Uniformed/look for easy way out	Be informed/look for options
14. Communication	Nonverbal	Use verbal communication. Be direct, clear, specific, accurate, and honest in communication patterns
15. Approach issues	Avoid dealing with issues	Approach issues directly
16. Style	Make demands	State preferences

Individuation occurs by desensitizing troublesome complex reactions until the ego is able to assimilate contents of the complex without being overwhelmed. It is the use to which complexes are put, not their existence, that can cause difficulty. Individuation is a process of self-reflection and understanding. It is meant to free one from unnecessary bondage to complexes that are dominant in one's personal psychology in order to find a meaningful life. Only a strongly developed personality can withstand the tensions of seeing deeply into the unconscious. The successful exploration of one's unconscious returns one to the world as a deeper and more integrated person able to use mature judgment in day-to-day emotional life (Hall, 1986).

Practicing life enhancing behaviors accompanied by a sound financial plan can lead one to financial security. The ten steps in a sound financial plan include:

1. Maintain financial records.
2. Control cash flow
3. Manage credit and debt wisely
4. Insure adequately
5. Establish/contribute to savings regularly
6. Pay necessary taxes but not more
7. Maintain current lifestyle at retirement
8. Have an up-to-date estate plan
9. Have an up-to-date financial statement
10. Use money as an object of exchange

Managing money is managing one's self with regard to the way one spends money. A strong sense of self-identity combined with a sound financial plan can lead to optimal financial quality of life. Optimal quality of life can be achieved by identifying self-defeating behavior; identifying and naming the source of stress that causes self-defeating behaviors and by identifying behavioral and financial strategies to reduce financial stress.

NOTE

[1] Personality – the total qualities and traits, including character or behavior, of an individual (Berube, 1985).

REFERENCES

Berube, M. A.: 1985, American Heritage Dictionary (Houghton Mifflin Company, Boston).

Bloomfield, H. H.: 1983, Making Peace with Your Parents (Ballantine Books, New York).

Bradshaw, J.: 1988, Healing the Shame that Binds You (Health Communications, Inc., Deerfield Beach, FL).

Bradshaw, J.: 1992, Homecoming (Bantam Books, New York).
Bradshaw, J.: 1990, 'Shopping until you can't stop', Lear's (October), p. 75.
Brehony, K. A.: 1996, Awakening at Midlife: Realizing Your Potential for Growth and Change (Riverhead Books, New York).
Calhoun, J. F. and J. R. Acocella: 1978, Psychology of Adjustment and Human Relationships (Random House, New York).
Campbell, J.: 1971, The Portable Jung (Viking Penguin Inc., New York).
Consumer Credit Counseling Service: 1998. Don't Let Financial Problems Ruin Your Relationships. News Release, April 30.
d'Astous, A.: 1990, 'An inqury into the compulsive side of "Normal" consumers', Journal of Consumer Policy 13, pp. 15–31.
Davidson, L.: 1998, 'Conflict can be a blessing', Horizons (May/June) 11(4), pp. 13–14.
Faber, R. J. and T. C. O'Guinn: 1989, 'Classifying compulsive consumers: advances in the development of a diagnostic tool', Advances in Consumer Research 16, pp. 738–744.
Faber, R. J. and T. C. O'Guinn: 1988. 'Compulsive consumption and credit abuse', Journal of Consumer Policy 11, pp. 97–109.
Florida Starting Points Initiative: June, 1998, Maximizing our Brain Power: We Need to Use It or Lose It (Florida State University, Tallahassee).
Gardner, M. P. and D. W. Rook: 1988, 'Effects of impulse purchases on consumers' affective states', Advances in Consumer Research 15, pp. 127–130.
Gordon, T.: 1975, Parent-Effectiveness Training (New American Library, New York).
Hall, J. A.: 1986, The Jungian Experience: Analysis and Individuation (Inner City Books, Toronto, Canada).
Hoffman, Bob: 1979, No One is to Blame: Getting a Loving Divorce from Mom and Dad (Science and Behavior Books, Inc., Palo Alto, CA).
Ilg, F. L., L. B. Ames and S. M. Baker: 1982, Child Behavior (Harper & Row, New York).
Kerr, M. E.: 1988, 'Chronic anxiety and defining a self', The Atlantic Monthly (September), pp. 35–58.
Krych, R.: 1989, 'Abnormal consumer behavior: a model of addictive behaviors', Advances in Consumer Research 16, pp. 745–748.
Langrehr, V. B.: 1991, 'Financial counseling and planning: similarities and differences', Financial Counseling and Planning 2, pp. 155–168.
Lasater, L.: 1988, Recovery from Compulsive Behavior (Health Communications, Inc., Deerfield Beach, FL).
Lerner, H. G.: 1985, The Dance of Anger (Harper & Row, New York).
Lieberman, C: 1988, 'Compulsive spending, how it develops, how to curb it', Privileged Information (February 15), pp. 5–6.
May, G. M.: 1992, Care of Mind, Care of Spirit (HarperCollins, New York).
McNeal, J. U. and C. H. Yeb: 1993, 'Born to shop', American Demographics (June).

Morris, W. (ed.): 1971, The American Heritage Dictionary (Houghton Mifflin Company, Boston).
O'Guinn, T. O. and R. J. Faber: 1989, 'Compulsive buying: a phenomenological exploration', Journal of Consumer Research 16 (September), pp. 147–157.
Peck, M. S.: 1983, People of the Lie: The Hope for Healing Human Evil (Simon & Schuster, New York).
Perry, B. D.: 1995, Incubated in Terror: Neurodevelopmental Factors in the Cycle of Violence, Children, Youth and Violence: Searching for Solutions (New York: The Guilford Press, New York).
Quint, B. G.: 1981, 'Why families fight about money', USAir (June).
Pittman, F. S.: 1987, Turning Points (W. W. Norton Company, New York).
Rook, D. W.: 1987, 'The buying impulse', Journal of Consumer Research 14, pp. 189–197.
Satir, V.: 1972, Peoplemaking (Science and Behavior Books, Inc., Palto Alto, CA).
Scherhorn, G.: 1990, 'The addictive trait in buying behavior', Journal of Consumer Policy 13, pp. 33–51.
Vernon, Ann: 1989, Thinking, Feeling, Behaving: An Emotional Education Curriculum for Adolescents, Grades 1–6 (Vol I). Research Press, 2612 North Mattis Avenue, Champaign, Illinois 61821.
Vernon, Ann: 1989, Thinking, Feeling, Behaving: An Emotional Education Curriculum for Adolescents, Grades 7–12 (Vol II). Research Press, 2612 North Mattis Avenue, Champaign, Illinois 61821.
Viscott, D.: 1976, The Language of Feelings: The Time-and-Money Shorthand of Psychotherapy (Arbor House, New York).
Waddell, F. E.: 1989, 'Compulsive spending addiction', Professional Counselor (May/June), pp. 48–51.
White, B. L.: 1985, The First Three Years of Life (rev. edn.) (Prentice Hall, New York).
Woititz, J. G.: 1983, Adult Children of Alcoholics (Health Communications, Inc., Deerfield Beach, FL).

Maddux Financial Services
125 Wakefield Drive
Athens, GA 30605-4384
E-mail: emaddux101851@msn.com

ROBERT OWEN, ALFRED NTOKO, DING ZHANG and JUNE DONG

PUBLIC POLICY AND DIFFUSION OF INNOVATION

ABSTRACT. Marketers have traditionally studied diffusion of innovation with a primary focus on the individual consumer as a unit of analysis, the major types of findings being characteristics of adopter categories and opinion leadership. We propose that this perspective is not adequate from a macromarketing perspective, in which the goals are to set public policy for societal good or to create an environment which enables the diffusion of an innovation in a way that no single marketer could do alone. In setting public policy which can enable (or inhibit) diffusion of innovation for societal good, a system composed of a mass social infrastructure, a competitive infrastructure, and a technical infrastructure should be considered.

INTRODUCTION

After the Soviet break-up, the same Ukrainian people who designed and built high-technology missiles during the Cold War years with the U.S. could not gain access to Internet technology that is available to many U.S. pre-school children. A time-limited (a few hours per week) World Wide Web account in Ukraine costs a half-month's salary for a professor (Nick, 1998); in contrast, American college students generally get an unlimited account "free" with tuition. How can the Ukraine, for all of its cold war era scientists and engineers, maintain any economic or technical momentum in such an environment? How can public policy be set to provide a solution?

The United States, on the other hand, is currently concerned that high-technology information encryption is suddenly available to anyone with a Web browser, making it difficult to monitor the activities of spies and terrorists. China is concerned that this new technology will put culturally-undesirable wants and information in the hands of anyone, causing undesirable social and cultural changes. How can public policy be set which *slows* the diffusion of an innovation or which changes public perception regarding the desirability (or undesirability) of an innovation?

Social Indicators Research **60:** 179–190, 2002.

Marketing research in the study of diffusion of innovation has maintained a pro-innovation focus with the individual consumer as the unit of analysis. This bias is only natural: are we not, after all, in a business that attempts to understand the needs and wants of consumers for the purpose of selling more stuff? Such a focus does not necessarily serve us well, however, if our concern is of a macro-marketing perspective, where the needs of a single marketer are secondary to the needs of a social system. The present manuscript reviews some different perspectives on the diffusion of innovation that might present different perspectives on the management of diffusion with respect to setting public policy. Specifically, we look (1) at the traditional approach, that of the diffusion of an innovation through different adopter categories, (2) at an approach which views diffusion from a mass marketing rather than adopter category perspective, (3) at an approach which views diffusion as occurring in an environment competitors, assisting or stifling diffusion, and (4) at an approach which views diffusion as occurring in an environment which is technologically enabling or inhibiting.

Much of the work in the area of diffusion in marketing is based on the ideas proposed in Rogers' (1962) original text on the subject and continued through the most current edition (Rogers, 1995). Rogers (1995: Table 2-1) classifies marketing and management diffusion studies as using individual consumers as the main unit of analysis, with the major types of findings being characteristics of adopter categories and of opinion leadership in diffusion. We believe that to be useful, a macromarketing perspective must take a more holistic view, with the unit of analysis being larger components of the system, of which individual consumer or consumer segments are only a part.

THE PROCESS OF DIFFUSION THROUGH INDIVIDUALS IN A SOCIAL SYSTEM

Diffusion theory as based on the approach of Rogers is focused in large part on the communication between individual members of a social system:

The main elements in the "classical model" of the diffusion of new ideas . . . are

(1) the *innovation* . . .
(2) which is *communicated* through certain channels
(3) over *time*
(4) among members of a *social system*

(Rogers, 1976; italics and numbers are original, indents are added for emphasis).

Indeed, summaries of diffusion theory by marketers have maintained that "diffusion theory's special focus is on interpersonal communications within social systems" (Gatignon and Robertson, 1985), that its "main focus is on communication channels, which are the means by which information about an innovation is transmitted to or within the social system" (Mahajan et al., 1990).

There has been much criticism of diffusion research for what is often a pro-diffusion focus (cf., Rogers, 1995). Marketers, for example, naturally have an interest in increasing sales of new products. We therefore are very interested in how "innovators" differ in needs and wants from "laggards" and in how to help prospective buyers to better understand how a new product can fill a need. This perspective leads to an interest in understanding how to better target consumers so that an innovation will diffuse faster and how to develop marketing strategies aimed at potential adopters (cf., Mahajan et al., 1990). From this perspective, then, interest is in focusing first on innovators and opinion leaders, then on to early adopters, and then on successive adopter categories until the product has diffused.

If opinion leaders, innovators, and such influence successive categories of adopters, then understanding how each of these entities plays an influential or gatekeeping role can provide insights into how to control the diffusion of an innovation. That is, it can be used not only to assist diffusion, but to impede it as well. This approach, viewing diffusion as a process to be modeled, could be useful if the idea or product is adopted as a result of the existence of different types of adopter categories or as a result of the existence and influence of opinion leaders.

A Social Process vs. Mass Diffusion

Perhaps most children in a school district can be persuaded that cigarette smoking is bad if a rock star says so, influencing some local students to quit or to not start, further influencing other students. This is the social process approach – that diffusion slowly spreads through a social system. From a public policy perspective, however, it seems just as reasonable to believe that ideas or products could diffuse rather rapidly *en masse*. Might the death of a popular school teacher through cancer be just as likely to influence the *majority* of students, giving them *all at once* a perception that there is a certainty in the cause and effect relationship between smoking and health?

UNCERTAINTY AND RISK IN A MASS MARKET

Sheth (1981) proposed that our interest should be less in the *minority* of people who *adopt* an innovation, and more in the *majority* of people who *resist* an innovation. Sheth implies that the likelihood that an innovation will successfully diffuse is dependent on the changes in habit and perceived risks that a *mass* market associates with an innovation. That is, the focus of Sheth's "Less Developed Concept in Diffusion Research" (LDC) is less on the individual or a particular segment as a unit of analysis, and more on how an innovation may or may not have value to the vast majority of members of a social system.

Sheth's LDC posits two fundamental factors with respect to the propensity of people to resist or adopt an innovation: (a) habit toward an existing practice or behavior, and (b) perceived risks associated with innovation adoption. Some innovations are "discontinuous" because they require altogether new habits by the consumer, and therefore represent high perceived risks. Lowered perceived risk and less change in habit to a *mass* market should increase the likelihood of consumer adoption.

In a study of ATM (automatic teller machines) adopters and nonadopters, Stevens et al. (1989) found that laggards did not appear to have a strong resistance to ATMs, but merely lacked confirmation of the innovation's utility. However, nonadopters and rejecters of ATM usage appeared to have specific reasons for resistance. Frambach (1993) proposes that the uncertainty surrounding an innovation might make a potential adopter postpone the decision to either adopt or reject an innovation. Simply lowering uncertainty to a majority of adopters by confirming an innovation's advantages would, then, seem to be a strategy to increase adoption without necessary regard to a process involving a sequential passage through a series of adopter categories.

Perhaps the best example of how a focus on innovators impeded the adoption of a product is the automotive industry in the U.S. The tradition of the automotive industry in the U.S. during the first decade of the century was to cater almost exclusively to the wealthy (cf., Owen, 1991). The first commercial vehicles designed under the direction of Henry Ford were said to be high-priced racing models (cf., Sward, 1948; Pound, 1940). Mr. Ford was twice involved in failures in the automotive industry, first with the Detroit Automobile Company in 1899 and again with the Henry Ford Automobile Company in 1901. Both organizations were dissolved by investors after Ford had expended their resources on high-powered racing models. The Ford Motor Company, formed in 1903, also came close to disaster by making expensive, heavy cars before introducing cars for a wider "mass market" (Pound, 1940). Our current thinking, that efforts in launching an innovation should be focused on "innovators," was not appropriate in the diffusion of the U.S. automobile.

The Model T, as a "universal car," was finally launched in 1908 and sold very well. Designed as a farmer's car and looking very much like a horse and buggy, but without the horse, the Model T drove very well on roads traveled by horse and buggy, contrary to the more luxurious products made for the rich "innovators." The Model T was very reliable and very low in price. By making a car that was reliable and low in price, and which traveled on roads used by the majority of people in the social system, the Model T lowered risks and change in habit to the *masses* of prospective adopters, not just an "innovative segment," and this one product was no doubt an important factor (albeit not the only one) in the diffusion of the automobile.

The traditional social process approach to diffusion would attempt to understand the diffusion of ATM usage and automobile purchase through a succession of different adopter categories, each with its own needs and wants, whereas Sheth's approach would define all adopter groups as the mass majority, with the nonadopters and rejecters as a minority. From a macromarketing perspective, Sheth's approach is simpler: find out what are the perceived risks and changes in habit that the *majority* of people feel toward ATM usage, automobile ownership, or any other new innovation. The traditional focus on adopter categories might actually *slow* diffusion, if more rapid diffusion is what is desired. On the other hand, the social process approach might be a more desirable strategy if, from a public policy perspective, it is desirable that an innovation diffuse in a more slow and systematic manner.

MARKETERS AND COMPETITORS AS FACTORS IN DIFFUSION

Gatignon and Robertson (1985) proposed that Rogers' basic elements of innovation, communication channels, time, and social system, be extended to include:

– the role of *marketing* (change agent) actions
– the role of *competitive* actions

with further discussion of competitive effects on technology diffusion in Robertson and Gatignon (1986).

The factors proposed by Gatignon and Robertson are a departure from the approach of most marketers in that these are factors associated more with a system that can enable or inhibit diffusion, rather than a focus on a process by which an idea or innovation diffuses among individual members of a social system. These are factors which are under the control of marketers (or of competitors who are marketers) and which can affect individual consumers. For example, the marketer can promote the product heavily in an effort to create demand. America Online, for example, promoted heavily on television and mailed offers of free online time to encourage American consumers to use the World Wide Web. Direct mailings of software with fee online time by the marketer (America Online) no doubt caused many people to become users of the Web without any direct influence by opinion leaders.

On the other hand, the actions of another competitor are not directly under the control of any one marketer. The actions of another competitor can affect the diffusion of the marketer's product, but do not necessarily affect the diffusion of the product class. Many Web browsers were introduced and failed to diffuse after the introduction of the first graphical browser, Mosaic, but graphical browsers as a technology still diffused. The U.S. Department of Justice case against Microsoft, which wanted to bundle its Explorer browser with the Windows operating system (among other similar issues with other products and competitors), potentially blocking Netscape as a competitor, did not have a direct relationship with the diffusion of Web browsers; this case had to do with how particular *products* might have greater or lesser advantages as the *technology* diffused. Nonetheless, the argument has been raised with regard to these legal proceedings that the dominant position of Microsoft and its competitive behaviors have served to stifle innovation (and therefore diffusion) in the affected industries (cf., Wolffe and Kehoe, 1998).

TECHNOLOGICAL INFRASTRUCTURE CONSTRAINTS ON DIFFUSION

With its focus on the communication channel and on consumer adopter categories, the marketing perspective on diffusion has generally ignored issues of a technological infrastructure as an enabling factor. Consider, for example, the invention of the incandescent lamp, or "light bulb" as the sort of issue that is *not* studied by marketing researchers. Of what good is a light bulb without electricity? Popular focus has been on Thomas Edison's search for materials that could be used as a filament in the incandescent lamp, but that project was far from his only concern in developing this innovation. Realizing that his incandescent lamp had little consumer appeal without an electrical distribution system, Edison set forth to invent or design all of the equipment needed for commercial use of the Edison lamp even before a useful filament material had been found, including sockets, switches, fuse elements, wiring systems, dynamos, etc. (Jones, 1931). By considering the commercial distribution of electricity before perfecting the incandescent lamp, Edison ensured that a product of great commercial value on a mass scale would diffuse rapidly.

Consider, on the other hand, the failed diffusion of interactive television and videotex technologies of the 1970s and 80s in the U.S. These technologies bear remarkable resemblances to the features currently offered on the Web, and yet these technologies were never commercially successful. These technologies promised that consumers would be able to use a television or computer terminal to do shopping, banking, travel reservations, and such from the comforts of home. Describing a system very much like telephone- and cable-based Web connections that evolved several years later, Arlen (1988) describes how the videotex system was supposed to work: electronically stored information would be accessed by "households with office-quality PCs (probably with 256 kilobytes of memory) and 1200-baud modems" for a "monthly fee [that] approaches that of cable TV," not including a "proposed $5-per-hour 'data access fee,' to be collected by local phone companies."

So why did interactive TV and videotex not diffuse? For the same reason that expensive touring and racing cars did not cause rapid diffusion of the automobile. These technologies required that users purchase proprietary software, accounts, and connection boxes. Not everyone could afford to spend so much money at the risk that the proprietary supplier might not continue the service. Additionally, the quality and speed of information and graphics that could be delivered with a 256 KB computer and a 1200-baud modem left much to be desired – the user interface was far from natural. Only an "innovator" would want such a limited system at such an expense and risk, as would only an innovator want one of the early luxury or racing automobiles.

On the other hand, the Mosaic graphical browser became available in the U.S. at a time when PC computers had the capacity to handle the graphics and information loads. Importantly, the Internet provided a non-proprietary public roadway on which to ride this browser. Mosaic was free, and the commercial company that was founded on its ideas, Netscape, was free to educational users and offered as free on a trial basis to anyone else. A technological infrastructure existed for the Web which hadn't existed for videotex: powerful but low cost general purpose PCs that were already owned by many people, an Internet system that was non-proprietary and owned by no single entity, a browser that was essentially free, and relatively easy access to the Internet by many people.

CONCLUDING REMARKS

We have looked at four different perspectives on the diffusion of innovation which might present different perspectives on the management of diffusion from the perspective of public policy:

(1) *slow diffusion of innovation through different adopter categories* – a process whereby different segments of a social system adopt an innovation at different points in time for different reasons.
(2) *rapid diffusion through a mass market* – diffusion of an innovation to the majority of a mass market by lowering perceived risk and change in habit to all members of a social system.
(3) *diffusion in a competitive and regulated marketplace* – diffusion in which a monopolistic or a competitive situation exists, allowing greater or lesser innovation.
(4) *diffusion in an environment which is technologically enabling* – diffusion in an environment which has the technical infrastructure that is supportive of the innovation.

The traditional approach in marketing has been to view diffusion as a communication process and as a problem of appropriately targeting individual consumer segments (adopter categories). This approach is, perhaps, appropriate if indeed the different adopter segments have different needs and will adopt an innovation at different points in time. Such an approach might be appropriate to public policy makers (whether government or industry) if it is desirable that the diffusion of a product or idea is to be slow and controlled.

An alternative perspective that could be suggested by Sheth's (1981) LDC is that a majority of prospective adopters might all have the *same* reasons for initially resisting the innovation. If a common point of resistance with regard to perceived risk and change in habit can be found, then perhaps an innovation can be enhanced by launching an innovation which appeals to the majority of members of a social system rather than merely appealing to the "innovator" segment of adopters. In retrospect, this appears to have worked to enable the diffusion of the automobile. If the public policy maker wants to enhance (or inhibit) the diffusion of an innovation, then an appeal is not made through a series of steps through opinion leaders, innovators, and such, but is made to a mass market in which the majority of members share perceptions of risk and change in habit associated with adopting the innovation.

These two approaches focus on the social system composed of adopting units. A third perspective looked at the potential impact of competition and regulation within an innovative industry. In the current proceedings associated with several Microsoft products and practices in the U.S., arguments have been raised that the dominant position of the software maker could be stifling innovation of technology associated with microcomputers; Microsoft has provided arguments that the opposite is true.

Government regulation could also provide for competitive factors that are important to society even when large corporations are not involved. Consider a simple idea such as mixed crops, as when pumpkins are planted with corn. The mixing of such crops makes greater use of land and helps to insure against losses (to the individual farmer) if one crop should fail. Although such a system works well if crops are tended and harvested by hand, this system makes it difficult or impossible to tend and harvest crops with machinery. If government makes machinery available to farmers as a way to increase productivity for all of society, but government crop insurance is not available, individual farmers might still prefer to use labor intensive mix crop agricultural methods as a way to reduce personal financial risk. That is, there are competitive factors that are part of a larger social system that cannot be controlled by a single marketer.

A fourth perspective looked at the way a technological environment might enable the diffusion of a technology, creating an environment in which it is physically possible for the innovation to diffuse in a way that presents low perceptions of risk and change in habit to members of a social system. This approach considers diffusion not just in the context of a social system, but in the context of a system which includes a technological infrastructure which interacts with a social infrastructure. The incandescent lamp could not diffuse without a system for electrical distribution; the stuff of the World Wide Web could not diffuse without powerful, low priced computers and a non-proprietary Internet backbone. Had a government institution never created an Internet for public consumption, then the ideas originally launched as videotex in the 1970s might never have been able to diffuse to the masses.

We do not mean to propose that these four perspectives are the only ways to view diffusion of innovation as it relates to public policy for societal good. However, we do mean to propose that the traditional marketing approach to diffusion, with a focus on the individual as part of a social process, is, alone, not adequate in the setting of public policy. Our hope is that we can raise some initial awareness for other approaches to the study of diffusion which might help us to better understand a variety of strategies that might be used to both assist and impede the diffusion of innovation for the better good of society rather than an individual marketer.

REFERENCES

Arlen, G.: 1988, 'People still don't know just what they're missing', Channels, 7(11), p. 123.

Frambach, R. T.: 1993, 'An integrated model of organizational adoption and diffusion of innovations', European Journal of Marketing 27(5), pp. 22–41.

Gatignon, H. and T. S. Robertson: 1985, 'A prepositional inventory for new diffusion research', Journal of Consumer Research 11(March), pp. 849–867.

Jones, F. A.: 1931, The Life Story of Thomas Alva Edison (Grosset & Dunlap Publishers, New York).

Mahajan, V., E. Muller and F. M. Bass: 1990, 'New product diffusion models in marketing: a review and directions for research', Journal of Marketing 54(January), pp. 1–26.

Nick: 1998, Personal Internet conversations with a professor in Ukraine.

Owen, R.S.: 1991, 'Serendipity, diffusion, then foresight: hindsight supporting Sheth's "LDC" from the marketing of the model T and other discontinuous innovations', Marketing History: Its Many Dimensions, pp. 324–341. C. R. Taylor, S. W. Kopp, T. R. Nevitt and S. C. Hollander (eds.), Proceedings of the fifth Conference on Historical Thought in Marketing, sponsored by the Academy of Marketing Science and Michigan State University.

Pound, A.: 1940, The Turning Wheel (Doubleday, Doran, & Company, Inc., Garden City, New York).

Robertson, T. S. and H. Gatignon: 1986, 'Competitive effects on technology diffusion', Journal of Marketing 50(July), pp. 1–12.
Rogers, E. M.: 1962, Diffusion of Innovation (The Free Press, New York).
Rogers, E. M.: 1976, 'New product adoption and diffusion', Journal of Consumer Research, 2(March), pp. 290–301.
Rogers, E. M.: 1995, Diffusion of Innovations, fourth edition (The Free Press, New York).
Sheth, J. N.: 1981, 'Psychology of innovation resistance: the Less Developed Concept (LDC) in diffusion research', Research in Marketing 4, pp. 273–282.
Stevens, R. E., W. E. Warren and R. T. Martin: 1989, 'Nonadopters of automatic teller machines', Akron Business and Economic Review 20(3), p. 55.
Sward, K.: 1948, The Legend of Henry Ford (Rinehart and Company, Inc., New York).
Wolffe, R. and L. Kehoe: 1998, 'Microsoft on trial', Financial Times (London), (19 OCT 98), p. 23.

Texas A&M University – Texarkana Robert Owen
P.O. Box 5518
Texarkana, TX 75505-5518
USA
E-mail: robert.owen@tamut.edu

Texas A&M University at Texarkana Alfred Ntoko

State University of New York at Oswego Ding Zhang

State University of New York at Oswego June Dong

SECTION III

DETERMINANTS AND CORRELATES OF WELL-BEING AND QUALITY OF LIFE

DAVID M.S. KIMWELI and WILLIAM E. STILWELL

COMMUNITY SUBJECTIVE WELL-BEING, PERSONALITY TRAITS AND QUALITY OF LIFE THERAPY

ABSTRACT. In this study, factors that are instrumental in improving individuals' as well as communities' subjective well-being (SWB) and Quality of Life (QOL) such as positive and negative relationships, personality characteristics or traits as defined by family members or spouse, perceptions of the future as looking good, and psychological factors (such as congruency, thriving/resilience personality, belongingness, external and internal power and psychoallostasis), demographic variables, and religion were examined. The findings indicate that congruency with one's community values and expectations, belongingness, thriving personality, psychoallostasis and positive relationships or closeness to people in one's community, and the perception of the future both for the individual and for the community as bright, are important indicators of Quality of life and increased Subjective well-being. Additionally, family or spousal ratings of personality characteristics as desirable affected SWB only if the ratings corresponded to the individuals' rating. Path analysis indicate that the high levels of happiness experienced by people living in Individualistic-sub-collectivistic cultures such as Appalachia is strongly linked to communal homeostasis and psychoallostasis lifestyles prevalent in these communities. Implications of these findings to Quality of life therapy (QOLT) and healthy psychology at both the individual level and community level are discussed.

KEY WORDS: Appalachia, anxiety, clinical, cognitive-restructuring, community well-being, coping, counseling, cross-cultural, culture, depression, disasters, enmasse, inoculation, intervention, treatment, happiness, healthy psychology, Kentucky, mental health, optimism, other, personality traits, positive affect, power, prevention, psychiatrist, psychodynamic, psychotherapy, quality of life, relationships, religion, resilience, satisfaction, self, subjective well-being, technology, therapy, trauma, thriving

Practice of psychology, just like other dynamic fields, does not always keep pace with theory. Current theoretical developments from all branches of psychology that have utility need to be synthesized and incorporated into the practice of psychology. Specifically, clinicians, healthy psychologists, and psychiatrists need to recognize the potential contributions of quality of life, degree of

Social Indicators Research **60:** 193–225, 2002.

excellence in life (QOL) and subjective well-being, life satisfaction, and personal happiness (SWB) constructs to mental health (Frisch, 1998; see Deiner and Larsen, 1993 for definitions of SWB; Veenhoven, 1984 for definitions of QOL). Conversely, the practice of Quality of Life Therapy (QOLT) will be enhanced by assimilating to its application knowledge gained from advances in cross-cultural studies, Maslow's theory, learned optimism theory, and advances in technology. Specifically, application of these synthesized constructs to mental health service delivery to applicable target communities such as Appalachia, will not only cut down costs, but will reduce redundancy and duplication of effort.

The implications to the practice of psychology of synthesizing advances in psychology and technology can be enormous if applied appropriately to self-improvement techniques. With such synthesis it is plausible that self-improvement techniques can be applied en masse (through group therapy, community consciousness raising efforts, through the use of satellites, Internet, etc) rather than the one on one individual therapy.

Specifically, the enmasse application of psychotherapy, treatment and interventions is vital, cuts costs, and fits the exigency of needed interventions for natural disasters and for the effects of war and terrorists acts. The perpetual focus on mental disorders from the ill-being model rather than well-being model has continued to hinder psychotherapy by limiting therapy to individuals and amelioration of negative factors. The failure of psychotherapy to focus on prevention has proven costly in terms of diminished well-being, poor health living and deterioration of communities' quality of life. Research in optimism (Seligman, 1991) indicates that individuals can be inoculated against helplessness by teaching them learned optimism. By using appropriate technology, by focusing on well-being and learned optimism, communities can be inoculated en masse against pathology. In spite of these advances and possible utilization of technology for outreach, practice of psychology has not only continued to focus on individuals rather than communities, but also on psychopathology from the ill-being model. As psychologists, we have done little to promote community action groups, mental health inoculation consciousness and the promotion of quality of life of people or groups of people that are at risk of deteriorating psychological well-being despite the accumulation of psychological treatment interventions, breakthroughs in technology and the advancement of service delivery methods of the 21st century.

As a result of this lack of synthesized and appropriate application of modern research, measures of non-pathological conditions have been missing in mental health practice, despite research calling for use of such measures to augment measures of ill-being (see Strupp, 1996). Such measures are needed because positive affect (well-being) and negative affect (ill-being) are independent emotions, and causes of well-being are not regained by treating ill-being. For example, by treating a patient's helplessness concomitant with depression does not automatically unleash the client's fountains of optimism! Specifically, lost psychological health is not retrieved by amelioration of symptomatology. Indeed, emotions responsible for psychological wellness (positive) and the emotions responsible for ill-being (negative) activate different parts of the brain (George et al., 1995).

Consequently, the goal of therapy should not be only to reduce negative symptoms, but should be also to increase quality of life and subjective well-being of clients, and more importantly, to prevent the inception of mental and psychological illnesses. In quality of life theory, subjective well-being, satisfaction with life, and quality of life are equated and defined as "a person's subjective evaluation of the degree to which his or her most important needs, goals, and wishes have been fulfilled" (Frisch, 1998: p. 24).

In order to effect efficacious service delivery to clients, clinicians and psychologists will need to measure clients' daily life functions, interactions with other community members, coping mechanisms, resilience-thriving-educing factors and psychogenesis of well-being and mental health. Indeed, these stated areas and aspirations constitute a determination of a part of the individual's satisfaction or dissatisfaction with life; their assessment of past failures and enjoyment of life; anticipation of future impediments; pursuit of psychological health goals; and reorientation of life pursuits towards optimized psychological health state. Such an assessment is necessary because clients do not live in isolation, nor do they live in states devoid of past, present or future Psychodynamic forces and

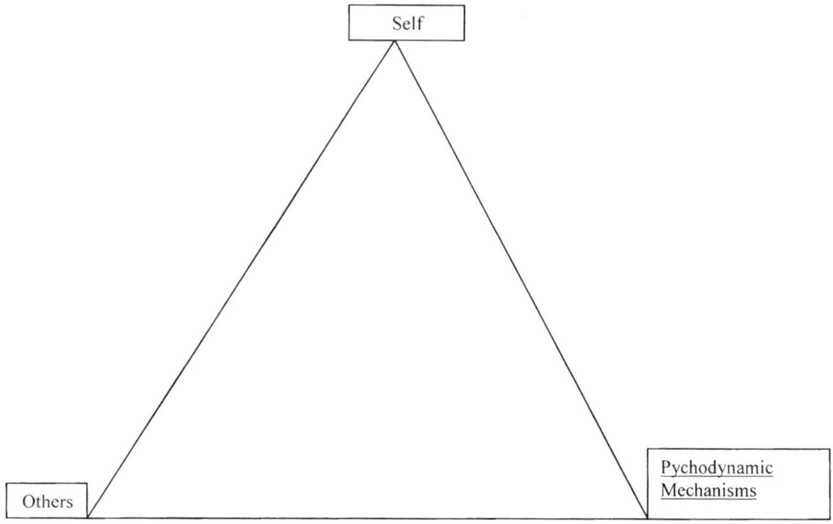

Figure 1. Quality of life assessment model. The self-other-pschodynamic-congruent index. *Note.* To capture the scope of clients' problems, we need to assess not only the effects of self, but the effects of others as well as the dynamic environmental and situational effects that continuously affect clients' QOL.

underpinnings, but in fact, clients are just as subject to bifurcations that produce sudden changes in behavior as other dynamic systems (see Glass and Mackey, 1988). Clients' feelings and daily activities are affected by not only the evaluation of their own lives, but by the evaluation of other people who live in the same community and by other unanticipated factors that if anticipated could contingently be handled differently to ensure a positive outcome. Such evaluations are driven in part by personality characteristics and by their acceptance as norms within a given community. Consequently, the "individual-self" is influenced positively or negatively by the "community-self," by "other-selves" and by external dynamic forces (see model displayed as Figure 1). Indeed, Seligman (1991) states that "the waxing of the self in our time coincides with a diminished sense of community and a loss of higher purpose; these together proved rich soil for depression to grow in" (p. 284).

Clients' interactions with their relatives, neighbors, friends, and external psychodynamic forces form an intertwined web of dependence that serves not only as a coping system through social comparison mechanisms, but also as a psychological breakdown mechanism. The "individual-relative-neighbors-psychological forces-intertwined web of dependence" determines how clients view their personality characteristics or traits, their current and future life {note that personality as is used here includes personality levels 1 and level 2 as formulated by McAdams (1994)}.

Meanings of personality characteristics/traits evolve through socialization processes whereas the impacts of external psychodynamic forces shape behaviors, perceptions, aspirations, experiences, and goals through exposure and encounters. Once meanings of personality characteristics have been negotiated, these personality traits in turn gird interrelationships.

Over an extended period of time, some personality traits/characteristics such as "adaptability," "dominant," "aggressive," "willingness to take risks" and "independent" take positive connotations whereas traits/characteristics such as "moody," "jealous," "tender," "compassionate," "sensitive to needs of others" and "conventional" take negative connotations (see Bem, 1975).

Although this dichotomy of negative/positive understanding of the preceding traits/characteristics is not universally accepted, a community's definition and the individual's definition, depending on if they are in harmony or not, may affect SWB. Diener et al. (1999) identify one's family, one's group, and significant others' views of one's life, as components of subjective well-being. It is therefore important, on the one hand, when assessing individual's SWB to obtain from family members ratings not only of their perception of the individual's well-being, but also of how the family members perceive the individual's personality traits. These perceptions determine the quality of interrelationships in one's group because one's group is not entirely separated from one's culture or community. On the other hand, psychodynamic forces can not be overlooked in spite of how they are viewed. The impacts resulting from encounters with psychodynamic systems may be viewed as sources of stress, or as anchors of a thriving personality or may even be viewed as neutral. For instance, the effects of abuse on a child may cement the determination to be a loving and caring parent, or may cause the victim to perpetuate the cycle of abuse – victim-victimizer-victim phenomena or cause the individual to live a traumatized lifestyle. Therefore the forgoing argument underscores the need for a holistic approach to Quality of Life (QOL) therapy both in terms of assessment and treatment.

To our knowledge, studies in SWB that examine family ratings of individuals' SWB, personality traits, communality factors as well as tertiary psychodynamic factors have not been conducted. Consequently, this study aims to fill this gap by examining the effects of family/relative views on respondent's SWB, personality characteristics and how these ratings affect the respondent's views on their own SWB. Additionally, we seek to untangle psychodynamic predictors of the three measures postulated by Kimweli (2002) to constitute SWB, i.e., Satisfaction with Life Scale (SWLS), Health Opinion Survey (HOS) and the Affect Balance. The uniqueness of this study is underscored by the fact that respondents are drawn from a culture that values kinship norms. Cultures that value community or in group norms are termed collectivistic. Interrelationships are particularly vital in these collectivistic cultures. Western cultures however, are considered individualistic and the role of self is deemed paramount whereas the role of others and that one of psychodynamic systems tends to be ignored especially in therapy.

In the following section, literature that ties the concepts and constructs stated in the preceding paragraph will be reviewed vis a vis the failure to approach QOLT holistically. First, cultural dichotomy will be addressed, followed by a discussion of individualistic-sub-collectivistic cultures as well as a discussion on individualized valued areas of life and finally, a review of individualistic-sub-collectivistic and individualized coping skills will be offered.

CULTURAL DICHOTOMY

Cross-cultural research has identified two dichotomous cultures, the individualistic and the collectivistic cultures corresponding to western cultures and non-western developing societies (Triandis, 1985, 1988, 1994, 1995). These cultures result in distinct "selves" that have different corresponding needs. For example, individualistic selves have interpersonal needs that are self-centered and focus on self-identity, independence and self-sufficiency (see Markus and Kitayama, 1994). On the other hand, collectivistic "selves" have

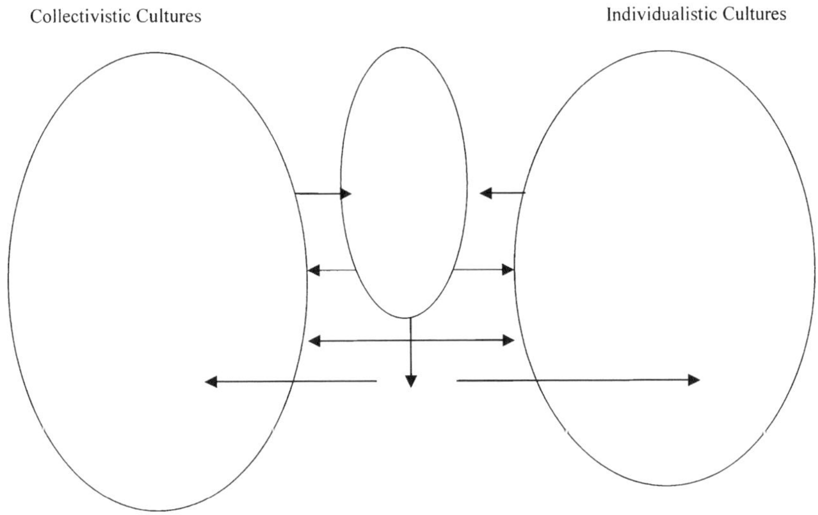

Figure 2. A model of psychological transformation to individualistic-sub-collectivistic cultures. *Note.* Continuous exchange of values, ideas, experiences occur thus the dichotomy cannot be static.

needs that are centered on respect from others; status, acceptance and success come from both possession of socially accepted attributes and socially ascribed goals (Katayama et al., 1997). Not surprising, the practice of psychotherapy has tended to pursue goals that elevate self in the expense of "others."

Some researchers are beginning to argue for the possibility of interchangeability of cultural selves due to the psychological transformation from collectivistic orientations to individualistic tendencies as developing cultures espouse westernization (see Yang, 1998 for a review). This psychological transformation is assumed to be unidirectional. However, we present a new view of this transformation (refer to Figure 2).

According to this Kimweli/Stilwell new proposed model, psychological transformation is viewed as occurring constantly in both directions, thus it is bi-directional. Technology and movement back and forth between and among cultures, make this model tenable. This "both direction transformation" results into "individualistic sub-collective cultures and collective sub-individualistic cultures" (we adapt the former name as the appropriate one and hence applicable to both types). In other words, none of the cultures is static and isolated from the dynamic influence of the other.

Consequently, collectivistic cultures are constantly getting a dose of individualism whereas individualistic cultures are assimilating some collectivistic aspects at the same time – this is true both at the community and individual level. Thus, cultures are becoming more homogenous in a sense; that is, we are getting closer and closer to the "global village" phenomena. As values that are amendable to some of the cultures in the extreme poles of the individualistic verses collectivistic dichotomy are assimilated, an "in between group" is formed which continues to grow and further influences the surrounding cultures resulting in the expansion of the "in-between group" – comprising of individuals that value not only the self but "others." It is the "in-between group" that we refer to as individualistic-sub-collectivistic culture.

Individualistic-Sub-Collectivistic Cultures

Definition and examples. Individualistic sub-collectivistic cultures are not fully collective but espouse collective ideals within an individualistic worldview. The kinship relations that bind people together especially in rural areas make the up-holding of collectivistic ideals possible. People in these rural communities refer to themselves as "family."

Usually in these rural communities, beliefs (especially religious beliefs) and communal values are held commonly while individual members pursue individual goals. A working definition of an individualistic-sub-collectivistic culture is "a culture that is thriving in a capitalistic-individualistic society, and at the same time espousing commonly held norms, values and beliefs strongly enough to collectively define its identity." Examples of such cultures in the United States include the Appalachian culture, Mormonism, ethnic cultures such as recent American Hispanic immigrants, recent Asian immigrants, some Native American tribes, concentrated Jewish communities and to a lesser degree, "American far right conservatism" in specific concentrated areas of the country, especially the South. Only Appalachian culture will be addressed in detail in this paper.

Appalachian culture/community. Although Appalachian culture is western by all means, its core values are different from those of the rest of the United States. Appalachian culture values (to a very high degree) kinship relations, dependency, trust and closeness to people and adherence to norms valued by their community (Browner and Leslie, 1996). These "Appalachian norms and values" comprising "Appalachianism" are characteristic of social and relational needs that are important for the cohesion of their society/culture. Consequently, Appalachians' well-being stems from the fulfillment of interpersonal and belongingness needs. In other words, Appalachians define themselves in terms of what Triandis (1994) calls "in-group/family membership." In this respect, belongingness serves as self-definition. Additionally, community norms become individual norms, in-group aspirations become self aspirations, community well-being begins to constitute individual well-being and individual ill-being with time begins to formulate the construction of communally defined psychopathology (see Kimweli, 2002).

According to Kitayama et al. (1997) belongingness needs are adaptive and important for psychological well-being. In this respect, we post that Appalachia is an individualistic – sub-collective culture. Subsequently, in order to improve individualistic – sub-collectivistic cultures' (such as Appalachia's) Quality of Life (quality of life as defined by the community norms and values), through quality of life therapy, personal happiness, satisfaction, affect and adjustment to the collectively held standards must be addressed as models of treatment (cf. Ogles, Lambert and Masters, 1996; Strupp, 1996). The preceding components of quality of life both for the individual and for the community members as a whole need to be addressed. Additionally, relationships, day to day interactions, external influences and accepted personality traits must be addressed.

Conversely, at an individual level, when endeavoring to improve quality of life of members of an individualistic-sub-collective culture, ignoring the clients' feelings of contentment or lack thereof, belongingness, emotions and experiences (that make people's life worth while and enjoyable as well as make them attractive to friends and potential mates who in turn offer them social support within their culture), minimizes the expansiveness of the client's presenting problem. Rarely are presenting problems limited to the clients' understanding or perceptions. More often the clients' larger world and larger worldview also bears on their problems. This larger view needs to be assessed and addressed in therapy.

Additionally, measures of QOL and SWB are predictors of not only subsequent illnesses or disorders but also of treatment costs (Baruffol et al., 1995; Moreland et al., 1994). Measures of QOL and SWB are predictors of those who might be at risk for psychological disturbance (Frisch, 1998). Knowing factors that predispose individuals and by extension their communities to low quality of life is important. Such knowledge provides insight on how to execute treatment outcomes. Factors that affect SWB are usually in areas that are most valued by the individual within community norms or culturally prescribed ideals – since self is an extension of the cultural-self and culture is an extension of the self – the self-other-dimension.

Individualized Valued Areas of Life

Individuals differ in domains of value in their lives. Some individualized valued areas of life include security, affection, happiness, pride, religious activities, love, family life, health (see Frisch, 1998). Other domains that have not been examined include the following: friendships, communality, community aspirations, influence over people as well as influence by other people, being trusted and loved by friends, acceptance or stigmatization of behaviors resulting from secondary gains due to a particular worldview, staticity or fluidity of attitudes and values, and the degree of acceptance as well as permeation of emerging selves and trends.

Satisfaction in a valued life area results in high SWB for the individual as well as for the community. Dissatisfaction on a domain area may result, for example, in *dissatisfaction-rejection-depression* caused by constant negative self-evaluation, hopelessness, and community deevaluation. Negative self-evaluation, may be precipitated by non-acceptance or criticism by one's group members. Low levels of QOL may result in sub-clinical levels of anxiety and low positive affect or high unpleasant affect as well as generalized unhappiness. Diener et al. (1999), list guilt and shame, anger, stress and envy, among others, as comprising unpleasant affect. Consequently, these individualized valued domains may be affected by the disharmony resulting from different perceptions or interpretations of personality characteristics by both the individual and his/her community.

Individualistic-Sub-Collectivistic Culture and Individualized Coping Skills

The collective values of individualistic-sub-collective cultures provide adaptively defined psychological well-being for that particular community. For the individual members, on the other hand, adaptability or coping mechanisms depend on constructed comparisons. The manner, in which an individual compares him/herself with others in that community and fits in, affects their SWB and also provides a way to deal with the resulting QOL. For example, reduction of stress or anxiety.

The comparison standard may be based on an individual's feelings of deservingness, expectations or ideals from the community (Sirgy et al., 1995), ability to adhere to culturally prescribed norms or ideals, goals, affective reactions, alternative world views or imaginary standards (see Miller and Prentice, 1997). Indeed, individuals with low SWB tend to make unfavorable comparisons with other people in their lives.

Furthermore, an individual's perception of health, rather than objective health, due to a downward comparison, influences SWB. The influence of other people to an individual's Quality of life could be unconscious (Diener and Fujita, 1997). This unconscious response to other people's influence may break down cognitive, affective, or behavioral coping mechanisms as well as the ability to adapt to psychologically health behaviors. Thus, adherence to cultural norms or ideals could as well be adaptive or malfunctional.

The purpose of this study therefore is three fold. The first purpose is to partial out valued domains and aspects of cultural ideals or community norms that are essential to an individuals' subjective well-being or overall QOL. Knowledge of these culturally or communally defined valued domains that are predictors of improved QOL and SWB for individualistic-sub-collectivistic cultures will provide mental health professionals with strategies that are essential for service delivery of QOLT. This investigation is guided in part by the work of Frisch (1998) on (QOLT) as well as hypotheses that we have formulated under the auspices of current advances in SWB, QOL studies and the models developed by Kimweli (2002) to guide future studies in SWB.

Frisch (1994) identified 16 specific domains that constitute people's overall QOL. Although Frisch's 16 domains include community, his work did not untangle communality factors that might contribute to QOL. In this research, we hypothesize, that, interpersonal relationships, be they negative or positive, a sense of beloingingness, a sense of the future for the community as being favorable or bright, and the ability to adhere to and the desire and willingness to live by the values of the community (a condition we refer to as communalhomeostasis), constitute the "community aspect" of quality of life. Additionally, other individual psychological characteristics such as present and future perceived psychological health condition, religiosity (individuals and families') are used in this research as predicators of subjective well-being (see also Kimweli and Stilwell, 1997).

The second purpose of this study is to obtain family (spouse, parent or relatives such as siblings or grant parents) ratings of the individuals' SWB and personality characteristics. These ratings will help in determining whether an individual's assessment of his/her personality traits and levels of SWB, correspond to others' ratings as well as help determine personality pathways that influence SWB (see Figures 3 and 4).

This part of the study is guarded by the hypothesis that, individual's favorable rating of a personality trait/characteristic corresponds to the individual's high levels of positive affect and subsequent high levels of SWB. The individual's positive rating may or may not be influenced by others' ratings. Formulation of this hypothesis is guided by the fact that one's happiness is noticeable to people with whom one associates and the hypothesized role of communalhomeostasis.

The third purpose of this study is to determine possible linkages between measures of SWB/QOL and psychological variables derived from the model displayed in Figure 1 as formulated in the literature review section – the self-other-psychodynamic congruent index. Specifically, the linkage of SWB/QOL and the congruency with community values and norms, ability to thrive in the midst of

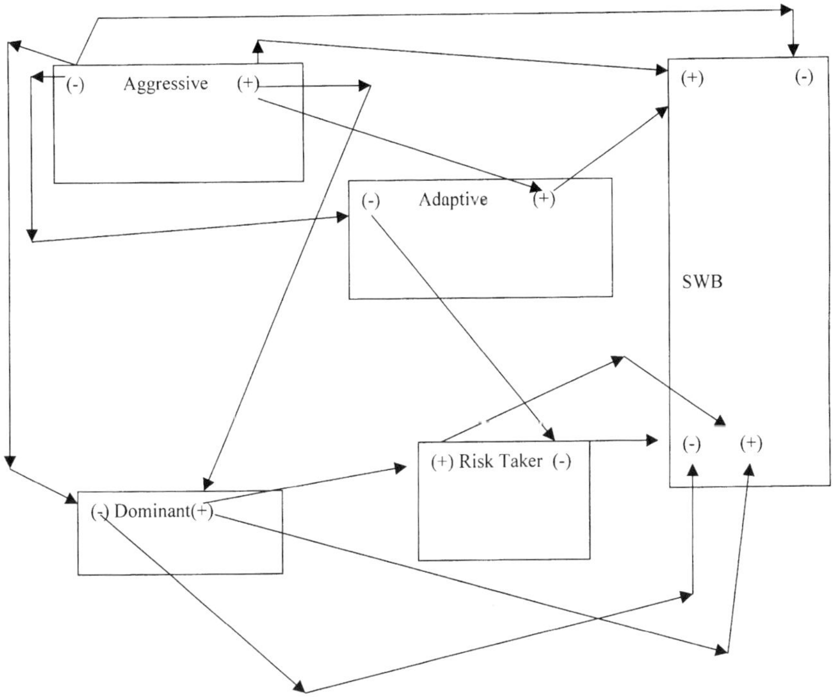

Figure 3. A model depicting the agreement of an individual's and community's assessment of traits considered positive and the hypothesized relationship to SWB.

adversity and future unpredictable events such as death in the family, lose of employment and possible natural disasters will be examined.

METHODS

Sample

The data for this study was obtained from Appalachian communities. The participants were drawn from regions officially designated as comprising the Appalachian region in parts of Eastern Kentucky, Tennessee and Western Virginia. For the first analysis, the sample included 470 Caucasian community members (150 males and 320 females) with a mean age of 25 years of age. A demographic questionnaire with several psychological health indices developed by the authors in addition to measures of subjective well-being i.e. the Satisfaction with Life Scale (SWLS), the Health Opinion Survey

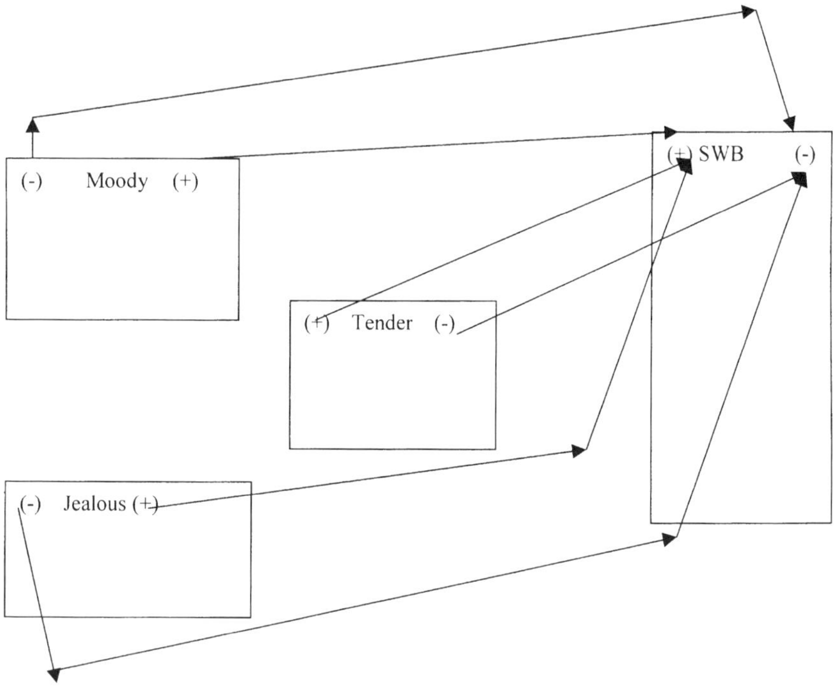

Figure 4. A model depicting the agreement of an individual's and community's assessment of traits considered negative and the hypothesized relationship to SWB.

(HOS), the Affectometer 2 (Positive and Negative Affect Scale) and personality/traits questionnaire with items adapted from Bem were administered.

Dependent Measures

The use of dependent measures was guided by advances in subjective well-being and Quality of life research (Frisch, 1998). Subjective well-being has three hallmarks: a cognitive, the positive/negative affect and mood aspects (Diener, 1994). Each of the three aspects was measured separately following a model developed by Kimweli (2002). The cognitive component was measured by the Satisfaction with Life Scale (Diener et al., 1985), the positive/negative affect component by the Affectometer 2 (Kammann and Flett, 1983) and the mood aspect by the Health Opinion Survey (Murphy, 1986).

Satisfaction with life scale. The SWLS was developed to measure the hallmark of subjective well-being referred to as satisfaction with life, which is judged to be important by the respondent (Diener et al., 1985). The SWLS is a five-item-Likert questionnaire with a scale ranging from *1-strongly disagrees to 7-strongly agree.* According to the authors, the scale has high temporal stability, high item correlations (0.81, 0.63, 61, 75 and 0.66), and a high coefficient alpha of 0.87. The summation of the respondents' endorsement of the items of this scale constitutes the satisfaction with life dependent variable.

Affectometer 2. The Affectometer 2 measures positive and negative feelings in recent experience. The Affectometer 2 measures frequency of affect (Diener, 1994). Additionally, the Affectometer 2 assesses well-being as conceptualized by an individual's feelings (Chamberlain and Zika, 1990). The Affectometer 2 has an alpha of 0.72 and correlates highly with several other measures of subjective well-being (Kammann and Flett, 1983). The Affectometer 2 is a 40 item, *5 point-Likert scale, 1 not at all to 5 all the time.* The summation of the respondents' endorsement of the items of the Affectometer 2 constitutes the positive/negative dependent variable and the difference constitutes an Affect Balance Scale.

The health opinion survey. This scale is a 20 item survey that is usually used to compare groups (particularly rural groups) on anxiety and depression symptoms (see Abbott and Klein, 1979; Mitchell and Abbott, 1987; Murphy, 1986). The Health Opinion Survey items are constructed in non-technical/clinical terms and thus it is easy for respondents to understand. The HOS categories are the same as Beck's Depression Inventory. The HOS is *Likert scale, 1 for never, 2 for sometimes, 3 for often.* The summation of the respondents' endorsement to the items of the HOS constitutes the anxiety dependent variable.

Independent Measures

Independent measures comprised of sex, family income, and religiosity of both the respondent and their families (a Yes/No response). In addition, the following psychological indices were developed using Oblique factor rotations. The resulting scales used in the study had high internal consistency with Cronbach alpha coefficients that ranged from 0.92 to 0.98.

Congruency with community values. This scale was constructed from items *anchored 1 for not at all to 5 for all the time*. The following are examples of the items that were used to construct this scale: (a) I believe and do things as expected by my community; (b) I feel like my behaviors are accepted by my friends, relatives and community members; (c) My life style is in conformity with the values, aspirations and expectations of my family and community. The alpha for this scale was 0.92.

Thriving index. The items for this scale were anchored *1 for not at all to 5 for all the time*. Example items include: (a) I can handle adversity; (b) I have dealt satisfactory with hardships in the past; (c) I am strong enough to continue with my life no matter what happens to me; (d) I can be strong even if I had a death in the family; (e) I can go on with my life even if I were to loose my job. The Cronbach's alpha for this scale was 0.96.

Belongingness index. The items for this scale were anchored *1 for not at all to 5 for all the time*. Example items include: (a) My community accepts me; (b) I feel like I belong to my community; (c) I am just as happy as other members of my family, community and church; (d) I feel like my community values me and the things I do. The Cronbach's alpha for this scale was 0.94.

Power and control over unpredictable life events. The alpha for this scale was 0.98. Example items include: (a) No matter what curve ball life may through at me, I will go on with my life; (b) I do not let accidents in life and mistakes that I do deter me; (c) Bad things do happen but what I do about them is the most important thing. The items for this scale were anchored *1 for not at all to 5 for all the time*.

Power and control over internal process. The alpha for this scale was 0.96. This scale constituted items that deal with the inner self and the ability to utilize inner resources. Example items include: (a) I can get motivated when I want to (b) I can change negative thoughts to positive ones; (c) I have strong faith; (d) I look foreword to changing situations and circumstances around me. The items for this scale were anchored *1 for not at all to 5 for all the time.*

Other people's influence. This scale which displayed good internal consistency (alpha = 0.96) consisted of items that were indicative of willingness to defer to others. Example items include: (a) I do let people's opinion affect my life and the way I do things; (b) I care of what other people think of me; (c) It is very important that I get a long with other people. *The items for this scale were anchored 1 for not at all to 5 for all the time.*

Bright future for individual and for the community. The items for this scale tapped the future outlook the respondent had for him/herself as well as for the community. Items included: (a) My future looks good; (b) My community's future looks good; (c) My life's future looks good; (d) I do not see a reason to expect problems in the future; (e) I am optimistic of my future. The Cronbach's alpha for this scale was 0.98. The items for this scale were anchored *1 for not at all to 5 for all the time.*

Subjective psychological health. This scale (alpha of 0.94) measured the respondent's subjective evaluations of their psychological and over all health condition. Example items include: (a) I am healthy enough to do things; (b) I am psychologically health; (c) I do not have a mental health problem; (d) I do not consider my self to be all that stressed; (e) I consider myself a happy and outgoing person; (f) I could be happier. *The items for this scale were anchored 1 for not at all to 5 for all the time.*

Positive relationships. The alpha for this scale was 0.96. Example items are: (a) I feel loved by my family and friends; (b) I feel trusted by my family and friends; (c) I have people that can help me if I were in trouble; (d) I feel close to people around me; (e) I have not lost any friendships recently. The items for this scale were anchored *1 for not at all to 5 for all the time.*

Negative relationships. The items for this scale were anchored *1 for not at all to 5 for 1ll the time*. Example items for this scale include: (a) I seem to be left a lone when I don't want to be; (b) I have no interest in people; (c) I do not care about people any more; (d) I have recently lost friends that I cared for. The Cronbach's alpha for this scale was 0.93.

Psychoallostasis. Items that were used to construct this scale measured respondents' ability to adapt and behave in a healthy conscious way despite the possibility of health crises or risks and the willingness to live a lifestyle that promotes a health living. Some of the items used in the construction of the scale are: (a) I exercise to reduce my weight, blood pressure and cholesterol; (b) I find ways to reduce stress in my life; (c) I fear that my health may be getting worse; (d) No matter what the doctor may tell me, I am positive I can make my health better; (e) I try to prepare and deal effectively with situations that may stress me, and increase my blood pressure; (f) I carefully select and watch what I eat; (g) I expect to live a long and a health life; (h) I enjoy (or plan to enjoy) sex with my partner in a marriage relationship; (i) I regularly go for medical checkups; (j) I consider use of drug and alcohol to be a bad lifestyle. The items for this scale were anchored *1 for not at all to 5 for all the time*. The Cronbach's alpha for this scale was 0.96.

Personality questionnaire. A personality questionnaire adapted from Bem (1984) listing positively considered personality characteristics (adaptability, dominant among others) and negatively considered personality characteristics such as moody, compassionate etc. was administered. The principal respondent was to indicate whether he/she considered the trait negative or positive and then indicate the extend the characteristic was applicable to them. Respondents' family members or relatives (such as spouse, siblings, grant parents or uncles etc.) were required to rate whether they considered the trait negative or positive and to what degree they considered the trait to apply to the principal respondent (to what degree the principal respondent exhibits it). Items are anchored 1 *for never or almost never true to 7 for always or almost always true*.

TABLE I

Descriptive statistics

Variable	N	Mean	STD
Anxiety	470	28.69	5.89
SWL	470	26.65	6.99
Affect Balance	470	2.65	0.99

Note. Appalachian sample studied here has significantly higher satisfaction with life and Affect Balance than any group studied so far using these instruments.

RESULTS

Analysis 1

Relations between variables

Descriptions statistics are presented in Table I and bivariate correlations are presented in Table II.

The correlations indicate that there is a higher correlation between SWB and congruency with one's community ($r = 0.39$, $p < 0.01$), with ability to thrive in face of adversity ($r = 0.20$, $p < 0.01$), belongingness ($r = 0.25$, $p < 0.01$), with power over external events ($r = 0.41$, $p < 0.01$), with power over internal thoughts ($r = 0.49$, $p < 0.01$). Subjective well-being (SWB) is negatively related with other people's influences over one's life ($r = -0.35$, $p < 0.01$), is positively related to a bright future for the individual and the community ($r = 0.39$, $p < 0.01$), is positively related to subjective psychological health ($r = 0.22$, $p < 0.01$), and positively related to positive relationships ($r = 0.36$, $p < 0.01$) whereas it is negatively related to negative relationships ($r = -0.20$, $p < 0.01$).

Multiple Regression

To investigate which variables are predictors of SWB (Satisfaction with life, anxiety/depression and positive affect), multiple regressions were run. The results are displayed in Table III.

The results indicate that males are less likely to experience anxiety/depression ($\beta = -0.13$, $p < 0.05$). People who perceive their future and their communities' as looking good are more satisfied

TABLE II

Bivariate correlations between variables

Variables	1	2	3	4	5	6	7	8	9	10	11	12	13	14	15	16	17	18
Sex																		
Income	0.02	–																
HOS	−0.13	−0.9																
SWLS	0.08	0.05	−0.63*	–														
Affect Balance	0.11	0.04	−0.56*	0.68**	–													
Congruency	−0.05	−0.1	−0.39**	0.49**	0.43*	–												
Thriving	0.08	−0.01	0.09	0.2**	0.18**	0.34*	–											
Belongingness	0.20	0.18	0.21	0.25**	0.26**	0.38**	0.41*	–										
Power external	0.09	0.24*	−0.39*	0.41*	0.38*	0.24*	0.1*	0.32*	–									
Power internal	0.19	0.13	−0.41*	0.49*	0.32*	−0.35*	0.48*	0.41*	−0.8*	–								
Other's influence	0.03	−0.29*	−0.36*	−0.35**	−0.37*	0.21	0.19	0.31*	−0.32*	−0.32*	–							
Bright future	0.02	0.3	−0.19**	0.39**	0.47**	0.58*	0.47**	0.42*	0.36*	0.36*	0.43*	0.19	–					
Psychological health	0.07	−0.29*	−0.40**	0.22**	0.24**	0.49*	0.46**	0.36*	0.21	0.46**	−0.39*	0.37*	0.38*	–				
Positive relationships	0.04	0.10	0.13	0.36**	0.40**	0.32*	0.36*	0.41*	0.32*	0.39**	0.41*	0.35*	0.28*	0.38*	–			
Negative relationships	0.3*	−0.2	−0.9	−0.20**	−0.18**	−0.29*	−0.21*	−0.30*	−0.32*	−0.32*	−0.36*	−0.28*	−0.32*	−0.21*	0.02	–		
Psychoallostasis	0.5	0.09	−0.45*	0.56*	0.49*	0.39*	0.69*	0.35*	0.34*	0.73*	0.19	0.89*	0.81*	0.29*	0.35*	−19	–	
Respondent's religion	0.12	0.19	−0.21*	0.31*	0.35*	0.40*	0.38*	0.41*	0.37*	0.37*	0.43*	0.32*	0.30*	0.27*	−0.35*	0.38*	0.41*	–
Family's religion	0.02	0.03	−0.9*	0.25*	0.14*	0.21*	0.22*	0.38*	0.33*	0.02	0.03	0.09	0.25*	0.14*	0.21*	0.22*	0.38*	0.33*

Note. Sex is coded 0 = *female*, 1 = *male*, income is combined family income mean income is 30,000.000. Respondents' and family's religiosity are dummy variables 1 = *Yes*, 0 = *No*.

*$p < 0.05$, **$p < 0.01$

TABLE III

Multiple regression for subjective well-being

Predictor variable	Satisfaction	Anxiety/ depression	Affect balance
Demographics			
Sex	−0.9	−0.13*	0.8
Income (Family)	0.05	−0.10	0.1
Religiosity			
Family's	0.17*	−0.12*	0.16*
Respondent's	0.15*	−0.19*	0.20*
Subjective psychological health	0.15*	−0.35***	0.13*
Communalhomeostasis			
Congruency	0.37***	−0.28***	0.39***
Belongingness (collectivity*)	0.23***	−0.20**	0.21***
Bright future	0.35**	−0.24**	0.38**
Other people's influence	−0.21***	0.25***	−0.36***
Relationships			
Positive relationships with other people	0.24*	−0.17*	0.19*
Negative relationships	−0.21*	0.18*	−0.06
Psychodynamic factors			
External power	0.27*	−0.23*	0.25**
Internal power	0.26**	−0.21**	0.21**
Psychoallostasis	0.37**	−0.32**	0.35**
R square	0.57**	0.53*	−0.51***
F-value	0.33	0.32	0.34
	27.6***	19.9***	18.8***

Note. Unlike Moslow's (1987) concept of belongingness and love needs, Alderfer (1969, 1972) makes a distinction between relatedness needs (relation with another person) and belongingness needs (relation with a group (collectivity). In this paper, belongingness is used in the context of collectivity.
Sex is coded 0 = *female*, 1 = *male*.
$^{*}p < 0.05$, $^{**}p < 0.01$, $^{***}p < 0.001$.

with life ($\beta = 0.35$, $p < 0.001$) and are more likely to experience positive affect ($\beta = 0.3$, $p < 0.001$), but less likely to experience anxiety/depression ($\beta = -0.24$, $p < 0.01$). Having subjective psychological healthy condition reduces satisfaction with life ($\beta = -0.15$, $p < 0.05$), and reduces anxiety ($\beta = -0.35$, $p < 0.001$).

Indeed, communalhomeostasis factors were all strong predictors of SWB. Specifically, congruency was the highest predictor of Satisfaction with Life ($\beta = 0.37$, $p < 0.001$), Affect Balance ($\beta = 0.39$, $p < 0.001$), and a strong predictor of reduced anxiety ($\beta = -0.28$, $p < 0.001$).

Similarly, the psychodynamic factors were strong predictors of SWB with psychoallostasis showing the strongest predictive effect, ($\beta = 0.37$, $p < 0.001$) for Satisfaction with Life, ($\beta = -0.32$, $p < 0.001$) for anxiety/depression, and ($\beta = 0.35$, $p < 0.001$) for Affect Balance.

In summary, as displayed in Table III, all the variables were strong predictors of SWB with the exception of family income. Even the families' religion (as well as the individuals) was a strong predictor of SWB and reduced levels of anxiety/depression ($\beta = -0.12$, $p < 0.05$).

Analysis 2

Sample

The sample for the second analysis was reduced when pairs of either a parent, a relative or a spouse to the principal respondent were extracted (N = 235, with 71 males, 164 females). The combination of mother/sister or mother daughter or daughter/grandmother had 83 participants.

PATH ANALYSES

Hypotheses and procedures. Path analyses were used to examine the relationships among personality characteristics and subjective well-being. The conceptual models in Figures 2 and 3 propose that positive ratings of either positive or negatively considered traits increases SWB, whereas negative ratings of either positive or negative traits lowers SWB; but the effects of other people's ratings on SWB are not known. None the less, we predicted that others' ratings will only have effect on the principal respondent's SWB only if the ratings affect the principal respondent's self-ratings. LISTREL 8 (Joreskog and Sorbom, 1993) was used for data analysis.

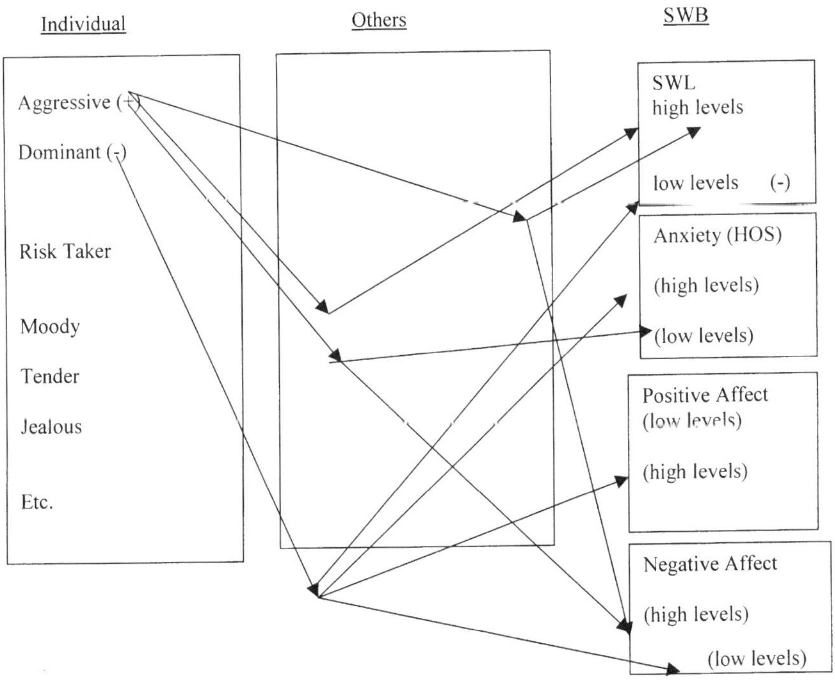

Figure 5. A model depicting the results of the path analysis. *Note*. The results displayed in this model confirm that an agreement on a trait as being positive resulted in high levels of SWL and Affect Balance while an agreement of the trait as being negative resulted in the converse. All the coefficients are higher than 0.35 and are significant at the 0.01 level.

Results of Analysis 2. Figure 5 shows the path diagrams and directions of the effects.

The Normal Fit Index (NFI) was 0.95 and Bentler's Comparative Fit Index (CFI) was 0.99. In both indices, values greater than 0.90 are indicative of overall fit of the data to the model.

The results of the model-testing procedures confirmed the hypothesis represented in Figures 2 and 3 with all the total effects falling between 0.35 to 0.41 at the 0.01 significance level. Thus, for individuals who consider any of the traits as negative, their SWB was correspondingly low, whereas for those who considered any of the traits as positive, their SWB was correspondingly high. Specifically, as one's positive ratings increased even in negatively perceived individual characteristics, the ratings corresponded to higher level of satisfaction with life (SWL), positive affect, lower levels of negative affect, but did not affect anxiety levels.

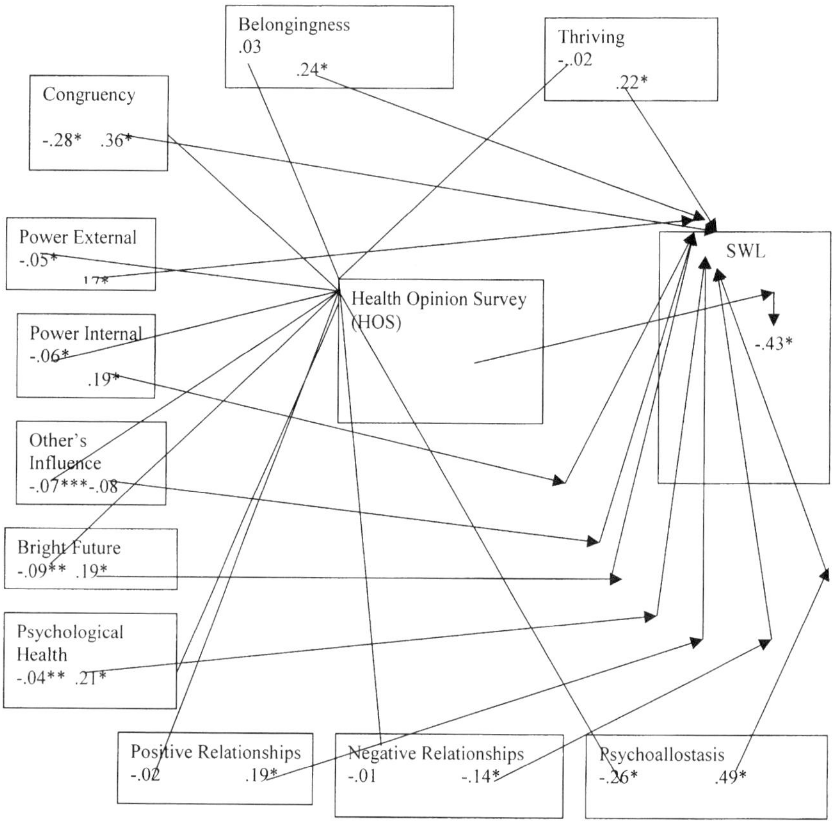

Figure 6. A path model of predictors of Health Opinion Survey (HOS) and Satisfaction with Life (SWB). *Note.* $^{*}p < 0.05$, $^{**}p < 0.01$, $^{***}p < 0.001$.

Higher negative ratings corresponded to lower SWL and positive affect, but higher levels of anxiety. Additionally, other's negative ratings corresponded to increased negative affect, anxiety and lower positive affect but not SWL. Conversely, the results indicate, that, if a negative individual trait or characteristic is viewed by his/her relatives as a positive characteristic, the individual's and the families' assessment of their SWB will be positive (high SWB) as displayed in Figure 5.

Analysis 3. Several other path analyses were conducted in order to determine probable linkages among the predictor and dependent variables. Results are displayed in Figures 6, 7 and 8.

Examination of these path models reveals the dynamics of how subjective well-being is experienced. Since the coefficients between

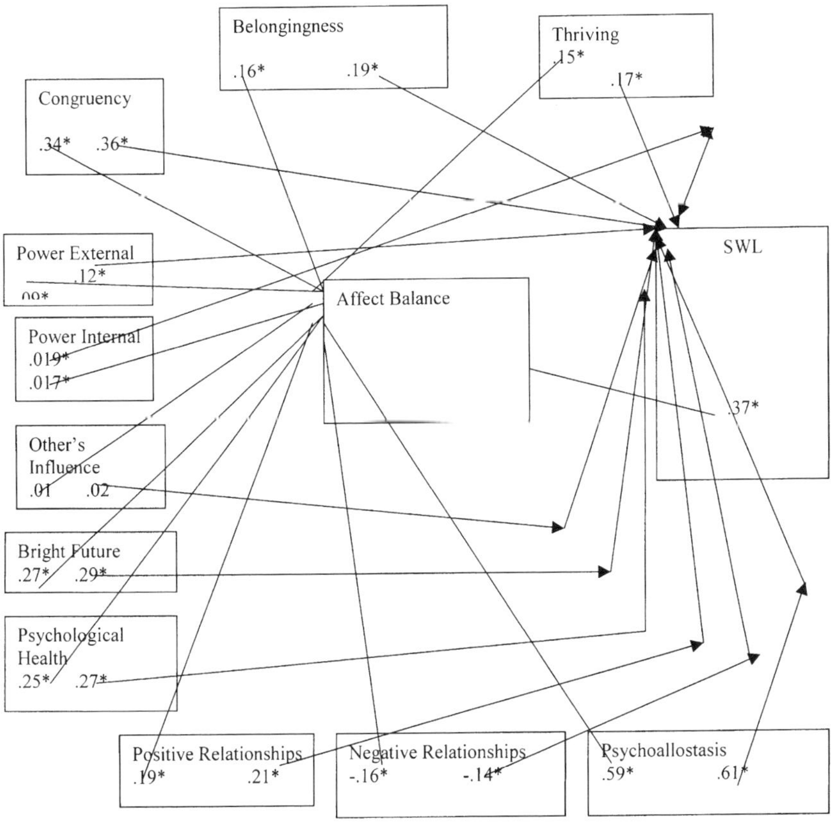

Figure 7. A path model of predictors of Affect Balance and Satisfaction with Life (SWB). *Note.* $^{*}p < 0.05$.

each of the components of SWB are larger than the coefficients between the SWB components and the various predictor variables, these components act as mediating variables between the predictors and the Satisfaction with Life Scale.

However, psychoallostasis predictor is an exception with larger coefficients (0.49 for SWL, 0.46 for HOS, and 0.59 for the Affect Balance) demonstrating that it is a major intervening variable to an individual's subjective well-being.

Indeed, as data displayed in Figures 6, 7, 8 demonstrate, there is a strong linkage between subjective well-being and the various predictor variables namely, congruency, thriving, belongingness, both internal and external power, bright future, subjective psycho-

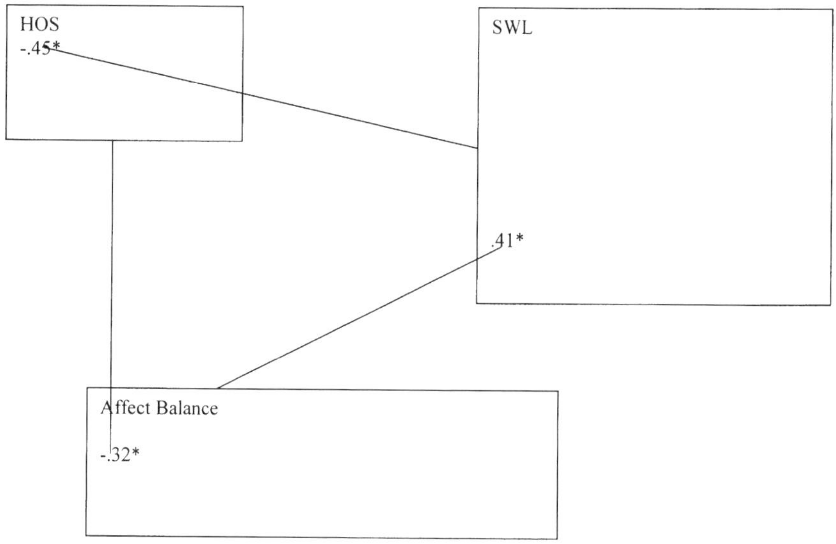

Figure 8. A path model for subjective well-begin components. *Note.* $*p < 0.05$.

logical health, relationships and psychoallostasis. Please refer to the figures for the specific magnitude of the coefficients.

DISCUSSION

Possessing the ability to mirror one's aspirations, needs, lifestyle and personality characteristics and to live congruently with one's family and community is indeed linked to high levels of subjective well-being.

Additionally, a thriving personality, belongingness, the perception of having power and control of both external and internal events and the inner underpinnings of life events, limited circumscription of the influence of other people, and possession of psychoallostasis are psychological mechanisms or even predispositions for increased psychological well-being as well as increased subjective well-being or happiness.

Indeed, people who possess psychologically healthy attributes not only experience high levels of Satisfaction with Life, Affect Balance and experience low levels of anxiety/depression, but also consider their future and their communities' as bright and thereby experiencing high levels of SWB. Additionally, when these respondents' understanding of themselves corresponded with the relative's, the result was increased Satisfaction with Life, increased Affect and decreased anxiety/depression. In other words, all aspects of SWB are affected (for a detailed understanding of these components of SWB, see Kimweli, 2002). These interrelationships indicate that QOL is *a function of belongingness and a constellation of community bound homeostatic systems as well as self-integration and synchronization with others.*

The importance of belongingness for individualistic-sub-collectivistic cultures such as Appalachia is underscored by the fact that isolation is debilitating. This finding of the connection between QOL and collectivistic psychological syndrome as Triandis et al. (1985) calls it, is significant in that it points to means of improving QOL by interpersonal interventions.

Additionally, the finding that looking forward to a good and bright future increases subjective well-being and thereby improves the quality of life of individuals and their communities, is a new addition to Frisch's 16 areas of life that constitutes individuals' overall {QOL} (1994). This aspect of people's life is controllable and can be addressed in Quality of life therapy (QOLT). Indeed, the results are consistent with Frisch's (1998) conclusions that management, alleviation or eradication of physical or psychological disorders does not necessary result in improved QOL. More is needed to project people's aspirations to improve QOL.

As can be extrapolated from the results, if one were to treat the anxiety/depression and ignored the communalhomeostasis, psychoallostasis and the psychodynamic factors, the end result would be reduced anxiety/depression and not increased SWB. Indeed, whereas psychological treatment may result in increased satisfaction, reduced anxiety, increased positive affect (better quality of life), that would be but the beginning of the story. *A favorable perception of the future, congruency with one's community, belongingness, psychoallostasis, both internal and external perceptions of power and other people's influence over one's life were stronger contributors to most of the domains of SWB and Quality of life considered in this research* (refer to Tables II and III) and would need to be addressed to achieve optional functioning.

The implications of this finding for Quality of life therapy (QOLT) is that cognitive restructuring can be used to help clients refocus their life so that they can obtain the desired results of a good future and greater compatibility or harmony with their community.

Cognitive restructuring may also reveal "in-build-competencies" hitherto undiscovered that can be utilized as "future-forward-looking-strategy building blocks." This approach ensures that clients take responsibility of the direction their future life takes rather than obsessing and dwelling on the past or the present. Once clients are "refocused on their future lives," strategies can be formulated that enable clients to discover ways to get their needs met and thereby increasing their satisfaction with life projectively by focusing, preparing and anticipating future contingencies. Therapy goals can be targeted to specific areas of need with the aim of empowering the client to control "future directions" of their lives to the extent that they can "perceive their life in the future as looking good" and are living accordingly.

Another area that has emerged as important in this research is interdependence what is probably closely related to Markus and Kitayama's social centricism (Markus and Kitayama, 1991). According to the findings of this research, there is indeed a strong linkage between subjective well-being and the ability to live a lifestyle that is congruent with one's community rules, expectations, and aspirations as well as living a lifestyle that fosters positive relationships. Indeed, as the results indicate, negative relationships are linked to high levels of anxiety (HOS) and low levels of Satisfaction with Life as well as Affect Balance. Positive relationship with other people are correlated with Quality of life. Positive relationships' greatest effect is in buffering anxiety and increasing positive affect and thereby increasing SWB (see also Kimweli and Stilwell, 1997). QOLT can then focus in ways that aim at fostering good relationships with one's family and community members. Although traditionally therapy has focused in helping self develop ways to individualize – kind of stand-alone phenomena, the findings of this research indicate that the role of others is a stronger predictor of SWB. This finding is pointing to the need to help clients' find ways to enhance the quality of relationships they are involved in.

The most important finding of this research is the discovery of the strong linkage between what is here referred to as *psycho-allostasis and the components of SWB. This term is here defined as psychological stability through change that is accompanied by a positive outlook despite the looming possibility of health problems and risks*. This definition emanated from the indices that comprised this concept and scale. Since this scale tapped individuals' current lifestyle as well as an indication of how they may live their lives in the future and is strongly linked to increased levels of SWB, inducing this concept needs to be a major goal of QOL therapy.

Individuals' as well as their communities' QOL can be increased by having them focus on a healthy and preventative lifestyle. As the indices comprising the psychoallostasis scale indicate, a preventive health lifestyle focuses on the future but does not ignore current life circumstances. It follows from the findings of research that prolonged psychological wellness, resilience and the ability to thrive can be maintained through psychological inoculation despite the presence of adverse psychological factors.

Consequently, QOLT therapy can focus on these aspects of clients' life. Specifically, the findings of this study indicate that *clients' perceptions of the relationships and his/her actions towards the relationships* rather than "other people's reactions" seems to be the issue. These perceptions can be altered through cognitive restructuring, behavioral modification techniques, and assertive skill training – all of which can actually be conducted with large groups of people – enmasse.

Additionally, the finding that individuals tend to perceive themselves as mirrors of their culture, i.e. value similar personality characteristics as their relatives and family members, and that this mirroring affects people's SWB, has QOLT implications. QOLT can seek to harmonize individuals' versus families'/communities' interpretations of how personality traits are perceived in interrelationships. This intervention may help individuals anticipate their family members and relatives' expectations. Indeed, just as the results indicate, what is considered a positive trait and results in better interactions, and by extension a source of increased SWB, ends up, being viewed by the individual as a positive trait even where it is considered a negative trait by individualistic cultures.

In relation to Appalachian culture, relationships, a good bright future and congruency to its cultural values are important issues – a fact that is evidenced by the significantly higher levels of satisfaction with life and Affect Balance experienced by the Appalachian sample studied here than any other group studied so far using these instruments (see also Kimweli, 2002). Appalachians live in close kinship communities and even tend to live together after migrating to cities (see Obermiller, 1978). Additionally, the Appalachian region as a whole is poor. Consequently, a better future and broken relationships bear more weight for Appalachians.

In conclusion, although the interpretation of these results should reflect the Appalachian community context, the findings have a wider application. The implications are that specific domains that are linked to increased SWB and improved QOL can be implemented (taught, induced etc.) to inoculate individuals and communities against ill-mental health. Just as impoverished communities are inoculated against poverty by appropriation of funds, these communities can be inoculated against concomitant ill-mental health by application of strategies that tackle and bring about the QOL factors discussed above. Inoculation can also be achieved by focusing the community to issues that point to their improved future preventative lifestyle that increases their psychoallostasis and communalhomeostasis discovered in this research. Indeed, given the current advances in technology and psychology, enmasse inoculation of communities against ill-mental health by application of the well-being principles untangled here should not be perceived as an illusive goal.

REFERENCES

Abbott, A. and R. Klein: 1979, 'Depression and anxiety among the Kikuyu in Kenya', Ethos 7, pp. 161–188.

Alderfer, C. P.: 1969, 'An empirical test of a new theory of human needs', Organizational Behavior and Human Performance 4, pp. 142–175.

Alderfer, C. P.: 1972, Existence, Relatedness, and Growth (Free Press, New York).

Baruffol, E., L. Gisle and P. Corten: 1995, 'Life satisfaction as a mediator between distressing events and neurotic impairment in a general population', Acta Psychiatrica Scandinavica 92, pp. 56–62.

Bem, S. L.: 1975, 'Sex Role Adaptability: one consequence of psychological androgyny', Journal of Personality and Social Psychology 31, pp. 634–643.

Bem, S. L.: 1984, Bem Sex Roles Inventory: Professional Manual (Mind Garden, Palo Alto, CA).

Browner, C. H. and J. Leslie: 1996, 'Women, work and household health in the context of development', in C. F. Sargent and C. B. Brettell (eds.), Gender and Health: An International Perspective (Prentice Hall, New Jersey).

Chamberlain, K. and S. Zika: 1990, 'Stability and change in subjective well-being over short time periods', Social Indicators Research 26, pp. 101–117.

Diener, E.: 1994, 'Assessing subjective well-being: progress and opportunities', Social Indicators Research 36, pp. 107–127.

Diener, E., R. A. Emmons, R. J. Larsen and S. Griffin: 1985, 'The satisfaction with life', Journal of Personality Assessment 49, pp. 71–75.

Diener, E. and F. Fujita: 1997, 'Social comparisons and subjective well-being', in B. Buunk and R. Gibbons (eds.), Health, Coping, and Social Comparison (Erlbaum, Hillsdale, NJ).

Deiner, E. and R. J. Larsen: 1993, 'The experience of emotional well-being', in M. Lewis and J. M. Haviland (eds.), Handbook of Emotions (Guilford Press, New York), pp. 405–415.

Diener, E., E. M. Suh, R. E. Lucas and H. L. Smith: 1999, 'Subjective well-being: three decades of progress', Psychological Bulletin 125, pp. 276–302.

Evans, D. R.: 1994, 'Enhancing the quality of life in the population at large', Social Indicators Research 33, pp. 47–88.

Frisch, M. B.: 1994, Quality of Life Inventory (QOLI) (National Computer Systems, Minneapolis, MN).

Frisch, M. B.: 1998, 'Quality of life therapy and assessment in health care', Clinical Psychology: Science and Practice 5(1), pp. 19–40.

George, M. S., J. A. Ketter, P. L. Parekh, B. Horowitz, P. Herscovitch and R. M. Post: 1995, 'Brain activity during transient sadness and happiness in healthy', American Journal of Psychiatry 152, pp. 341–351.

Glass, L. and M. Mackey: 1988, From Clocks to Chaos, the Rhythms of Life (Princeton University Press, Princeton, NJ).

Joreskog, K. G. and D. Sorbom: 1993, LISTREL 8: Structural Equation Modeling with the SIMPLIS Command Language (Scientific Software, Chicago).

Kammann, R. and R. C. Flett: 1983, 'A scale to measure current level of general happiness', Australian Journal of Psychology 35, pp. 259–265.

Kimweli, D. M. S.: 2002, The Relationship of Gender-Role Development, College Level and Subjective Well-Being among Appalachians. Unpublished doctoral dissertation, University of Kentucky, Lexington.

Kimweli, D. M. S. and W. E. Stilwell: 1997, Subjective Well-Being as an Individual Construction. Paper presented at the International Society for Quality-of-Life Studies Conference, Charlotte, NC, November.

Kitayama, S. M., H. R. Markus, H. Matsumoto and V. Norasahkunkit: 1997, 'Individual and collective processes in the construction of the self: self-enhancement in the United States and self-criticism in Japan', Journal of Personality and Social Psychology 72, pp. 1245–1267.

Markus, H. R. and S. Kitayama: 1991, 'Culture and self: implications for cognition, emotion, and motivation', Psychological Review 98, pp. 224–253.

Markus, H. R. and S. Kitayama: 1994, 'A collective fear of the collective: implications for selves and theories of selves', Personality and Social Psychology Bulletin 20, pp. 568–579.

Maslow, A. H.: 1987, Motivation and Personality, 3rd edn. (Harper and Row, New York).

McAdams, D. P.: 1994, 'Can personality change? Levels of stability and growth in personality across the life span', in T. F. Heatherton and G. J. L. Weinberger (eds.), Can Personality Change? (American Psychological Association, Washington, DC), pp. 299–313.

Miller, D. T. and D. A. Prentice: 1997, 'The construction of social norms and standards', in E. T. Higgins and A. W. Kruglanski (eds.), Social Psychology: Handbook of Basic Principles (Guilford, New York).

Mitchell, S. and S. Abbott: 1987, 'Gender and symptoms of depression and anxiety among the Kikuyu secondary school students in Kenya', Social Science and Medicine 24, pp. 303–316.

Moreland, K. L., R. D. Fowler and L. M. Honaker: 1994, 'Future directions in the use of psychological assessment for treatment planning and outcome evaluation: recommendations and predictions', in M. E. Maruish (ed.), The Use of Psychological Testing for Treatment and Outcome Assessment (Erlbaum, Hilldale, NJ), pp. 581–602.

Murphy, J.: 1986, 'Trends in depression and anxiety: men and women', Acta Psychiatrica Scandinavica 73, pp. 113–127.

Obermiller, P. J.: 1978, 'On the question of appalachian ethnicity', in S. Weiland and P. J. Obermiller (eds.), Perspectives on Urban Appalachians (Appalachian Awareness project, Cincinnati, Ohio).

Ogles, B. M., M. Lambert and K. Masters: 1996, Assessing Outcome in Clinical Practice (Allyn and Bacon, Boston).

Seligman, M. E. P.: 1991, Learned Optimism (Alfred. A. Knopf, New York).

Sirgy, M. J., D. Cole, R. Kosenko, H. L. Meadow, D. Rahtz, M. Cici, G. X. Jin, D. Yarsuvat, D. L. Blenkhorn and N. Nagpal: 1995, 'A life satisfaction measure: additional validational data for the congruity of life satisfaction measure', Social Indicators Research 34, pp. 237–259.

Strupp, H. H.: 1996, 'The tripartite model and the consumer reports study', American Psychologists 51, pp. 1017–1024.

Triandis, H. C., K. Leung, M. V. Villareal and E. L. Clack: 1985, 'Allocentric versus idiocentric tendencies: convergent and discriminant validation', Journal of Research in Personality 19, pp. 395–415.

Triandis, H. C.: 1988, 'Collectivism and individualism: a reconceptualization of a basic concept in cross-cultural psychology', in G. K. Verma and C. Bagley (eds.), Personality, Attitudes and Cognitions (Macmillan, London), pp. 60–95.

Triandis, H. C.: 1994, Culture and Social Behavior (McGraw-Hill, New York).
Triandis, H. C.: 1995, Individualism and Collectivism (Westview, Boulder).
Veenhoven, R.: 1984, Conditions of Happiness (Reidel, Boston).
Yang, K. S.: 1998, 'Psychological transformation of the chinese people as a result of societal modernization', in M. H. Bond (ed.), The Handbook of Chinese Psychology (Oxford University Press, Hong Kong), pp. 479–498.

Educational and Counseling Psychology Department
College of Education
The University of Kentucky
249 Dickey Hall
Lexington KY 40506-0017
E-mail: dmkimw00@pop.uky.edu; westil2@pop.uky.edu

MEGAN CLEAVER and THOMAS E. MULLER

I WANT TO PRETEND I'M ELEVEN YEARS YOUNGER: SUBJECTIVE AGE AND SENIORS' MOTIVES FOR VACATION TRAVEL

ABSTRACT. Subjective age–as distinct from chronological age–is a relatively recent area of scientific inquiry within quality-of-life studies. The purpose of this empirical study was to see whether the size of the gap between actual and self-perceived age could be predicted from a knowledge of a senior's reasons for wanting to travel on vacation, and his or her value priorities and sense of physical well-being. A survey of 356 Australian seniors ranging in age between 56 and 93 yielded data on their subjective age, measured in terms of (a) how old they felt; (b) the activities they would choose to experience or enjoy while on a vacation; and (c) the age they wished to be treated and recognized as–as well as their psychological motives for vacation travel, personal values, and self-rated health. The results of multivariate analyses indicate that the gap between actual age and subjective age is a function of seniors' particular motives for travel and what they value in life, and, for certain aspects of subjective age, how healthy they feel and their gender.

THE PSYCHOLOGICAL CONSTRUCT OF SUBJECTIVE AGE

Subjective age (sometimes referred to as self-perceived age, and operationalized or measured as "cognitive age") is the element of self-concept that reveals how old one feels, irrespective of one's chronological age (Blau, 1956; George et al., 1980; Wylie, 1974). This perception of one's age indicates how people position themselves within their life cycles. Subjective age may contribute, more than chronological age, to understanding how seniors view themselves and behave (Wilkes, 1992).

Neugarten and Neugarten (1986: p. 42) note that "A person uses age as a guide in accommodating to the behavior of others, in forming and re-forming the self-image, in giving meaning to the life course, and in contemplating the time that is past and the time that is left ahead."

Social Indicators Research **60:** 227–241, 2002.

People of all ages assess their subjective ages as different from their chronological ages and commonly perceive themselves to be younger than their chronological age (Bultena and Powers, 1978; Markides and Boldt, 1983). Apparently, the gap widens between subjective age and chronological age, as people grow older. Middle-aged adults place their self-perceived ages as 5–15 years younger than their chronological age, while more than half of adults over 60 feel 16–17 years younger (Underhill and Caldwell, 1983). Other studies support the significance of subjective age, reporting that 60–75 percent of people aged over 60 feel younger than their chronological ages (Blau, 1956; Bultena and Powers, 1978; Markides and Boldt, 1983).

Socio-economic background explains a portion of self-perceived age variance, but psychological factors also contribute to subjective age differences (Henderson et al., 1995). Moreover, younger subjective age correlates with life satisfaction and lifestyle (Bultena and Powers, 1978; McTavish, 1971; Wilkes, 1992). Studies show that older people who are self-confident, outgoing, socially venturesome, physically active, and influential in dealing with others possess younger subjective ages than their less confident, risk-averse peers (Day et al., 1988; Sorce et al., 1989). Furthermore, people driven to sustain their independence, and outwardly directed to seek social involvement, are more satisfied with their lives and enjoy a younger self-image (Gollub and Javitz, 1989).

Subjective age attributes also seem to affect economic behavior. Older people who perceive themselves to be younger than their chronological age are sophisticated and discerning shoppers (Age Wave, Inc., 1990). They are comparison shoppers (Schiffman and Sherman, 1991) who actively gather merchandise information and consider shopping as a recreational opportunity for healthy exercise (Tongren, 1988). Stephens (1991) notes that the cognitively younger elderly are affluent and consequently less averse to consumer experimentation and readily accept new products and services. And cognitively younger consumers show a higher interest in clothing fashion (Wilkes, 1992). Wilkes (1992) also found that cognitively younger women in the 60–79 age range were more likely to participate in entertainment and culturally related activities.

PERSONAL VALUES, LIFESTYLE AND TRAVEL MOTIVES

Another factor which drives human behavior and, specifically, consumption patterns and desired lifestyle, is a person's system of value priorities (Feather, 1996; Kahle, 1996; Rokeach, 1973; Schwartz, 1996). While the influence on travel behavior of both personal values (Muller, 1991; Pitts and Woodside, 1986) and life-styles (Shih, 1986) has been studied, the relationship between values and subjective age has not been properly explored.

Gerontologist Neugarten's (1968) landmark studies of aging have established that, as people approach the latter part of their lifetimes, they reveal a sense of competence and mastery and a preoccupation with self-utilization. There is a tendency to search for self-fulfilling activities and experiences. As older people contemplate the reality that there is "only so much time left to live," the recurrent theme in their minds is expressed well by one such person: "It adds a certain anxiety, but I must also say it adds a certain zest in seeing how much pleasure can still be obtained, how many good years one can still arrange, how many new activities can be undertaken ..." (Neugarten, 1968: p. 97). One would therefore expect not only a shift in value orientation as people reached retirement age, but also a synergistic effect of values and subjective age on the decision to travel and explore the "world" as a tourist.

Given this evidence, we would hypothesize that an older person's self-perceived age, relative to his or her actual age, is associated with (and can be predicted from) the person's deep-seated reasons for wanting to travel on vacation. Ryan and Glendon (1998) showed that distinct groups of holiday travelers can be identified on the basis of their psychological motives for travel. However, the link between travel motives and subjective age has, to our knowledge, not been empirically tested.

From a practical standpoint, the nature of the association between subjective age and travel motives would seem to be a useful piece of knowledge for organizations and policymakers who wish to promote tourism among seniors and retirees as a means of enhancing the subjective well-being of this segment of the population. A large proportion of Australia's 2.9 million seniors (people aged 60, or over) undoubtedly want to continue travelling for pleasure for as long as they are able. For one thing, 49 per cent of Australians aged

60 or more have no disability or physical impediment to mobility (Australian Bureau of Statistics, 1993). Yet, while older adult travelers in countries such as Canada (Duncombe, 1994; Zimmer et al., 1995), Germany (Romsa and Blenman, 1989) and the United States (Javalgi et al., 1992; Vincent and de los Santos, 1990) have been the subject of empirical research, Australian seniors were, until very recently, largely ignored as a tourism segment worth studying (Presland and Matthews, 1998).

THE SCOPE OF THIS STUDY

Synthesizing the research evidence reviewed, we hypothesize that the gap between subjective age and chronological age can be predicted from an older person's deep-seated (psychological) reasons for travel, personal values, and self-assessed state of health. Thus, the purpose of this study was to establish empirically the association between subjective age and these predictor variables within the 60-plus age segment of the population.

RESEARCH METHOD

A sample of 356 people aged between 56 and 93 was identified for us by the Office of Aging, in the Queensland Department of Families, Youth and Community Care. Interviews were conducted in group settings that varied between 10 and 30 persons in community halls and seniors citizens' clubs around Southeast Queensland; they filled out a self-completion questionnaire after listening to instructions from the researchers.

Vacation travel motives were measured with 48 items that were culled from three sources and adapted for this study of seniors. First, several items were adapted from Beard and Ragheb's (1983) leisure motivation items, which cover four components of leisure motives: intellectual, social, competency/mastery, and stimulus avoidance. Second, other items were constructed from the 28 travel benefit statements used in Moscardo et al.'s (1996) study of travel motivation. Finally, additional items were taken from studies of factors likely to motivate the behaviors of aging Baby Boomers (see Cleaver et al., 2000; Muller, 1997; Muller and Cleaver, 2000). The 48 travel motivation items were presented as "My own reasons for holiday travel are . . ." and respondents indicated on a 10-point rating scale whether they agreed or disagreed with each reason.

The List of Values (Kahle, 1996) was chosen because it is short as well as being adequate for the scope of this study. Respondents rated the relative importance of each of the nine terminal values on 10-point rating scales. Self-rated overall health was assessed with a 10-point rating scale anchored at "poor" and "excellent." Also recorded were year of birth and gender.

Subjective age was measured in three ways: (a) Felt age ("I *feel* as though I am in my . . ."); (b) Activities age ("While on a travel holiday, the *activities* I would choose to experience or enjoy would be those of a person in their . . ."); and (c) Recognition age ("When on a travel holiday, I expect to be *treated and recognised* as a person in their . . ."). For all three questions, 14 half-decades (from "early-20s or younger" to "late-80s or older") were provided as response categories. These measures are a refinement of the subjective (cognitive) age scales developed by Barak and Schiffman (1981) and were adapted after evaluating Wilkes' (1992) research findings on cognitive age.

The magnitude of the gap between actual and subjective ages was computed for each person by subtracting subjective age from actual age. In order to convert the 14 discrete subjective-age categories (early-60s, late-60s, early-70s, etc.) into interval data so that these gaps could be computed, we arbitrarily set each subjective-age category at either the 3rd or 7th year of that decade (e.g., early-60s was recoded as 63, and late-60s as 67). For about eight percent of respondents, these gaps were negative integers, meaning that they considered themselves to be older than their chronological age.

FINDINGS

Factor Analysis of the Motives

The purpose of this step was data reduction of the 48 travel motive items. Principal components factor analyses were performed to extract groups of travel motives where the individual items were highly intercorrelated, but distinct from other groups of motives.

The overriding objective was interpretability of the resulting varimax-rotated factor matrix, not maximum explained variance or the inclusion of all factors with eigenvalues of 1.0 or higher. On the basis of our theoretical expectations and the interpretability of the factor-item loadings, seven factors were extracted (explaining 60 percent of the variance in the 48 items). They clearly reflected most of the underlying dimensions of travel motives that we expected and we labeled the factors accordingly. Table I identifies the seven factors and the individual items comprising each factor.

The next step was to average each respondent's scores on the items within each of the seven factors. We did this after first cleaning up the factors by removing seven items which loaded similarly on more than one factor (factor-item correlations within 0.05 of one another).

Multiple regression served as the principal statistical technique, with the gap between actual and subjective age being the dependent variable. The predictor variables were seven travel motive factors, nine personal values, self-rated health, and gender. Since subjective age was measured in three ways, three sets of regressions were run. In each regression the dependent variable was the gap between actual age and either felt age, activities age, or recognition age.

Felt Age

Table II gives the main statistics for the regression analysis, where the dependent variable is the gap between actual age and felt age. The results are reported for the 256 cases with no missing data on any of the predictor or dependent variables. Four of the independent variables are significant predictors of the difference between actual and felt age. They are tabled in descending order of strength as predictors (betas).

The importance of the personal value, *fun and enjoyment in life*, is positively correlated with the difference between actual and felt age. Thus, seniors for whom this is an important goal in life tend to feel younger than those for whom fun and enjoyment is less important. Self-assessed health is the second strongest predictor of the magnitude of the gap between actual and felt age. People who give themselves a better health rating put a greater distance between their actual age and the age they feel. Conversely, seniors who rate

TABLE I

Individual Items Loading on the Seven Extracted Vacation Travel-Motive Factors

Nostalgia
To visit a friend or relative
To make pilgrimages to places which have memories for me
To visit a place where my family's roots are
To try to achieve family togetherness on a holiday
To be able to relive some of the good memories and good times from my past
To enjoy surroundings that are comforting and reassuring
Friendship
To meet new people and make new friends
To become better friends with someone, by holiday-making together
To travel together with a group of people who share my interests and values
Learning
To collect new and different experiences
To satisfy my curiosity or increase my general knowledge
To keep me well informed and on top of what's going on
To learn new things and enrich my life
To become a more cultured person
To feel connected with other people and experience a sense of community
To experience the fun of discovery
To feel I am actively involved in the world around me
To be a little adventurous
To improve or renew my skills as a traveler
Escapism
To get away from the demands at home and in daily life
To relax and do nothing at all
To indulge in a bit of luxury
To get away from doing too much thinking
To avoid boredom
To be entertained and looked after by others
To change my surroundings for the sake of change
Thinking
To help me think about who I am and what life means
To raise my self-esteem

TABLE I

Continued

To challenge my mental abilities
To share my thoughts and feelings with my travelling companion
To go to a place where I can feel safe again
To find simplicity, certainty, or peace of mind and soul
Because I sometimes like to be alone
Status enhancement
To enable me to go to places where my friends or rivals have not been
To gain the respect of others
To keep up with all the holiday travelling that I see others doing
To be able to tell stories of my holiday adventures and mishaps to my grand-children
To be able to tell others about where I have been and what I have seen
Physical stimulation
To give me a chance to participate in a sport I am fond of
To find thrills or excitement
To obtain some form of physical invigoration

their own health more poorly tend to feel closer to their actual age. If perceived good health is positively correlated with life satisfaction, then this result supports Sherman and Schiffman's findings (Wolfe, 1990: p. 212) that a greater sense of life satisfaction is associated with a lower cognitive age.

The escapism factor, which captures the stimulus-avoidance component of travel motivations (getting away from a demanding home environment, relaxing and doing nothing, etc.) has a negative coefficient. Thus, seniors who travel for the purpose of escaping from day-to-day duties and winding down are more likely to feel their actual age. Also, those for whom *security* is important as a value tend to feel closer to their actual age (and subjectively older than seniors for whom security is not so important).

TABLE II

Regression Results, Based on How Old Seniors *Feel*

Predictor variable	B	Beta	p ≤
Fun and enjoyment in life	0.995	0.258	0.001
Self-rated health	1.026	0.220	0.001
Escapism	–0.754	–0.185	0.05
Security	–0.602	–0.160	0.05
(Constant)	3.938		
$F(18, 237) = 2.963, p < 0.001$			
$R^2 = 0.184$			

Activities Age

Table III gives the regression results for the gap between actual age and activities age, the age seniors would *act*, in terms of chosen activities while on a travel vacation. These results are based on the 248 cases with no missing data on any of the variables. Ten of the independent variables are significant predictors of the gap between activities age and actual age, and they are tabled in descending order of predictive strength.

Gender is the strongest predictor of the gap between actual and activities age. Males have a tendency to desire vacation activities associated with much younger age groups, whereas females tend to prefer activities that are seen as closer to their own chronological age. In other words, females want to act their age while on vacation. The next strongest predictor is the travel motive of status enhancement. Seniors who travel on vacation partly to impress significant others prefer the activities of people who are closer to their own actual age. Conversely, non-status-driven travel vacationers want to act younger than their actual age by a bigger margin than their status-driven age peers.

Once again, preoccupation with *security* as a personal value is negatively correlated with the desire to experience or enjoy vacation activities associated with chronologically younger people. Conversely, seniors for whom the value security is relatively unimportant tend to want to act much younger than they actually are.

TABLE III

Regression Results, Based on What Age Seniors Would *Act* When Choosing Vacation Activities

Predictor variable	B	Beta	p ≤
Gender	6.089	0.261	0.001
Status enhancement	–1.011	–0.254	0.01
Security	–0.887	–0.229	0.005
Self-respect	0.872	0.209	0.01
Being highly regarded by others	0.589	0.197	0.01
Friendship	–0.741	–0.187	0.05
A sense of belonging	–0.674	–0.182	0.07
Fun and enjoyment in life	0.655	0.311	0.05
Warm relationships with others	0.721	0.161	0.07
Physical stimulation	0.602	0.145	0.07
(Constant)	1.731		
$F(18, 229) = 4.283, p < 0.001$			
$R^2 = 0.252$			

The personal values *self-respect* and *being highly regarded by others* are positively correlated with the difference between actual and activity age. Thus, seniors for whom either of these values are an important goal in life tend to be interested in "younger" activities. The travel motivation factor friendship and the personal value *a sense of belonging* are both negatively correlated, therefore those seniors who are motivated to travel for friendship or hold a sense of belonging as an important life goal are more likely to be interested in activities of their actual age rather than activities associated with younger age groups.

The final three predictor variables, the personal values, *fun and enjoyment in life* and *warm relationships with others*, and the travel motivation factor, physical stimulation are also able to help predict the age related activities that seniors might involve themselves in while on a travel holiday. Those seniors who value fun and enjoyment in life, or warm relationships with others, or are motivated to travel for physical stimulation are more likely to involve themselves in activities associated with younger age groups than their actual chronological age.

TABLE IV

Regression Results, Based on What Age Seniors Would Like To Be *Recognized and Treated as* While on Vacation

Predictor variable	B	Beta	$p \leq$
Physical stimulation	0.480	0.152	0.07
Self-rated health	0.516	0.141	0.05
(Constant)	8.416		
$F(18, 232) = 11.612, p < 0.058$			
$R^2 = 0.111$			

Recognition Age

Table IV presents the regression results for the gap between actual age and recognition age–the age a senior expects to be *recognized and treated as*, while on a travel vacation. These results are based on the 251 cases with no missing data on any of the variables.

Just two variables are predictive of this gap between actual and subjective age, and both are barely significant; thus these findings are only suggestive. The travel motivation factor, physical stimulation, is the stronger predictor of the two. Seniors who want to travel for physical stimulation are less likely to expect to be treated in accordance with their actual age and don't mind being treated as a younger person. This also appears to be the case for seniors who perceive themselves to be in relatively good health. Conversely, seniors who give themselves lower overall health ratings tend to expect, during their vacation travel, to be treated and recognized in a way that befits their actual age.

SUMMARY AND IMPLICATIONS

The aim of this study was to discover whether the size of the difference between a senior's subjective age and actual age could be predicted from data on his or her travel motives, personal values, feeling of physical well-being, and gender.

We believe that this is still uncharted territory within the field of quality-of-life studies. The relationships we studied are important because the theory of subjective age is still incomplete and the concept of subjective age has both intuitive appeal and practical implications for organizations and policymakers whose goal is to improve the subjective well-being of the 60-plus population. If the correlates of subjective age are better understood, then perhaps the link between felt age–or activities age–and satisfaction and happiness can be established.

We found that the mean difference between felt age and actual age is 10.2 years. The mean difference between activities age and actual age is 11.2 years. Thus, the seniors in our study typically felt a decade younger than they were, and were attracted to vacation activities that were associated with people who were on average, more than a decade younger than themselves. The mean difference between recognition age and actual age is 7.2 years. This difference was found to be only mildly significant and therefore the findings for feel age and activities age will be concentrated on.

Our findings indicate that certain travel motives and personal values are associated with a senior's perceptions of how old she or he feels and wishes to act. We found that the importance attached to the value *fun and enjoyment in life* is a reliable predictor that a senior feels younger than his or her actual age and would prefer to experience or enjoy vacation activities associated with younger people. Self-rated health also provides predictive value, as those who rate their health highly are more likely to feel younger than their actual age. On the other hand, seniors who are security conscious and whose reasons for holiday travel are to get away from domestic duties and find an occasion to relax and do nothing tend to feel closer to their actual age.

Gender is the strongest predictor of the gap between actual and activities age. Males have a greater tendency than females to desire vacation activities associated with much younger age groups. Seniors who travel on vacation partly to impress significant others prefer the activities of people who are closer to their own actual age.

Security is also negatively correlated with the desire to experience or enjoy vacation activities associated with chronologically younger people, therefore seniors who do not value security tend to want to act much younger than they actually are. The personal values, *self-respect, being highly regarded by others, fun and enjoy-*

ment in life and *warm relationships with others* and the travel motivation factor, physical stimulation are positively correlated with the difference between actual and activity age. Thus, seniors for whom any of these values are an important goal in life or are motivated to travel for physical stimulation tend to be interested in "younger" activities. Those seniors who are motivated to travel for friendship or hold a sense of belonging as an important life goal are more likely to be interested in activities of their actual age rather than activities associated with younger age groups.

Further research is needed to establish the validity of our findings, and it looks as if there are some theoretically exciting and strategically useful relationships to be tested further. By and large, the seniors we interviewed are the parents of the post-war Baby Boom Generation in Australia. If the correlates of subjective age found in this study are confirmed in future research, the next stage would be to search for the same effects within samples of aging Baby Boomers–who represent a very sizeable portion of the populations of the United States, Canada, Australia and New Zealand.

REFERENCES

Age Wave, Inc.: 1990, Marketplace 2000 (Author, Emeryville, CA).

Australian Bureau of Statistics: 1993, Disability, Ageing and Carers Australia, 1993 (Catalogue No: 4430.0) (Commonwealth of Australia, Canberra).

Barak, B. and L. G. Schiffman: 1981, 'Cognitive age: a nonchronological age variable', in Kent B. Monroe (ed.), Advances in Consumer Research, Vol. 8 (Association for Consumer Research, Ann Arbor, MI), pp. 602–606.

Beard, J. G. and M. G. Ragheb: 1983, 'Measuring leisure motivation', Journal of Leisure Research 15(3), pp. 219–228.

Blau, Z. S.: 1956, 'Changes in status and age identification', American Sociological Review 21, pp. 198–203.

Bultena, G. L. and E. A. Powers: 1978, 'Denial of aging: Age identification and reference group orientations', Journal of Gerontology 33, pp. 748–754.

Cleaver, M., B. C. Green and T. E. Muller: 2000, 'Using consumer behavior research to understand the Baby Boomer tourist', Journal of Hospitality & Tourism Research 24(2), pp. 274–287.

Day, E., B. Davis, R. Dove and W. French: 1988, 'Reaching the senior citizen market(s)', Journal of Advertising Research 27, pp. 23–30.

Duncombe, R.: 1994, How to Prepare for and Better Serve the Seniors Customer Segment. Presentation speaking points dated February 1 (Tourism Canada, Marketing–U.S.A., Ottawa).

Feather, N. T.: 1996, 'Values, deservingness, and attitudes toward high achievers: research on tall poppies', in C. Seligman, J. M. Olson and M. P. Zanna (eds.), The Psychology of Values: The Ontario Symposium, Vol. 8 (Lawrence Erlbaum Associates, Mahwah, New Jersey), pp. 215–251.

George, L. K., E. J. Mutran and M. R. Pennybacker: 1980, 'The meaning and measurement of age identity', Experimental Aging Research 6, pp. 283–298.

Gollub, J. and H. Javitz: 1989, 'Six ways to age', American Demographics 11, pp. 28–57.

Henderson, K. V., R. E. Goldsmith and L. R. Flynn: 1995, 'Demographic characteristics of subjective age', Journal of Social Psychology.

Javalgi, R. G., E. G. Thomas and S. R. Rao: 1992, 'Consumer behavior in the U.S. pleasure travel marketplace: an analysis of senior and nonsenior travelers', Journal of Travel Research 30(Fall), pp. 14–19.

Kahle, L. R.: 1996, 'Social values and consumer behavior: research from the list of Values', in C. Seligman, J. M. Olson and M. P. Zanna (eds.), The Psychology of Values: The Ontario Symposium, Vol. 8 (Lawrence Erlbaum Associates, Mahwah, New Jersey), pp. 135–151.

Markides, K. S. and J. S. Boldt: 1983, 'A structural modeling approach to the measurement and meaning of cognitive age', Journal of Consumer Research 19, pp. 292–301.

McTavish, D. G.: 1971, 'Perceptions of old people: a review of research methodologies and findings', The Gerontologist 11, pp. 90–101.

Moscardo, G., A. M. Morrison, P. L. Pearce, C-T. Lang and J. T. O'Leary: 1996, 'Understanding vacation destination choice through travel motivation and activities', Journal of Vacation Marketing 2(2), pp. 109–122.

Muller, T. E.: 1991, 'Using personal values to define segments in an international tourism market', International Marketing Review 8(1), pp. 57–70.

Muller, T. E.: 1997, 'The benevolent society: value and lifestyle changes among middle-aged Baby Boomers', in L. R. Kahle and L. Chiagouris (eds.), Values, Lifestyles and Psychographics (Advertising and Consumer Psychology Series, Society for Consumer Psychology) (Lawrence Erlbaum Associates, Mahwah, NJ), pp. 299–316.

Muller, T. E. and M. Cleaver: 2000, 'Targeting the CANZUS Baby Boomer explorer and adventurer segments', Journal of Vacation Marketing 6(2), pp. 154–169.

Neugarten, B. L.: 1968, 'The awareness of middle age', in B. L. Neugarten (ed.), Middle Age and Aging (University of Chicago Press, Chicago), pp. 93–98.

Neugarten, B. L. and D. A. Neugarten: 1986, 'Changing meanings of age in the aging society', in A. Pifer and L. Bronte (eds.), Our Aging Society: Paradox and Promise (W. W. Norton, New York), pp. 33–51.

Pitts, R. E., Jr. and A. G. Woodside: 1986, 'Personal values and travel decisions', Journal of Travel Research 25(Summer), pp. 20–25.

Presland, A. and A. Matthews: 1998, 'A golden opportunity', Seniors Card Tourism Scheme Bulletin, April, 1–2.

Rokeach, M.: 1973, The Nature of Human Values (The Free Press, New York).

Romsa, G. and M. Blenman: 1989, 'Vacation patterns of the elderly German', Annals of Tourism Research 16(2), pp. 178–188.
Ryan, C. and I. Glendon: 1998, 'Application of leisure motivation scale to tourism', Annals of Tourism Research 25(1), pp. 169–184.
Schiffman, L.G. and E. Sherman: 991, 'Value orientations of new-age elderly: the coming of an ageless market', Journal of Business Research 22, pp. 187–194.
Schwartz, S.: 1996, 'Value priorities and behavior: applying a theory of integrated value systems', in C. Seligman, J. M. Olson and M. P. Zanna (eds.), The Psychology of Values: The Ontario Symposium, Vol. 8 (Lawrence Erlbaum Associates, Mahwah, New Jersey), pp. 1–24.
Shih, D.: 1986, 'VALS as a tool of tourism market research: the Pennsylvania experience', Journal of Travel Research 24(4), pp. 2–11.
Sorce, P., P. R. Tyler and L. Loomis: 1989, 'Lifestyles of older Americans', Journal of Consumer Marketing 6, pp. 53–63.
Stephens, N.: 1991, 'Cognitive age: a useful concept for advertising?' Journal of Advertising 20, pp. 37–48.
Tongren, H. N.: 1988, 'Determinant behavior characteristics of older consumers', Journal of Consumer Affairs 22, pp. 137–157.
Underhill, L. and F. Caldwell: 1983, ' "What age do you feel?" . . . Age perception study', Journal of Consumer Marketing 1(Summer), pp. 18–27.
Vincent, V. C. and G. de los Santos: 1990, 'Winter texans: two segments of the senior travel market', Journal of Travel Research 29(Summer), pp. 9–12.
Wilkes, R. E.: 1992, 'A structural modeling approach to the measurement and meaning of cognitive age', Journal of Consumer Research 19, pp. 292–301.
Wolfe, D. B.: 1990, Serving the Ageless Market (McGraw-Hill, New York).
Wylie, R. C.: 1974, The Self Concept (University of Nebraska Press, Lincoln, NE).
Zimmer, Z., R. E. Brayley and M. S. Searle: 1995, 'Whether to go and where to go: identification of important influences on seniors' decisions to travel', Journal of Travel Research 33(3), pp. 3–10.

Hagoromo University of International Studies
1-89-1, Hamadera Minami-machi Sakai
Osaka 592-8344
Japan
E-mail: muller@hagoromo.ac.jp

JOANNE BRYANT, ANNETTE J. BROWNE, SYLVIA BARTON and BRUNO D. ZUMBO

ACCESS TO HEALTH CARE: SOCIAL DETERMINANTS OF PREVENTIVE CANCER SCREENING USE IN NORTHERN BRITISH COLUMBIA

ABSTRACT. The purpose of this study was to examine the extent to which social factors are influential in determining women's access to cancer screening services in Prince George, British Columbia. Specifically, this study evaluated the association of age, income, education, work status, disability, marital status, and immigrant status with previous use of screening mammography and Pap tests. Data was obtained from the 1994 National Population Health Survey, which contains a sample of 416 women from the Prince George area. A series of logistic regression analyses were used to distinguish *ever* versus *never* been screened as well as recency of previous screening. Participation rates in screening mammography in Prince George are comparatively high; however, no association was found between social factors and previous mammography use. This suggests women in Prince George are participating in mammography services regardless of social background. Participation rates in Pap test screening in Prince George are high and are similar to provincial averages; however, while a large percentage of women have been screened, this percentage varies across social groups. Immigrant women, single women, and women with less education are over represented among women who have never had a Pap test. In addition, older women are less likely to obtain a recent Pap test when compared to younger women. This study suggests that certain groups of women in northern British Columbia experience low participation in health services, resulting in a higher risk for poor health and a poor quality of life.

Universal access is one of the five founding principles of the Canadian health care system, a system that permits many Canadians an outstanding health-related quality of life. In the formative years of the Canadian health care system, the term "universal access" meant, quite simply, free financial access; the belief being that free financial access would eliminate inequities in participation in the health care system, and consequently, inequities in health outcome. However, recent years have demonstrated health, and participation in the health care system, are complicated phenomena. No longer

Social Indicators Research **60:** 243–262, 2002.

simply about the absence of disease, health is now understood to be a comprehensive concept with social, economic, environmental, psychological and cultural determinants. With this new recognition of health determinants, policy makers have had to reconsider the meaning of universal access. The effects of age, race, class and gender have real effects on an individuals' ability to participate in the health care system. It is for this reason that, despite free financial access to health programs, socio-economic inequities remain associated with poor health and low participation in the Canadian health care system. The purpose of this study is to determine the extent to which selected social and economic factors are influential in determining participation in preventive cancer screening programs (namely screening mammography and Pap tests) in Prince George, a large community in northern British Columbia.

Disease prevention has gained considerable attention in recent years. Clearly, the most proactive approach to improving health in populations is to prevent the occurrence and/or proliferation of disease. Preventive screening practices such as mammography and Pap tests are classified as secondary prevention measures; that is, emphasis lies in early diagnosis and prompt intervention in order to lessen the duration and severity of disease (Pender, 1987). Advances in preventive screening technology have made it possible to substantially reduce morbidity and mortality due to cancer among women. It is estimated that regular mammography screening can reduce breast cancer mortality up to 40% (Center for Disease Control and Prevention, 1996). Similarly, regular cervical cancer screening can prevent almost all cases of invasive cervical cancer (Health Canada, 1998). Nevertheless, a reduction in cancer mortality and morbidity through preventive screening can only be reached if a significant portion of the target population accesses screening services on a regular basis.

British Columbia (BC) has extensive and well-established screening programs. The BC Cervical Cytology Screening Program was the first population-based cervical cancer screening program. Since 1955 the program has provided free Pap tests to all female residents of BC (Deschamps et al., 1992). Similarly, the Screening Mammography Program of BC was the first province-wide breast cancer screening program in Canada and has provided free mammography screening since 1988. Recent program expansions have included a number of mobile mammography vans allowing more than 95% of women in the province to be within an hour's drive of a screening facility (Clay et al., 1994). Both programs keep detailed records with linkages to the BC Cancer Registry. This allows for a comprehensive follow-up system in which a cancer screening history can be maintained for every woman participating in screening programs.

Despite the presence of comprehensive cancer screening programs, women in BC exhibit low participation rates. Only 39% of women 40 to 79 have ever had a mammogram, and 85% of women over the age of 20 have ever had a Pap test (BC Provincial Health Officer's Annual Report, 1996) indicating that a large proportion of women in BC have never been screened. Clearly the reasons why women do or do not participate in preventive screening practices are complex. Previous researchers have supported the notion that social and economic factors are influential in determining an individual's ability to access health services (Pender, 1987; Labonte, n.d.). Those from socially disadvantaged backgrounds participate in the health care system to a lesser extent than those from socially advantaged backgrounds. Certainly, efforts to improve accessibility to cancer screening services for women in BC must involve more than providing free financial access.

It is important to emphasize the relevance of socio-economic determinants to the health of women and thereby the importance of studying socio-economic determinants in evaluating screening accessibility for women. In comparison to men, women have less education and lower incomes, are subjected to greater degrees of discrimination and are more likely to be affected by violence. This further highlights the complexity of accessibility to health services for women. From a socio-economic perspective, women from disadvantaged social groups are doubly at risk for low participation in the health care system and consequently, at a greater risk for poor health.

Previous studies have identified patterns of social and economic variables influencing the screening behaviors of Canadian women. A recent analysis of 1994 National Population Health Survey identified a higher proportion of non-users of preventive screening among women with lower incomes and less education (Snider et al., 1996). Similarly, the 1990 Ontario Health Survey indicated that women with higher incomes were 1.7 times more likely to have received a Pap test than women with lower incomes (Katz and Hofer, 1994). Further analyses of the 1990 Ontario Health Survey found that, compared to Canadian-born women, recently immigrated women (<10 years) were significantly less likely to have ever had a Pap test (Goel, 1994). Women working in the home and women over the age of 65 were also significantly less likely to have ever had a Pap test.

METHODS

The data for this study comes from the 1994 National Population Health Survey (Statistics Canada, 1994). The National Population Health Survey (NPHS) was a large national survey collecting information on a variety of Canadian health issues, including mammography and Pap test utilization. A sample of 436 women was collected from Prince George.

Women included in the mammography analysis were between the ages of 40 and 79 years. These ages are in accordance with the guidelines of the Screening Mammography Program of BC that stipulate women should receive mammography screening every two years after the age of 40 until the age of 79. The mammography sample consisted of 186 women whose average age was 50 years.

Women included in the Pap test analysis were between the ages of 18 and 69 years. This is in accordance with the Canadian Guide to Clinical Preventive Health (1994) which recommends screening for cervical cancer should begin annually at age 18 or following initiation of sexual activity; after two normal smears, screening should proceed every three years until age 69. Note that Canadian Guide to Clinical Preventive Health guidelines were used instead of BC Cervical Cytology guidelines (which recommends screening every 2 years after 3 normal smears) because the NPHS allowed data to be divided into 1, 3 or 5 year increments only. The Pap test sample consisted of 418 women whose average age was 35 years.

Outcome variables were derived from the preventive health practices component of the NPHS. Women aged 35 and older were asked if they had ever had a mammogram and the recency of

TABLE I

Levels of Final Outcome Variables

Mammography variables	Pap test variables
EVER received a mammogram	EVER received a Pap test
• received a recent mammogram (in the previous 2 years)	• received a recent Pap test (in the previous 3 years)
• received a non-recent mammogram (longer than 2 years ago)	• received a non-recent Pap test (longer than 3 years ago)
NEVER received a mammogram.	NEVER received a Pap test.

their latest mammogram. Similarly, women aged 18 and older were asked if they had ever had a Pap test and the recency of their last Pap test. These original mammography and Pap test variables were used to create a final outcome variable for each practice. The final outcome variables had 4 levels, which are described in Table I. These categories reflect the recommendations of provincial and national screening guidelines, as discussed earlier.

Seven social and economic variables were selected from the 1994 NPHS database as potential predictors of mammography and Pap test utilization. The predictor variables were selected based on a review of the literature and include age, income, education, immigrant status, disability, marital status, and employment status.

Data analysis consisted of modeling a series of logistic regression equations predicting mammography and Pap test utilization from the seven social and economic predictors. Eight separate regression equations were modeled using various combinations of the levels of the outcome variables, as outlined in Table II.

Comparing different combinations of outcomes allowed for the production of a more detailed picture of mammography and Pap test use. The analysis of each model consisted of one run of the multiple logistic regression with all of the predictors entered simultaneously. In this way the impact of all seven predictor variables was evaluated. This modeling strategy was chosen because interpreting the individual effects of predictor variables within the context of the other predictor variables allows for a more realistic representation of the true effect of each significant variable.

TABLE II

Eight Models for Analysis

Model	Dichotomous outcome variable
Mammography models	
Model 1	NEVER had a mammogram vs. EVER had a mammogram
N = 186	(recent and non-recent)
Model 2	NEVER had a mammogram vs. had a RECENT mammogram
N = 151	
Model 3	NEVER had a mammogram vs. had a NON-RECENT mammogram
N = 97	
Model 4	had a NON-RECENT mammogram vs. had a RECENT mammogram
N = 118	
Pap test models	
Model 5	NEVER had a Pap test vs. EVER had a Pap test
N = 418	(recent and non-recent)
Model 6	NEVER had a Pap test vs. had a RECENT Pap test
N = 318	
Model 7	NEVER had a Pap test vs. had a NON-RECENT Pap test
N = 76	
Model 8	Had a NON-RECENT Pap test vs. had RECENT Pap test
N = 357	

The results of each of the eight logistic regressions were analyzed in two steps: (1) an assessment of overall model fit, followed by (2) an assessment of parameter significance. If the overall measure of fit was not significant ($p > 0.05$), then it was concluded that the predictor variables as a group did not significantly predict mammography/Pap test utilization and analysis ceased. If the overall fit was significant ($p \leq 0.05$), parameter significance was examined. Significant parameters (main effects of predictor variables) were interpreted in terms of their contrast coding matrix.

TABLE III

Rates of Screening – Mammography

Mammography		N		% of sample	
Yes	In previous 2 years	118	86	63%	46%
	Longer than 2 years ago		32		17%
No		65		35%	
N/A		3		2%	

TABLE IV

Rates of Screening – Pap test

Pap test		N		% of sample	
Yes	In previous e years	357	300	85%	72%
	Longer than e years ago		57		13%
No		19		5%	
N/A		42		10%	

RESULTS

Proportion of Women Screened

Tables III and IV indicate the proportions of women screened in Prince George. Thirty-five percent of women between the ages of 40 and 79 reported *never* having had a mammogram and 17% had not had a *recent* mammogram. Similarly, 5% of women between the ages of 18 and 69 reported *never* having had a Pap test and 13% reported not having had a *recent* Pap test.

The relationship between mammography use and Pap test use was significant, as revealed by a Chi-square Goodness of Fit test ($\chi^2 = 10.9$, d.f. = 1). An examination of 2×2 tables revealed a risk estimate of 9.3 (CI 1.9, 44.5) indicating that those women to have ever had a mammogram are 9.3 times more likely to have ever had a Pap test.

TABLE V

Logistic Regression Analyses – Mammography

Model	χ^2	d.f.	p-value	Effect size pseudo-R^2
MODEL 1: NEVER vs. EVER	20.31	14	0.12	0.090 small-med
MODEL 2: NEVER vs. RECENT	20.28	14	0.12	0.104 small-med
MODEL 3: NEVER vs. NON-RECENT	12.36	14	0.58	0.107 small-med
MODEL 4: NON-RECENT vs. RECENT	13.22	14	0.51	0.101 small-med

*Effect sizes are according to Cohen (1992).

Association of Predictors with Screening Practices

Mammography models

Table V indicates the overall fit of each of the four mammography utilization models. The regression analyses on the mammography sample revealed that the seven predictor variables were not significantly associated with previous mammography use. All p-values are greater than 0.05 and the effect sizes (pseudo-R^2) indicate approximately 10% of variation in mammography use can be explained by the predictor variables. These effects are considered small to medium according to Cohen (1992).

Pap test models – Overall fit

In contrast, analyses on the Pap test sample indicate the predictors, as a group, are significantly associated with previous Pap test use. Table VI shows that all p-values are less than 0.05 and effect size measures vary from 0.10 (small effect according to Cohen, 1992) to 0.50 (large effect). In other words, the predictors, as a group, explain approximately 30% of the variation in women having *never* received a previous Pap test (Model 5). Further, the predictors explain approximately 10% of the variation in women not having received a *recent* Pap test (Model 8).

TABLE VI

Logistic Regression Analyses – Pap Test

Model	χ^2	d.f.	p-value	Effect size pseudo-R^2
MODEL 5:	39.80	15	0.00	0.278
NEVER vs. EVER				large
MODEL 6:	45.40	15	0.00	0.346
NEVER vs. RECENT				large
MODEL 7:	39.47	15	0.00	0.495
NEVER vs. NON-RECENT				large
MODEL 8:	28.80	15	0.02	0.100
NON-RECENT vs. RECENT				small-med

*Effect sizes are according to Cohen (1992).

Pap test models – Significant parameters

The parameter results of the four significant Pap test models can be found in Table VIII. Table VII explains the codes used in Table VIII. The complexity of Table VIII can be summed into two main points. First, women are more likely to have *never* had a Pap test if they are immigrants, single, and less educated. Second, women are less likely to have had a *recent* Pap test if they are older.

The most consistent predictor of having *never* had a Pap test proved to be immigrant status. In fact, for each model involving never having had a Pap test (Models 5 through 7), immigrant status was a consistent contributor. Model 5 (*never* vs. *ever*) indicates immigrant women are 7 times more likely to have never had a Pap test relative to non-immigrant women (OR = 7.1, CI = 1.9, 26). Models 6 and 7 further support this result.

Marital status was another consistently significant contributor in distinguishing those women who had *never* had a Pap test. Marital status was a significant predictor in two of the three models involving never having had a Pap test (Models 5 and 6). Model 5 indicates that single women (i.e., single, divorced, separated and widowed) are 10 times more likely to have never had a Pap test relative to married women (i.e., married women and women living common law) (OR = 10.1, CI = 2.3, 45). This pattern is repeated in

TABLE VII

Code definitions for Table VIII

Code		Definition
Age	AGE(1)	18–29 years vs. 60–69 years
	AGE(2)	30–39 years vs. 60–69 years
	AGE(3)	40–49 years vs. 60–69 years
	AGE(4)	50–59 years vs. 60–69 years
Income	INC(1)	lowest vs. highest
	INC(2)	lower-middle vs. highest
	INC(3)	middle vs. highest
	INC(4)	upper-middle vs. highest
Education	EDUC(1)	less than high school vs. greater than high school
	EDUC(2)	high school graduation vs. greater than high school
Immigrant status		immigrant vs. non-immigrant
Disability		restriction of activity vs. no restriction of activity
Marital status		live-in partner vs. no live-in partner
Employ status	EMP(1)	currently working vs. have not worked in previous 12 months
	EMP(2)	not currently working vs. have not worked in previous 12 months

Model 6 where women without a live-in partner are 22 times more likely to have never had a Pap test (compared to having had a recent Pap test) than women with live-in partners (OR = 22, CI = 3.4, 143).

Education played a smaller role in distinguishing those women who had *never* had a Pap test (since the education variable was significant in only one of the models involving never having had a Pap test). Women with a high school education were 7.5 times more likely to have never had a Pap test when compared to women with more than a high school education.

Finally, in terms of the recency of receiving a previous Pap test (Model 8), age was the only significant predictor. With increasingly older age groups, the likelihood of a woman having had a *non-recent*

Pap test increased. In fact, women aged 60 to 69 were over 10 times more likely to have not had a recent Pap test than women aged 18 to 29 (OR = 10.8, CI = 2.8, 41.6).

DISCUSSION

It is clear that certain social and economic factors are influential in determining participation in cancer screening in Prince George. This study has identified that social and economic factors are not associated with receipt of a previous mammogram; yet, in contrast, immigrant status, marital status, education and age are associated with receipt of a previous Pap test. Specifically, women are more likely to have *never* had a Pap test if they are immigrants, single or less educated. For those women who have had previous Pap tests, age is associated with the *recency* of the last Pap test.

Social Determinants of Mammography Use in Prince George

Participation in mammography screening in Prince George (63% of the target population) is considerably higher than that reported by 1996 BC Provincial Health Officer (37% of the target population). High participation rates in Prince George are possibly due to the long history and central location of Prince George's screening clinic. The Screening Mammography Program of BC (SMPBC) opened a permanent clinic at Prince George Regional Hospital in 1991 (personal communication, S. Ottesen, March 3, 1999). Therefore, at the time this data was collected (1994), the clinic had been in full operation for 3 years. Mammography clinics in many other parts of the province were not built until 1994–1995; therefore, participation in other regions were likely not as high as in Prince George, simply because screening services were not yet available in these areas. Higher participation in mammography screening in Prince George might also be due to the higher mortality due to breast cancer in this region, as discussed earlier. It is possible that education and recruitment strategies for mammography screening have been enhanced for Prince George and its surrounding areas, which have been identified as high risk areas for breast cancer.

None of the seven social and economic variables seem to be associated with previous participation in screening mammography. This

TABLE VIII

Odds Ratios for Significant Models – Association between social and economic factors and receipt of Pap test

Predictors	Model 5 NEVER vs. EVER			Model 6 NEVER vs. RECENT			Model 7 NEVER vs. NON-RECENT			Model 8 NON-RECENT vs. RECENT		
	p	OR	CI (95%)	p	OR	CI (95%)	p	OR	CI (95%)	p	OR	CI (95%)
Age	**0.91**			**0.82**			**0.60**			**0.01**		
AGE(1)	0.85	1.2	(0.2, 6.7)	0.57	0.57	(0.1, 3.9)	0.29	5.3	(0.24, 118)	0.03	3.5	(1.2, 10.4)
AGE(2)	0.73	0.00	(0.00, ∞)	0.73	0.00	(0.00, ∞)	0.73	0.00	(0, ∞)	0.01	4.8	(1.6, 14.7)
AGE(3)	0.80	0.78	(0.1, 5.5)	0.38	0.36	(0.04, 3.4)	0.89	0.81	(0.04, 14.8)	0.04	3.7	(1.1, 12.7)
AGE(4)	0.62	0.58	(0.7, 4.9)	0.27	0.27	(0.03, 2.8)	0.55	3.4	(0.06, 185)	0.00	10.8	(2.8, 41.6)
Income	**0.45**			**0.35**			**0.43**			**0.96**		
INC(1)	0.63	0.59	(0.07, 5.1)	0.52	0.47	(0.05, 4.7)	0.76	1.8	(0.04, 74.3)	0.82	0.81	(0.12, 5.5)
INC(2)	0.12	0.15	(0.01, 1.6)	0.05	0.06	(0.0, 0.98)	0.90	0.77	(0.01, 48.5)	0.48	0.60	(0.14, 2.5)
INC(3)	0.54	0.59	(0.1, 3.3)	0.26	0.33	(0.05, 2.2)	0.90	1.2	(0.07, 21.7)	0.47	0.68	(0.24, 1.9)
INC(4)	0.19	0.30	(0.05, 1.8)	0.25	0.33	(0.05, 2.2)	0.20	0.12	(0.00, 3.0)	0.58	0.77	(0.31, 1.9)

TABLE VIII

Continued

Predictors	Model 5 NEVER vs. EVER			Model 6 NEVER vs. RECENT			Model 7 NEVER vs. NON-RECENT			Model 8 NON-RECENT vs. RECENT		
	p	OR	CI (95%)	p	OR	CI (95%)	p	OR	CI (95%)	p	OR	CI (95%)
Education	**0.16**			**0.05**			**0.28**			**0.09**		
EDUC(1)	0.34	2.0	(0.5, 7.9)	0.14	3.1	(0.68, 14)	0.34	0.32	(0.03, 3.3)	0.03	2.4	(1.1, 5.1)
EDUC(2)	0.06	4.1	(0.97, 17)	0.02	7.5	(1.4, 39)	0.45	2.7	(0.21, 34)	0.90	1.1	(0.43, 2.6)
Immigrant status	0.00	7.1	(1.9, 26)	**0.01**	7.5	(1.8, 31)	**0.00**	62	(3.8, 1017)	**0.39**	0.63	(0.22, 1.8)
Disability	0.57	0.64	(0.13, 3.1)	**0.33**	0.37	(0.05, 2.7)	**0.99**	1.0	(0.1, 10)	**0.72**	1.1	(0.55, 2.4)
Marital status	**0.00**	10.1	(2.3, 45)	**0.00**	22	(3.4, 143)	**0.08**	0.07	(0.00, 1.4)	**0.67**	0.84	(0.38, 1.9)
Employ status	**0.38**			**0.35**			**0.15**			**0.22**		
EMPLOY(1)	0.33	0.50	(0.12, 2.1)	0.15	0.31	(0.06, 1.5)	0.92	1.2	(0.07, 18.5)	0.76	0.88	(0.39, 2.0)
EMPLOY(2)	0.65	1.5	(0.29, 7.4)	0.68	0.67	(0.10, 4.5)	0.09	16	(0.54, 401)	0.19	2.0	(0.71, 5.5)

implies that women are participating in mammography services regardless of their social background. Yet, 35% of women aged 40 to 79 years have never been screened for breast cancer, suggesting the presence of barriers other than those examined in this study. Other research has suggested that an important predictor of participation in regular mammography screening is a reminder (i.e., letter or telephone call from the screening facility or physician's office) of an upcoming recommended screening date. In fact, physician recommendation has been found to be the primary predictor of regular participation in mammography screening (Johnson et al., 1996; Potvin et al., 1995; Rimer et al., 1991). Physician recommendation plays such an important role in predicting participation in mammography screening that it is likely to overcome many of the factors associated with low participation, including socio-economic factors (Beaulieu et al., 1996).

Clearly, more research needs to be conducted in order to determine the existing barriers to mammography services. Still, it is important to remember that participation in mammography in Prince George is comparatively high; in fact, almost half of the women in the target population have had *recent* mammograms. Given the comparatively high participation in Prince George, it might be wise to study the factors that are *facilitators* to mammography screening in this population. This might allow insight into ways in which participation can be further improved.

Social Determinants of Pap Test Use in Prince George

Eighty-five percent of women in Prince George have *ever* had a Pap test, a participation rate that is the same as the BC average reported by the 1996 Provincial Health Officer. In fact, in Prince George, 72% of women reported having had a *recent* Pap test. It appears that women are being well served by Pap test screening services in Prince George. However, while a large percentage of women have been screened, this percentage varies across social groups. Immigrant women, single women, and women with less education are over represented among women who have *never* had a Pap test.

When compared to Canadian born women, immigrant women in Prince George are at higher risk of having *never* received a Pap test. This pattern has specific relevance for BC where almost one-third of the population is immigrant. Furthermore, BC has the fastest growing immigrant population in Canada, the population having grown 25% since 1991 (BC Statistics, 1996). In terms of Pap test screening, the large and fast growing immigrant population means a likely future increase in the numbers of women who are not receiving Pap tests. An appropriate course of action to curb this problem might involve the development of Pap test education and recruitment programs specifically for immigrant women; or more precisely, the development of programs for particular groups of immigrant women.

Marital status proved to be another important predictor of having *never* had a Pap test; single women had a much greater likelihood of *never* having had a Pap test when compared to married and common-law women. The interpretation of this finding is complex. If underuse of screening services is limited to single women who are *not* sexually active, then this may not pose a serious public health problem (Calle et al., 1993). Although all women should begin Pap test screening at age 18, in accordance with the Canadian Guide to Clinical Preventive Health (1994), the most important risk factor for cervical cancer is sexual activity. Therefore, it isn't vitally important for women who are not sexually active to be receiving Pap tests, especially if these women are young. However, certainly there are a large number of single women in the population who are sexually active, yet are not receiving Pap test screening. This poses a more acute public health problem since these women double their risk for cervical cancer if they are sexually active and not being screened.

Unfortunately, there was no ability for this study to include a measure of sexual activity. Therefore, the significance of the marital status variable in the context of this study is two-fold. First, in a positive sense, women in Prince George who are in married relationships and therefore probably participating in regular sexual activity are receiving Pap tests as recommended. Second, there is a large group of women in Prince George, over the age of 18 and therefore in the target population to have Pap tests, who have never had Pap tests. This group likely consists of (1) women who need to be receiving Pap tests, that is those who are sexually active and are not being screened and (2) women who do not necessarily need to be receiving Pap tests, that is those who are not sexually active. It is likely that the first situation is the more common since, according to the BC Provincial Health Officer (1995), fifty-two percent of girls age 17 years have had sexual intercourse.

The other predictor of having *never* received a Pap test was education; women with a high school education were more likely to have *never* had a Pap test when compared to women with more than a high school education. The education effect in this study was unusual since there is no effect when comparing women with less than a high school education to women with more than a high school education; however the general effect of education has been found in previous research (Katz and Hofer, 1994; Goel, 1994). This effect suggests that public health education regarding Pap test screening should be presented in a manner that is functional for those with less education. Previous research has suggested that educational literature regarding cancer screening should be written in a language equivalent to the sixth grade reading level and, in fact, that one-to-one personal contact is sometimes necessary to ensure participation when trying to encourage those with less education (Harper, 1993).

It is important to point out that only 5% of women in this sample have *never* had a Pap test. Therefore, significant social determinants of previous screening, such as immigrant status, marital status and education, are relevant for a small, specific group of women. This is not to negate the important role that these factors play in determining previous Pap test screening. Indeed, it is very clear that certain groups of women in Prince George need to be recruited into Pap test screening programs. However, in terms of overall participation in Pap test screening, most women in Prince George are receiving the screening that is recommended.

Finally, age was the only predictor associated with the *recency* of previous Pap tests; women in older age groups were less likely to have received a recent Pap test. Previous research has suggested that, with age, women are likely to become less sexually active and less importance is placed on reproductive health; thereby women attend screening examinations less frequently (Calle et al., 1993; Ives et al., 1996). However, other researchers suggest that the idea of women being less sexually active is false and simply reflects a larger encompassing social myth about older women (McKeever and Martinson,

1986). Older women are often stereotyped as inactive "grannies" who have poor health and are sexually inactive or uninterested (McKeever and Martinson, 1986). It is possible that older women internalize stereotypes such as this and consequently place less importance on their own sexual health. As a result, older women may participate in Pap test screening less regularly. It may be prudent for public education strategies to emphasize the importance of Pap test screening regardless of sexual activity, especially with respect to older women who are at increasingly higher risk of cancer, due to their age. Thirteen percent of women in this study had not received a recent Pap test; this represents a potentially large group of the Prince George population of women at increased risk for cervical cancer.

It is important to note that the predictors of Pap test screening are different for women who have *never* been screened versus women who have not been screened *recently*. This highlights the complexity of predictors for participation in screening practices and suggests that education and recruitment strategies should be tailored for different functions. In other words, to increase *re-screening*, older women should be targeted, yet to increase *screening in general*, immigrant, single and less educated women should be targeted.

Relationship Between Mammography and Pap Test Participation

A final element to the discussion about participation rates in preventive screening practices is the relationship between mammography and Pap test use. For example, in this study, women having had recent mammograms are nine times more likely to have also had recent Pap tests. It is not common for research in this field to examine determinants of *both* Pap tests and mammography, which seems to signify a gap in preventive health research considering that both practices are similar components of preventive health. There is a possible need to re-conceptualize participation in preventive screening practices: no longer should Pap test and mammography exist as separate entities, but as equal and related components of preventive health. For example, in light of the findings of this study, older women who do not participate in Pap tests on a regular basis may be encouraged to do so if they are participating in regular mammography screening. If the importance of both practices is emphasized, the factors determining the participation in one test may lead to the participation in the other also.

Unfortunately, the health care system is not designed to accommodate screenings for different types of cancer at one time. It is difficult for a woman to obtain a Pap test at the same time that she comes in for a mammogram, simply because these two screening tests are offered through different components of the health care system. Having to return for a second screening test creates time, transportation, and financial problems for women.

CONCLUSION

Clearly, an important determinant of a good quality of life is good health. Considering the complex determinants of health, improving health in the population is a complicated and difficult task. Improving access to health services is one means through which population health can be improved; however as this study suggests, improving access to health services is complicated and involves more than providing free financial access. This study has identified specific groups in the population that do not participate in cancer screening programs despite free financial access to these programs. For these groups, efforts should be made to encourage participation in order to ensure better health, and ultimately a good quality of life.

REFERENCES

Beaulieu, M. D., F. Beland, D. Roy, M. Falardeau and G. Hebert: 1996, 'Factors determining compliance with screening mammography', Canadian Medical Association Journal 154(9), pp. 1335–1343.

British Columbia Provincial Health Officer: 1995, 'Women's health feature report', in A Report on the health of British Columbians: Provincial Health Officers Annual Report 1995 (Ministry of Health and Ministry Responsible for Seniors, Victoria, BC).

British Columbia Provincial Health Officer: 1996, A Report on the Health of British Columbians: Provincial Health Officers Annual Report 1996 (Ministry of Health and Ministry Responsible for Seniors, Victoria, BC).

British Columbia Statistics: 1996, Special Feature: BC Immigrant Population, Ethnicity and Language [On-Line]. Available: http://www.bcstats.ca/reports

Calle, E. E., W. D. Flanders, M. J. Thun and L. M. Martin: 1993, 'Demographic predictors of mammography and pap smear screening in U.S. women', American Journal of Public Health 83, p. 53.

Canadian Task Force on the Periodic Health Examination, Health Canada: 1994, The Canadian Guide to Clinical Preventive Health Care (Minister of Supply and Services, Ottawa).

Center for Disease Control and Prevention: 1996, CDC Prevention Guidelines: Effectiveness [On-Line]. Available: http://hwcweb.hwc.ca/hpb/lcdc/hp_eng.html.

Clay, M. G., T. G. Hislop, L. Kan, I. A. Olivotto and L. J. Warren-Burhenne: 1994, 'Screening mammography in British Columbia: 1988–1993', The American Journal of Surgery 167, pp. 490–492.

Cohen, J.: 1992, 'A power primer', Psychological Bulletin 112(1), pp. 155–159.

Deschamps, M., P. R. Band, T. G. Hislop, H. F. Clarke, J. M. Smith, V. Ng and M. Math: 1992, 'Barriers to cervical cytology screening in native women in British Columbia', Cancer Detection and Prevention 16(5/6), pp. 337–339.

Goel, V.: 1994, 'Factors associated with cervical cancer screening: results from the Ontario Health Survey', Canadian Journal of Public Health 85, pp. 125–127.

Harper, P.: 1993, 'Mammography utilization in the poor and medically underserved', Cancer 72(4), pp. 1478–1482.

Health Canada: 1998, Cervical Cancer in Canada [On-Line]. Available: http://www.hc-sc.gc.ca/main/lcdc/web/bc/updates/cervix_e.html

Ives, D. G., J. R. Lave, N. D. Traven, R. Schulz and L. H. Kuller: 1996, 'Mammography and pap smear use by older rural women', Public Health Reports 111, pp. 244–250.

Johnson, M. M., T. G. Hislop, L. Kan, A. J. Coldman and A. Lai: 1996, 'Compliance with the Screening Mammography Program of British Columbia: will she return?' Canadian Journal of Public Health 87(3), pp. 176–179.

Katz, S. J. and T. P. Hofer: 1994, 'Socioeconomic disparities in preventive care persist despite universal coverage', JAMA: Journal of the American Medical Association 272, pp. 530–534.

McKeever, L. and I. M. Martinson: 1986, 'Older women's health care', in D. K. Kjervik and I. M. Martinson (eds.), Women in Health and Illness (WB Sanders, New York).

Pender, N. J.: 1987. Health Promotion in Nursing Practice (Appleton and Lange, Stanford).

Potvin, L., J. Camirand and F. Beland: 1995, 'Patterns of health services utilization and mammography use among women aged 50 to 59 years in the Quebec Medicare System', Medical Care 33(5), pp. 515–530.

Rimer, B. K., B. Trock, P. F. Engstrom, C. Lerman and E. King: 1991, 'Why do some women get regular mammograms?' American Journal of Preventive Medicine 7(2), pp. 69–74.

Snider, J., J. Beauvais, I. Levy, P. Villenueve and J. Pennock: 1996, 'Trends in mammography and pap smear utilization in Canada Chronic Diseases in Canada 17(3–4), pp. 108–117.
Statistics Canada: 1995, National Population Health Survey (NPHS): Public Use Microdata File Ddocumentation, 1994–1995 (Health Statistics Division, Statistics Canada, Ottawa).

University of British Columbia Bruno D. Zumno

University of Northern British Columbia Joanne Bryant
Annette J. Browne
Sylvia Barton

SYLVIA S. BARTON

ASPECTS OF THE EFFECT OF SUBSTANCE USE ON HEALTH, WELLNESS AND SAFETY OF EMPLOYEES AND FAMILIES IN NORTHERN REMOTE WORK SITES

ABSTRACT. The Northern B.C. Business Council on Substance Abuse, a non-profit organization in northern British Columbia, has been active in promoting healthy drug free workplace initiatives over the past six years. It has a membership of 71 business, industry and labour organizations throughout northern B.C. Many of its membership rely directly or indirectly on remote work site employment. In the past couple of years, a key issue raised by their membership is that an increase of substance availability and tolerance in remote work sites not only exists, but is having a negative impact on employee health and safety, increasing Workers' Compensation Board costs, increasing company sick time or leaves of absence, reducing productivity, with a trickle down affect into families and communities. The paper discusses aspects of the effect of substance use on health, wellness and safety of employees and families in northern remote work sites. A view of how the economic sectors of mining, oil and gas, forestry, transportation and exploration are affected is shared. Experiences of the ways northern families and communities are dependent and personally impacted by this type of work are raised. Some of the challenges and rewards inherent in addressing the costs of substance abuse in this type of workforce are voiced. The paper concludes with a description of a pioneer research initiative that intends to find "northern solutions" to address substance use and quality-of-work-life issues.

My interest in the effect of substance use on health and illness began early in my practice (nursing), where I cared for post-operative patients recovering from abdominal surgery and where withdrawal and addiction behaviours were a challenging component. It continued with emergency and intensive care patients who experienced alcohol and other drug-related injuries, accidents, acute illnesses and long-term disabilities. The issue was reflected in the community, as clients at home experienced chronic illness and mental health problems resulting from long-standing substance abuse. Most recently, through practice in outpost settings, I have viewed the world of addictions from a northern and remote perspective. Substances used may have changed as a result of

Social Indicators Research **60:** 263–274, 2002.

external patterns and pressures but the devastating outcomes to children, families and communities remain unchanged in terms of fetal alcohol effect/syndrome (FAE/FAS), children experiencing dysfunctional parenting, families torn by issues exacerbated by alcohol and other drugs, and communities struggling to deal with the aftermath.

Relative to this topic, my university appointment has offered me an opportunity to provide a research partnership with the Northern B.C. Business Council on Substance Abuse, a non-profit organization in northern B.C., which has been active in promoting healthy drug-free workplace initiatives over the past 6 years. It has a membership of 71 business, industry and labour organizations throughout northern B.C., many of whom rely directly or indirectly on remote camp work. Over the past few years, a key issue raised by their membership is that an increase of substance availability and tolerance in remote work sites not only exists, but is having a negative impact on employee health and safety, increasing Workers' Compensation Board costs, increasing company sick time or leaves of absence, reducing productivity, with a trickle down affect into families and communities.

In particular, the economic sectors of mining, oil and gas, forestry, transportation and exploration are dependent upon employment within remote work sites. Of grave concern are issues concerning the safety of employees and the use of alcohol, illicit drugs such as marihuana and licit drugs such as amphetamines being available and tolerated while on the job. For even the mildest degree of impairment existing within these workplaces could be catastrophic.

These remote work sites pose unique challenges, where employers and unions continue to look for guidance. For example, it is not unheard of for a company desperately in need of workers to drug test, find them all positive, and then hire them two weeks later because of the company's inability to recruit, and difficulties keeping within expected time-lines.

This paper examines aspects of substance use on the health, wellness and safety of employees in northern remote work sites. Shared is a view of how these economic sectors are affected. Experiences of the ways families and communities are dependent and personally impacted by this work are raised. Challenges and rewards inherent in addressing the costs of substance abuse in this type of workforce are voiced. The paper concludes with a description of a pioneer research initiative that intends to find "northern solutions" to address substance use and quality-of-work-life issues.

WORKPLACE PREVALENCE OF ALCOHOL AND OTHER DRUG PROBLEMS

Recalled from the past is the long-standing association of the workplace with the use and abuse of alcohol. British employers in the 18th century dispensed liquor to workers in lieu of wages, which became known as the "gin epidemic." British sailors continued to receive daily rations of rum into this century. More recently in the corporate workplace, the "liquid lunch" is an acceptable way of doing business. We have read about the transportation sector's use of amphetamines by cross-country truckers, which was not seriously discouraged as long as it meant getting products to their destination quicker than the competition. Then, on the coat-tails of a well-established pattern of permissiveness around licit drugs, came the illicit drug use of the '60s and '70s, which found its way into factories and boardrooms throughout Canada and the U.S.A. Employers are now confronted with different kinds of substances whose physical and psychological effects are more varied and unfamiliar than those of alcohol (Naegle, 1996).

Mounting Evidence

In Canada, recent national use surveys, provincial workplace research and industry-specific studies provide mounting evidence of the extent and consequences of substance abuse in our workplaces. In a survey of Canadian CEO's, 92% of respondents viewed substance abuse as having a significant impact in the Canadian workplace at large, with 16% viewing it as very significant. Alcohol was of most concern to 50% and one third felt that alcohol, illicit drugs and prescription drugs are of equal concern. Only 4% indicated that substance abuse was of no concern at all to their organization. Eighty-five percent believe substance abuse, if it exists in their workforce, will create a potential liability to their organization.

They frequently cite employee safety, employee morale and public safety as areas of potential liability (Hauserman, 1990).

Impairment due to drug and alcohol use by employees within the natural resource industries results in accidents, injury, anxiety and/or emotional distress. For example, responses to stimulant drugs such as cocaine and amphetamine-like substances result in restlessness, problems with task completion and irritability. However, health problems resulting from long term effects of heavy drinking usually are the precipitating factors in employees seeking consultation at the health service. These are typically disorders that include anxiety, gastritis, fatigue, and weight loss (Monfils, 1995).

A comprehensive Canadian survey of 18 000 people employed in transportation safety-sensitive positions in air, marine and surface (truck/bus) indicated that the percentage of people using drugs was similar to the general population. Public-sector marine employees were the exception, self-reporting a cannabis use rate of between 7 and 17% in the past 12 months. In each of the occupations studied, a relatively small group, usually under 5%, reported using substances while at work or just prior to work (Transport Canada, 1990).

The B.C. Trucking Association conducted a random survey and anonymous urine testing. On a typical work day, 2% reported they might drink during work hours or on a meal break. When asked about occasional use during their shifts or meal breaks, 17% indicated they sometimes have one or more drinks and 4% might use marihuana on work days (University of Toronto Faculty of Medicine, 1990).

A random national survey of people in positions critical to railway safety reported levels of alcohol use higher than those for the general public, with some workers reporting that they were coming to work either under the influence, or feeling the effects, of alcohol. While other drug use was comparatively small, most of those using illicit substances were doing so virtually every day. Over one-third felt that drug use by railway workers had, at some time, compromised safety on the job (Transport Canada, 1989).

In a major Imperial Oil study, 7% of employees reported that they had or currently have a substance abuse problem. Alcohol was seen by 78% of employees as the substance causing the greatest number of problems in the workplace. Accidents in which substance use by a member of the employee's work group was perceived to be a factor were reported by 3.3% and 41 "near misses" were reported by 7.2% of employees. Negative effects, other than accidents and "near misses," were reported by 22.5% of employees (Imperial Oil Limited, 1991).

Bringing together information about the many facets of substance abuse such as drug use, health and legal consequences of use, treatment, and law enforcement has recently been seen as essential for the development, implementation and evaluation of effective strategies. Fortunately, improved standards of living in North America have been accompanied by a desire to improve the overall quality-of-life, including the quality-of-work-life. Legislation, research and employer work practices have gradually supported efforts towards such objectives. However, quality-of-work-life depends on the provision of working conditions which match the employee as well as fulfilling production criteria. These include conditions that are not only promoted by humanitarian motives, but also by considerations of productivity and economy.

The economic sectors of natural resources need a view that reflects a company's philosophy, placing emphasis on basic workplace principles. These important principles include: work should take place in a safe and healthy work environment; conditions of work should be consistent with workers' well-being and human dignity; and work should offer real possibilities for personal achievement, self-fulfillment and service to society (Rice et al., 1997). No doubt there is a strong interest being shown by these sectors in improving working conditions. However, it is confounded by remote work sites that, for example, require workers to leave their communities and work 12 hour shifts and 42 days straight before having 14 days off. It is also severely hindered by the lack of knowledge, methods and techniques recommended by applied research in the behavioural sciences into organizational, management and technical solutions.

On that note, it is of no surprise that the 1995 World Competitiveness Report, prepared by the World Economic Forum and the International Institute for Management Development, showed that Canada moved up to 12th position among 48 countries in overall competitiveness, but ranked a distant 40th in the category of alcohol and drug abuse in the workforce as reported in the Toronto Star, September 6, 1995.

IMPACT ON FAMILIES AND COMMUNITIES

With substance availability and tolerance in the workplace and society so prevalent, there is a need to address substance use in northern remote work sites through a broad framework. One that not only includes the experiences of employees but includes the experiences of their families as well. Paramount to understanding substance use in the workplace, in my opinion, is the notion that there is a relationship between employee behaviours at work and their behaviours at home. The two environments are not separate but highly interdependent. Would investigating the relationship between work and home help us understand substance use in northern remote work sites?

Related Research

Some recent work through the Institute of Social and Economic Research at Memorial University of Newfoundland that addresses the relationships between home and work has been done relative to Newfoundland oil workers' responses to offshore employment (Storey and Shrimpton, 1993). Described in the Iser Offshore Oil Project (based primarily on North Sea oil and Canadian mining industry research) were the reactions of Newfoundland workers and their spouses to work on exploration rigs and supply boats, with discussions of the implications of this for social, psychosocial and cultural aspects of health and safety. In these and earlier studies by Eide et al. (1985), the relationships between work-related stress, health and safety were found to be complex.

Among the relationships were disorders such as cardiovascular diseases, gastrointestinal problems and depression associated with high levels of stress. Sutherland and Cooper (1986) found among most of their sample of North Sea workers a relationship between high levels of job dissatisfaction and anxiety, which they concluded could compromise mental and physiological health, and susceptibility to accidents. Subsequent research into the adoption of similar work patterns by the mining industry has provided additional information on what issues need to be addressed (Storey and Shrimpton, 1993). Possibilities for change focus on work scheduling, hiring and orientation, communications, counseling, personnel policies, and the work culture. Changes related to substance use was not mentioned.

A family life study by Storey et al., 1989, examined the needs of workers and families with respect to a variety of issues, including emotional problems associated with partings and reunions, mood swings, sleep loss and anxiety. Interestingly, there was only brief indication of marital, financial and alcohol-related problems. However, this was supported by Hellesøy (1985) in Norway, who revealed similar problems in other studies of offshore rig and platform workers.

An important theme in these studies is that strategies for coping with remote work site employment were recognized to vary considerably between families. And while they may have directly addressed the relationships between home and work, specific problems influenced by substance use were not examined. My conclusion is that workplace prevalence of alcohol and other drug problems in northern remote work sites is an area ripe for understanding and begs researching.

Substance Use as an Influence

In need of understanding are the areas where substance use could influence or be influenced by the nature and severity of the problems encountered. For example, these may include the rotational schedule of work, particularly its regularity and predictability; length of absence of the spouse; the nature and stress associated with partings and reunions; the family "type" and the degree to which separation upsets the family equilibrium; family experience of and preparedness for the separation; individual characteristics, particularly the ability to be alone; and levels of educational achievement.

Additionally, a study that looked at the outcomes of these problems and the role of substance use as a means of coping could focus on gender employee issues in remote work sites, as well as gender issues exhibited at home. Undoubtedly, these employees and their families face special adaptation issues that warrant investigation and understanding.

CHALLENGES AND REWARDS

There are many possible causes of impairment on the job, including illness, fatigue and emotional distress. The abuse of alcohol and other drugs is a major cause of impairment in Canada, affecting organizations both large and small (Inauqural National Report, 1997). Northern remote work sites are considered to be places where employees are affected particularly hard. It has been estimated that substance abusing workers cost Canadian industry two to three times more than other employees in terms of injuries, accidents and absenteeism (University of Toronto Faculty of Medicine, 1990).

Costs to Society

The extent to which alcohol and other drugs impact industry and workplace efficiency is evidenced by costs to society. The Canadian Centre on Substance Abuse estimates the public costs for alcohol, tobacco and illicit drugs in this country to be $18.45 billion or 2.7% of Canada's GDP. Productivity losses from illness and premature death account for $11.78 billion. The cost to the health care system is more than $4 billion, while law enforcement adds another $1.76 billion (Single et al., 1996). These and other consequences of substance abuse such as injury to others, theft, and employee morale pose real challenges for employers, employees, and the public in Canada.

Nature of the Work

Challenges are also found in the very nature of work in remote work sites that may actually contribute to problems. Employee stress, long hours, boredom and shift work have been identified as contributing to substance abuse problems (Transport Canada, 1990). In Alberta, a study of workers, employers and unions indicated some work design characteristics are positively associated with higher levels of alcohol consumption. Shift work, job-related travel, working at a remote site, and boredom on the job are associated with higher than average levels of drinking (Alberta Alcohol and Drug Abuse Commission, 1992).

Corporate Drug Policy

The rewards usually lie in a corporate drug policy being developed in a way that meets the needs of the employer, the public and the various employee groups, such as union representatives, work groups, front-line supervisors, senior managers, occupational safety and health divisions, security and the legal department. By integrating these needs, the goals of a comprehensive policy can then be established. The goals have the potential to reflect any one of a number of concerns such as improving productivity or reducing costs, improving employee and public safety, promoting employee health, reducing environmental risks or following industrial, community or union trends. Rewards also lie in Employee Assistance Programs that are based on the principle that both employees and employers gain from the program (Monfils, 1995). Employees have access to confidential assessment and referrals for professional treatment. Employees who seek help and regain satisfactory performance will have their job security and promotional opportunities protected. Employers gain from increased productivity and quality, lower absenteeism, fewer disciplinary actions, reduced accidents and less turnover.

A PIONEER RESEARCH INITIATIVE

The Northern B.C. Business Council on Substance Abuse has developed an advisory board representative of the community with a designated project coordinator. I am providing a research partnership through the University of Northern British Columbia. Together, we are working towards the development of a project that will explore the impact these northern remote work sites have on health, wellness and safety of employees and families in relation to substance use. To date, some preliminary interviews with wives of some of these employees, completed by the Business Council, have identified issues concerning the safety of their spouse while on the job with respect to illegal drugs being accepted and available in the workplace.

Purpose of the Study

The purpose of the study is to document the experiences of employees and their families as they define the problems of substance use in remote work sites and, where appropriate, to identify and develop recommended solutions to those problems. An attempt will be made to encompass a full range of work and family experiences and their manifestations in relation to substance use. We seek to consider the different reactions and adjustments to remote work site employment which depend on occupational, social and personal influences that may or may not result in substance use.

Research Approach

From a questionnaire survey of male and female employees and their families, personal interviews and focus groups, attitudes and responses to substance use will be explored. It is anticipated that the data collected will provide insight into many of the unique problems related to substance use experienced by workers who rely upon employment in remote work sites and which indirectly affect their families. It is intended that the overall findings will: enable some of the problems and issues identified to be prevented; propose measures that serve to mitigate the negative consequences of substance use; and serve to enhance already successful adaptive responses. With this information, many of the key stakeholders and partners with this project hope to see the "big picture" with respect to understanding the issues of substance use in remote work sites with an eye on implementing some "northern solutions."

CONCLUSION

Workplace prevalence of alcohol and other drug problems in remote work sites is not well understood. Information about the many facets of substance abuse such as drug use, health and legal consequences of use, treatment, and law enforcement needs to be brought together as essential elements for the development, implementation and evaluation of effective strategies. Many questions related to substance use in this area need to be raised by government, industry, labour, social and health agencies, as well as academia.

The extent to which alcohol and illicit drugs impact industries and workplace efficiency is beginning to be documented in certain areas by the criterion of cost to society. Today, the issue of increased substance availability and tolerance in remote work sites requires attention to and understanding of the influencing social, psychosocial and work culture factors. To this end, a pioneer research initiative in Prince George, B.C. is about to explore this high stakes domain.

REFERENCES

Alberta Alcohol and Drug Abuse Commission: 1992, Substance Use and the Alberta Workplace: Summary Report (Alberta Alcohol and Drug Abuse Commission, Edmonton, Alberta).

Eide, R., O. H. Hellesøy and A. C. Gogstad: 1985, 'Associations between experiences of environmental factors and health', in O. H. Hellesøy, (ed.), Work Environment Statfjord Field: Work Environment, Health and Safety on a North Sea Platform (Universitetsforlaget, Oslo, Norway), pp. 371–324.

Hauserman, J.: 1990, Substance Abuse in the Workplace – The Results of Mercer's Nationwide Opinion Survey of Canadian CEOs (William M. Mercer Ltd., Toronto, Ontario).

Hellesøy, O. H. (ed.): 1985, Work Environment Statfjord Field: Work Environment, Health and Safety on a North Sea Platform (Universitetsforlaget, Oslo, Norway).

Imperial Oil Limited: 1991, Substance Use and the Workplace Survey of Employees (Canadian Facts, Ottawa).

Inaugural National Report: 1997, Canadian Community Epidemiology Network on Drug Use (CCENDU) (Ottawa).

Monfils, M. K.: 1995; 'Needs assessment and implementation of an employee assistance program: promoting a healthier work force', AAOHN Journal 43(5), pp. 263–269.

Naegle, M. A.: 1996, 'Alcohol and other drug abuse: identification and intervention', AAOHN Journal 44(9), pp. 454–466.

McKenzie, D. and E. Single: 1997, Canadian Profile: Alcohol, Tobacco & Other Drugs (Canadian Centre on Substance Abuse & Addiction Research Foundation of Ontario, Chapters 2, 3, & 4, pp. 19–91).

Rice, C., R. Longabaugh and R. L. Stout: 1997, 'A comparison sample validation of "your workplace": an instrument to measure perceived alcohol support and consequences from the work environment', Addictive Behaviors 22(5), pp. 711–722.

Single, E., L. Robson, X. Xie and J. Rehm: 1996, The Cost of Substance Abuse in Canada (Canadian Centre on Substance Abuse, Ottawa).

Storey, K., M. Shrimpton, J. Lewis and D. Clark: 1989, Family Life Impacts of Offshore Oil and Gas Employment (Institute of Social and Economic Research Memorial University of Newfoundland, Iser Report No. 4).
Storey, K. and M. Shrimpton (eds.): 1993, Iser Offshore Oil Project: Social, Psychosocial and Cultural Aspects of Health and Safety in the Offshore Oil Industry (Institute of Social and Economic Research Memorial University of Newfoundland).
Sutherland, V. J. and C. L. Cooper: 1986, Man and Accidents Offshore: An Examination of the Costs of Stress Among Workers on Oil and Gas Rigs (Lloyd's List, Dietsmann International NV, Colchester, Essex).
Transport Canada: 1989, Task Force on the Control of Drug and Alcohol Abuse in the Railway Industry: Survey of Persons Employed in Positions Critical to Railway Safety: Final Report (Transport Canada, Ottawa).
Transport Canada: 1990, Substance Use in Transportation: Airports, Aviation, Surface (Bus/Trucking), and Marine: Integrated Report (Heffring Research Group, Toronto, Ontario).
University of Toronto Faculty of Medicine: 1990, Health News: Special Drug Issue (Toronto, Ontario).

University of Northern British Columbia
Prince George, BC
Canada

ABBOTT L. FERRISS

DOES MATERIAL WELL-BEING AFFECT NON-MATERIAL WELL-BEING?

ABSTRACT. Twelve measures of material well-being in the U.S. States were subjected to factor analysis. Four factors emerged: Security, Mastery, Harmony and Autonomy. Five self-reported measures of stress, mental health and general health are regressed upon the four quality of life measures. Only Harmony proved to be significantly associated with the stress-health factors. The elements of Harmony are shown to have a reasonable causative linkage to the stress-health factors. For another demonstration, money income of a representative sample of the U.S. population is shown to be associated with self-reported happiness, but with variation, enabling a classification of the population as to its Well-Being, Dissonance, Adaptation or Deprivation in the income-happiness relationship. Material well-being, thus, is shown to be linked to non-material, self-reported stress and health conditions.

The general purpose of this study is to find ways to improve the quality of life. Comprehending the material-non-material nexus will enable policy-makers to proceed with greater assurance when considering pathways to enhance subjective well-being.

Understanding well-being may be approached by studying material or non-material conditions of life. Material well-being refers to the physical support to life, to the attainments that make acquisition of physical attributes possible, such as education, economic power, good health, etc. Non-material well-being refers to the psychological dimension of living, satisfactions, happiness, enjoyment, etc. Studies have not shown these two dimensions of living to be highly associated (Diener et al., 1997). Material well-being does not always translate into non-material satisfactions. Research is needed to clarify the relationship and identify the conditions under which the material affects the non-material as well as vice-versa.

Measures of the quality of life in the United States by state that identify the material and the non-material conditions are examined. Owing to the paucity of non-material self-reported variables on a

Social Indicators Research **60:** 275–280, 2002.

state-by-state basis, we cannot expect a definitive result but only tentative suggestions, which may be useful in future studies.

In a previously reported study (Ferriss, 1998), twelve indicators were subjected to factor analysis, producing four factors. Identified as Security, Mastery, Harmony and Autonomy, these quality of life domains were then tested for possible association with external influences. An economic hypothesis held economic production to be the source of welfare (Moss, 1979). That was supported by statistically significant correlations between gross state domestic product per capita and Mastery, manufacturing production per capita and Harmony, Agricultural production per capita and both Security and Harmony. An increase 1980–1990 in the labor force was found to be associated with Harmony. Demographic hypotheses found no association between net migration during the past five years (1985–1990) and quality of life, but the percent of the population urban was associated with Security and Mastery.

A hypothesis was tested that the percent of the population of a state adhering to the Judeo-Christian faith would be associated with the quality of life. An association with the Harmony domain supported the hypothesis.

NON-MATERIAL VARIABLES

Turning now to measures of non-material or psychological dimensions of the quality of life, the following indicators are identified. A survey by Landau (Linsky et al., 1995) provides two state-by-state measures of stress: perceived stress, female, and perceived stress, male. From the Behavioral Risk Factor Surveillance System of the Centers for Disease Control and Prevention are three self-reports: average days mental health not good, 1994–1995, percent reporting mental health not good during the past 14 days, and, percent reporting health fair or poor (Centers for Disease Control and Prevention, 19996). These measures of stress, mental health and health do not meet requirements of the generally accepted definition of subjective well-being (SWB). For this reason, "non-material" and "psychological" are used to identify them. They are self-reports of health conditions that reflect well-being of the person.

TABLE I

Multiple regression and correlation (R-Square) of four quality of life components and self-reported health for U.S. states, circa. 1990–1995

	R-Square			
	Security	Mastery	Harmony	Autonomy
Perceived stress, female	0.0112	0.0002	0.1710	0.0008
Perceived stress, male	0.0031	0.0000	0.0005	0.0008
Mean, mental health not good	0.0000	0.0277	0.0092	0.0001
Percent mental health not good	0.0061	0.0032	0.0208	0.0002
Health fair or poor	0.0134	*	0.7207	0.0633
F-ratio of ANOVA	0.35	1.13	24.47	0.76
Probability	0.879	0.279	0.0000	0.586

* Not included in the regression because it is in the Mastery factor.

METHOD

The method of the analysis employs correlation and regression. These are ecological correlations. Relationships established by ecological correlations are not always reproduced with data from individuals (Robinson, 1950; Laughern and Lichtman, 1978). The procedure is to test whether the five self-reported health measures predict each of the four domains of the quality of life. Table I presents the results.

The table shows that the multiple regression produces no significant association between the self-reported health measures and Security, Mastery nor Autonomy, the percentages of the variances common to both being, in each instance, insignificant. The self-reported health measures, however, show a strong correlation with Harmony, owing to the high association of the female stress measure and the general self-report of health.

Harmony is so-named because it reflects a harmonious physical and social environment. The contributors to it are an index of environmental toxins, suicide rate, unemployment rate, crowded housing and income. Rationalizing this association one may say that a toxic environment may contribute to poor health, crowded housing and unemployment could produce stress, a low per capita income

TABLE II

General happiness and family income, U.S. householders, 1996 from general social survey percent of total sample

Family income	N	Very happy	Pretty happy	Not so happy	Total percent
Over $75k	328	5.3	7.0	0.6	12.9
$40k to 70k	685	8.9	15.9	2.2	27.0
$20k to 40k	802	9.4	18.8	3.3	31.5
$10k to 20k	429	4.2	9.9	2.8	17.2
Less than $10k	300	2.2	6.6	3.0	11.8
Total	2544				100.4

Note: The sum of the row totals exceeds 100.0 because of rounding.
Chi Square of frequency distribution = 114.2, df = 8, $P < 0.000$.

might carry with it both stress and poor health, and, finally, the ultimate consequence of these disabilities, suicide. A search of the stress and health literature would show these factors to contribute to poor health and stress (Linsky et al., 1995).

HAPPINESS AND INCOME

While the preceding establishes the domain of the QOL which appears to influence non-material well-being, it does not show the extent to which the population is affected. To gauge this effect, I turn to two widely accepted indicators of material and non-material well-being, namely, money income and happiness.

Table II presents a distribution of the percent of U.S. households (the population 18 years of age and over) in 1996 by general self-reported happiness and family income.

The table shows a statistically significant association between the three broad categories of happiness and family income. The middle income category may be separated into high and low income categories by using the median household income, which in 1996 was $35,492, as the break point. This produces a four-cell matrix of high/low income agains happy/not so happy. This results in the following:

	Happiness	
Income	Happy	Not So Happy
High	*Well-Being* 57.3	*Dissonance* 5.3
Low	30.9 *Adaptation*	6.5 *Deprivation*

While the happiness categories produce only a broad, gross classification, they nevertheless enable the conclusion that material *Well-Being*, as indexed by income, is associated with happiness and characterized more than half the U.S. population in 1996. At the other extreme are 6.5 percent of the population suffering *Deprivation*; their income is low and they are not happy. Some 30.9 percent have happily *Adapted* to their low income status, while 5.3 percent of the population are not happy despite their high income standing, characterized here as a state of *Dissonance*. These descriptors were contrived by Wolfgang Zapf, according to W. Glatzer (Glatzer and Mohr, 1987: p. 17).

SUMMARY

Twelve objective measures of the quality of life were distilled to four components: Security, Mastery, Harmony and Autonomy. Against these components of the quality of life, five stress, mental health and general health self-reported measures were regressed. Only Harmony proved to be significantly associated with the stress-health domain. The elements of Harmony appear to be causative of or consequence of stress and health conditions. The disaggregation of the quality of life index into (four) components illustrates the utility of research in considering separate domains in analysis. Within the limitation of this study, material conditions affect non-material, subjective reactions. To improve the quality o life attention to the material conditions of living should be the first step.

Using a rather gross indicator of happiness, the income-happiness relationship appears sufficiently strong to render a characterization of the U.S. population in 1996 into four categories: Well-Being, Adaptation, Dissonance and Deprivation. While income is but one indicator of material well-being, the use of other indicators in any analysis of the quality of life should consider the possibility of the three types of adaptation.

REFERENCES

Centers for Disease Control and Prevention: 1996, 'BRFSS Summary Prevalence Report' for 1994 and 1995 (Centers for Disease Control and Prevention, National Center for Chronic Disease Prevention and Health Promotion, Behavioral Surveillance Branch, Atlanta) (Mimeographed).

Diener, Ed., Eunkook Suh and Shigehiro Oishi: 1997, 'Recent findings on subjective well-being', Indian Journal of Clinical Psychology (March).

Ferriss, Abbott L.: 1998, 'The quality of life among U.S. states', Social Indicators Research 49, pp. 1–23.

Glatzer, Wolfgang and Hans-Michael Mohr: 1987, 'Quality of life concepts and measurement', Social Indicators Research 19(1), pp. 15–24.

Langern, L. and Allan J. Lichtman: 1978, Ecological Inference (Sage, Beverley Hills).

Linsky, Arnold S., R. Bachman and M. Straus: 1995, Stress, Culture and Aggression (Yale University Press, New Haven & London).

Robinson, William S.: 1950, 'Ecological correlations and the behavior of individuals', American Sociological Review 15 (June), pp. 351–357.

Emory University
1273 Oxford Road NE
Atlanta, GA 30306
U.S.A.
E-mail: aferris@emory.edu

MOHAMED ABDEL-GHANY and STEPHEN J. THOMA

DISTRIBUTION OF HOUSEHOLD INCOME IN AMERICA: EFFECTS OF SOURCE OF INCOME, INFLATION, AND COST OF LIVING DIFFERENTIALS

ABSTRACT. This study focuses on four aspects of the inequality of average household income among the American states. First, we document change in the inequality of nominal average household income between 1979 and 1990. Second, we identify states contributing to the observed inequality. Third, we examine the pattern in state income convergence-divergence when spatial and temporal state price differentials are accounted for. Fourth we provide estimates of impacts of alternative income components on income inequality. We find that inequality in real income is smaller than that in nominal income. Also, we conclude that traditional income measures that exclude transfer payments and other types of income overstate inequality.

INTRODUCTION

The convergence-divergence debate of income differences between the American States provides a continuing challenge to policymakers who must develop and implement policies to reduce these disparities. It has been alleged that faster income growth rates in the South and West in comparison with the Northeast and Midwest in the 1970s were due, in part, to the distribution of federal government funds [1]. These studies note that over a period of five decades beginning in the early 1930s, State differences in household income narrowed greatly. Coughlin and Mandelbaum (1988) [1] report that by 1978, State income inequality had fallen to less than one-third of its 1932 level. Since 1978, however, the trend toward income convergence among states has been reversed.

Many previous studies have attempted to examine interstate income disparity. These studies, however, assumed that spatial and temporal differences in state cost of living and inflation are negligible [2–18]. These studies have to a great extent, been restricted to

Social Indicators Research **60:** 281–297, 2002.

the use of nominal income due to a lack of a state-wide data on cost of living differentials.

Overlooking key differences in spatial and temporal price levels, a host of other studies have tried to assign inequality contributions to various components of income such as labor or property income [19–25]. In recent years, there have been a limited number of studies that attempted to address the issue of State spatial and temporal price differentials [26–29]. After adjusting for price differentials, these studies found much weaker evidence of income divergence among States.

The main purpose of this study is to supplement recent existing work by (1) examining the impact of adjusting for spatial and temporal price differentials on States income convergence-divergence pattern, and (2) providing estimates of impacts of alternative income components on income inequality.

METHODOLOGY

Data

The source of data for this study was the Woods & Poole Economics, Inc. Desktop Data Files [30]. The database on CD-Rom contains some of the Woods & Poole Economics, Inc. regional data and projections for the U.S., regions, Metropolitan Statistical Areas, states, and counties for every year from 1969 through 2020. The analyses in this study are confined to the year 1979 and 1990.

To adjust for cost of living differentials we used the 1979 cost of living index used by Bishop et al. (1994) [26]. Their index computation relies on the Bureau of Labor Statistics Index of Comparative Costs Based on Intermediate Budget for 1977. Unfortunately, this source of data has been discontinued since 1981. Therefore, we relied on a cost of living index developed recently by McMahon [31] for the year 1990.

To adjust for inflation we deflated nominal income by the Bureau of Labor Statistics Regional Consumer Price Index for each state within the specified region [32]. At the present time, there is no comprehensive data available on interstate inflation differentials.

Measure of Inequality

Coefficient of variation (CV) is used in this study as the basic measure of inequality. It is the ratio of the standard deviation of the distribution divided by its mean.

$$CV = \sqrt{v}/\mu$$

Where $v = (1/n)\sum_{i=1}^{51}(y_i - \mu)^2$. Where i = subscript denoting the individual states and y = state household income.

The larger the value of a CV, the more inequality.

Components of Income

Household income was used as the income measure unit. Household income includes:

1. **Wages and salaries** consist of monetary remuneration of employees, commissions, tips, bonuses, and receipts-in-kind that represent income to the recipients.
2. **Other labor income** consists primarily of employer contributions to private pension and private welfare funds.
3. **Proprietors' income** includes inventory valuation and capital consumption adjustments and is defined as the income, including income-in-kind, of proprietorships, partnerships and tax-exempt cooperatives.
4. **Dividend income** is the dividend income of persons from all sources.
5. **Rental income** is the income of persons from the rental of real property, and the royalties received by persons from patents, copyrights, and rights to natural resources.
6. **Personal interest income** is the interest income of persons from all sources.
7. **Transfer payments** are the income of payments to persons, generally in monetary form, for which they do not render services.
8. **Residence adjustment** is the net amount of personal income of persons residing in a specific geographic area but receiving the income outside that geographic area.

These components were grouped as follows: (1) **Earnings** is the sum of wages and salaries, proprietors' income minus residence adjustment, (2) **Other labor income**, (3) **Dividends, interest and rent**, and (4) **Transfer payments**.

Table I shows the percentage of the sources of household income for the fifty states and District of Columbia in 1979 and 1990. Earnings accounted for as low as 56.34% in the state of Montana and as high as 85.46% in the District of Columbia of total household income in 1990. The percentage of other labor income ranged from 3.8 in the District of Columbia to 6.51 in the state of Michigan of total household income in 1990. Dividends, interest, and rent represented only 4.96% of total household income in the District of Columbia, whereas the percentage was as high as 25.65% in the state of Florida in 1990. Households in the District of Columbia received 5.78% of their income in the form of transfer payments. On the other hand, transfer payments comprised 22.42% of total household income in the state of West Virginia in 1990.

EMPIRICAL RESULTS AND DISCUSSION

The results of our adjusting for spatial and temporal price differentials among the American States and District of Columbia are presented in Table II. Average household nominal income (unadjusted income) for 1979 and 1990 are shown in the second and fifth columns. Incomes in the third and sixth columns represent incomes adjusted for spatial price differences (cost of living differences) for 1979 and 1990. Entries in the fourth and seventh columns show real income (incomes adjusted for cost of living as well as the rate of inflation) for 1979 and 1990.

Adopting the classification framework of Coughlin and Mandelbaum (1988) [1], States are grouped according to their 1979-90 change in household income with respect to the national mean. States, in which household income increased (decreased) toward the mean during 1979–1990, are classified as upwardly (downwardly) convergent. On the other hand, those States in which household income increased (decreased) away from the mean are classified as upwardly (downwardly) divergent. As in earlier work [1], States

TABLE I

Percentage of the sources of household income

	1979				1990			
State	Earnings	Other labor income	Dividends, interest and rent	Transfer payments	Earnings	Other labor income	Dividends, interest and rent	Transfer payments
Alabama	68.54	5.96	9.70	15.80	62.73	6.01	13.89	17.36
Alaska	80.93	5.52	6.62	6.93	72.31	5.48	9.44	12.77
Arizona	66.33	5.49	15.08	13.11	61.13	5.11	18.27	15.49
Arkansas	66.40	5.20	11.78	16.61	60.69	5.58	14.99	18.74
California	67.59	5.60	14.35	12.47	65.66	5.74	15.91	12.69
Colorado	70.57	5.29	13.76	10.38	65.30	5.49	17.17	12.08
Connecticut	64.91	6.62	17.21	11.26	63.30	6.23	18.97	11.50
Delaware	70.83	6.75	11.92	10.51	66.74	6.32	16.17	10.77
Dist. of Columbia	85.54	3.17	4.04	7.26	85.46	3.80	4.96	5.78
Florida	58.46	4.70	21.09	15.75	54.22	4.67	25.65	15.46
Georgia	71.07	5.79	10.55	12.59	66.74	6.06	14.67	12.53
Hawaii	70.43	4.74	12.91	11.92	68.34	5.40	13.55	12.71
Idaho	69.04	5.14	13.57	12.25	65.09	4.93	15.58	14.40
Illinois	68.72	6.32	13.81	11.15	63.77	5.94	17.73	12.56
Indiana	69.54	6.96	12.52	10.97	63.54	6.44	16.23	13.79
Iowa	66.70	5.34	16.33	11.63	60.93	5.44	18.69	14.94
Kansas	66.73	5.69	15.18	12.40	60.84	5.55	19.15	14.46
Kentucky	68.12	6.75	10.69	14.44	61.25	6.09	15.61	17.05
Louisiana	70.82	6.44	10.51	12.24	61.93	5.80	15.13	17.14
Maine	64.80	5.51	12.76	16.93	61.24	6.03	16.48	16.25
Maryland	63.29	6.05	15.62	15.04	60.25	5.70	19.28	14.97
Massachusetts	66.06	5.68	13.89	14.38	64.21	5.61	16.38	13.80
Michigan	68.00	8.05	11.65	12.30	61.98	6.51	16.64	14.87
Minnesota	69.19	6.16	13.20	11.44	65.59	5.81	15.78	12.82
Mississippi	68.47	5.34	9.53	16.66	59.72	5.84	13.73	20.71
Missouri	68.96	5.55	13.47	12.01	62.85	5.51	18.07	13.56
Montana	65.62	4.77	16.17	13.45	56.34	4.45	20.39	18.82
Nebraska	68.78	4.84	15.25	11.13	65.11	4.94	17.00	12.96
Nevada	72.31	4.60	12.81	10.29	67.53	4.73	16.13	11.61
New Hampshire	63.07	6.58	16.51	13.84	59.75	6.37	21.18	12.70
New Jersey	62.92	6.56	16.71	13.81	60.94	5.71	20.54	12.81
New Mexico	69.11	5.43	11.71	13.75	61.53	5.57	16.16	16.74
New York	66.08	5.25	14.45	14.23	63.84	4.78	17.03	14.35
North Carolina	71.42	5.60	10.28	12.71	66.47	5.74	14.42	13.36
North Dakota	69.71	3.96	14.88	11.45	61.22	4.12	18.10	16.56
Ohio	69.33	6.48	12.02	12.17	62.68	5.60	15.89	15.83
Oklahoma	68.13	5.63	12.51	13.73	60.37	5.46	16.53	17.64
Oregon	67.92	5.53	14.08	12.47	62.48	5.46	17.40	14.67
Pennsylvania	66.15	6.56	12.08	15.21	60.32	5.81	17.54	16.33
Rhode Island	63.59	5.70	13.77	16.94	59.11	5.79	17.88	17.22
South Carolina	70.73	5.62	9.59	14.06	64.64	5.88	14.04	15.44
South Dakota	68.03	4.04	15.14	12.79	62.85	4.45	17.58	15.11
Tennessee	70.67	5.77	10.20	13.35	65.35	5.92	13.77	14.97
Texas	71.65	6.18	12.07	10.10	65.73	6.13	15.58	12.56
Utah	72.14	5.81	10.68	11.37	67.02	5.92	13.11	13.95
Vermont	65.80	5.39	14.67	14.14	62.24	5.63	18.47	13.67
Virginia	67.02	5.64	13.35	13.99	63.62	5.53	17.67	13.18
Washington	68.95	5.10	13.43	12.51	63.98	4.93	16.78	14.32
West Virginia	66.62	6.71	9.46	17.21	56.58	5.80	15.20	22.42
Wisconsin	67.79	6.08	13.26	12.87	61.62	6.23	17.23	14.91
Wyoming	73.75	5.70	12.66	7.90	61.70	5.01	20.01	13.28

TABLE II

Trend of average total household income

State	1979[1]	1979[2]	1979[3]	1990[1]	1990[2]	1990[3]
Alabama	40.00	43.01	59.41	44.25	49.28	38.53
Alaska	86.92	64.39	88.69	76.69	58.48	44.47
Arizona	48.56	48.56	66.89	48.50	54.19	41.21
Arkansas	38.78	43.09	59.52	41.81	47.15	36.86
California	56.19	54.03	74.42	66.83	56.15	42.70
Colorado	51.58	51.58	71.04	54.36	54.37	41.35
Connecticut	55.16	50.14	68.88	72.05	58.63	43.02
Delaware	57.17	61.47	84.90	66.68	61.79	48.31
District of Columbia	160.88	147.59	203.86	212.43	172.91	135.19
Florida	45.23	47.61	65.76	52.62	55.44	43.35
Georgia	44.84	48.21	66.59	52.80	57.02	44.58
Hawaii	62.83	47.60	65.56	72.99	53.61	40.76
Idaho	44.72	46.59	64.17	47.20	52.54	39.95
Illinois	56.30	56.87	78.33	62.06	60.49	47.48
Indiana	48.01	48.49	66.80	49.23	51.60	40.50
Iowa	48.28	50.29	69.27	48.47	50.86	39.93
Kansas	45.42	47.32	65.17	50.05	52.24	41.01
Kentucky	42.84	47.07	64.84	44.15	47.99	37.52
Louisiana	46.59	50.10	69.00	45.54	50.05	39.13
Maine	41.85	39.85	54.74	49.87	49.38	36.23
Maryland	43.40	45.20	62.44	54.60	51.51	40.27
Massachusetts	52.82	48.01	65.95	69.07	58.54	42.95
Michigan	54.39	54.39	74.92	55.87	57.01	44.75
Minnesota	51.45	52.50	72.32	58.15	58.15	45.64
Mississippi	37.58	42.71	58.99	38.12	44.32	34.65
Missouri	49.29	50.30	69.28	54.01	56.26	44.16
Montana	43.50	45.31	62.41	43.54	47.32	35.99
Nebraska	47.67	49.66	68.40	52.79	56.16	44.08
Nevada	58.96	58.96	81.21	59.89	61.74	46.95
New Hampshire	41.70	39.34	54.04	51.52	49.54	36.35
New Jersey	50.33	45.76	62.85	67.79	56.02	41.10
New Mexico	44.23	45.60	62.80	44.47	49.41	37.57
New York	56.41	51.28	70.44	72.90	65.68	48.18
North Carolina	42.23	45.90	63.40	48.69	50.20	39.25
North Dakota	48.08	50.61	69.71	47.44	52.14	40.92
Ohio	50.57	51.08	70.35	53.29	54.94	43.12
Oklahoma	43.49	46.76	64.59	43.51	46.79	36.58

TABLE II

Continued

State	1979[1]	1979[2]	1979[3]	1990[1]	1990[2]	1990[3]
Oregon	49.44	48.95	67.43	51.20	53.89	40.98
Pennsylvania	50.52	45.92	63.08	55.83	55.83	40.96
Rhode Island	46.39	41.79	57.41	53.60	50.10	36.76
South Carolina	40.85	43.93	60.68	46.21	51.34	40.14
South Dakota	43.61	46.39	63.90	47.63	52.92	41.54
Tennessee	43.01	46.25	63.88	47.93	52.10	40.73
Texas	51.38	54.66	75.50	52.89	56.26	43.99
Utah	48.12	48.12	66.29	50.46	57.34	43.60
Vermont	44.37	40.34	55.41	51.77	51.25	37.60
Virginia	45.42	48.84	67.45	55.21	50.66	39.61
Washington	51.39	49.89	68.72	55.38	55.94	42.54
West Virginia	43.04	47.82	66.05	40.57	44.10	34.48
Wisconsin	49.25	49.25	67.84	51.16	52.74	41.40
Wyoming	58.52	61.60	84.85	50.90	53.58	40.74

[1]Income is in thousands of dollars
[2]Income is in thousands of dollars adjusted for cost of living
[3]Income is in thousands of dollars adjusted for cost of living and inflation

in which change was less than 5% are classified as having no significant change.

The results of convergence/divergence analysis for nominal income are reported in Tables III through V and shown in Figure 1. Each State in the convergent groups contributed toward increasing equality (Table III). The States of Alaska, Colorado, Michigan, Nevada, and Wyoming contributed toward nominal household income equality during the period from 1979 to 1990 due to the downwardly convergent toward the national mean. The States of Maryland, New Hampshire, and Virginia also contributed to increasing equality of income during that period. Their incomes upwardly came closer to the national mean.

Table IV shows the States in the divergent groups. Each State in this group contributed toward household nominal income inequality during the 1979–1990 period. The incomes in the States of Arizona, Idaho, Indiana, Iowa, Kentucky, Louisiana, Mississippi, Montana, New Mexico, North Dakota, Ohio, Oklahoma, Oregon, Texas, Utah,

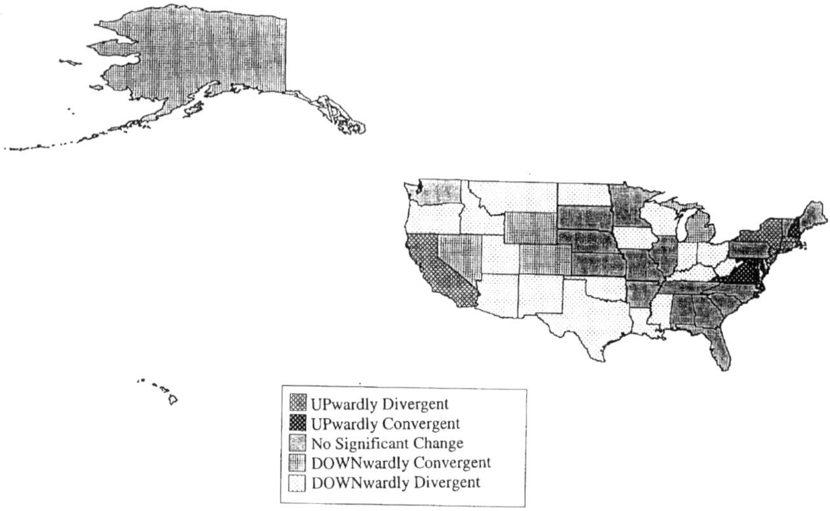

Figure 1. State per capita nominal income movement with respect to national mean 1979–1990.

TABLE III

Convergent states: Household nominal income as a share of national mean

State	Share of national mean (percent)		
	1979	1990	Change
Downward:			
Alaska	172.22	134.67	−37.55
Colorado	102.19	95.46	−6.73
Michigan	107.76	98.11	−9.65
Nevada	116.82	105.16	−11.66
Wyoming	115.95	89.37	−26.58
Upward:			
Maryland	85.98	95.87	9.88
New Hampshire	82.63	90.47	7.84
Virginia	89.99	96.95	6.96

TABLE IV

Divergent states: Household nominal income as a share of national income

State	Share of national mean (percent)		
	1979	1990	Change
Downward:			
Arizona	96.22	85.17	−11.06
Idaho	88.61	82.89	−5.73
Indiana	95.12	86.45	−8.68
Iowa	95.66	85.12	−10.54
Kentucky	84.87	77.97	−7.35
Louisiana	92.31	79.97	−12.34
Mississippi	74.46	66.93	−7.53
Montana	86.18	76.45	−9.73
New Mexico	87.63	78.08	−9.55
North Dakota	95.27	83.31	−11.96
Ohio	100.19	93.57	−6.62
Oklahoma	86.16	76.41	−9.76
Oregon	97.97	89.90	−8.94
Texas	101.80	92.86	−8.94
Utah	95.35	88.60	−6.76
West Virginia	85.27	71.24	−14.03
Wisconsin	97.58	89.83	−7.76
Upward:			
California	111.33	117.35	6.02
Connecticut	109.28	126.52	17.24
District of Columbia	318.76	373.02	54.26
Massachusetts	104.65	121.29	15.04
New Jersey	99.72	119.03	19.30
New York	111.77	128.01	16.24

West Virginia, and Wisconsin decreased away from the national mean. During the same period, however, the income in the States of California, Connecticut, Massachusetts, New Jersey, New York, and the District of Columbia increased away from the national mean.

States with no substantial change (less than 5%) of their nominal household income toward or away from the national mean during the 1979–1990 period are listed in Table V.

TABLE V

States with no significant change: Household nominal income as a share of national mean

State	Share of national mean (percent)		
	1979	1990	Change
Alabama	79.26	77.70	−1.56
Arkansas	76.84	73.41	−3.43
Delaware	113.27	117.09	3.82
Florida	89.61	92.39	2.78
Georgia	88.84	92.72	3.88
Hawaii	124.49	128.17	3.68
Illinois	111.56	108.98	−2.58
Kansas	90.00	87.88	−2.12
Maine	82.91	87.57	4.66
Minnesota	101.94	102.10	0.16
Missouri	97.66	94.83	−2.83
Nebraska	94.46	92.70	−1.76
North Carolina	83.68	85.50	1.82
Pennsylvania	100.09	98.04	−2.05
Rhode Island	91.91	94.12	2.21
South Carolina	80.95	81.14	0.19
South Dakota	86.84	83.63	−2.77
Tennessee	85.22	84.16	−1.06
Vermont	87.92	90.90	2.98
Washington	101.82	97.24	−4.58

Tables VI through VIII and Figure 2 show the convergence/divergence analysis of real household income (adjusted for spatial and temporal price differentials) during the 1979-90 years. The States of California and Delaware joined the previously listed states in the downwardly convergent group (Table VI). It should be noticed that prior to adjusting for spatial and temporal price levels, the State of California was classified among the upwardly divergent States.

The number of upwardly convergent States remained the same after converting nominal household income to real income.

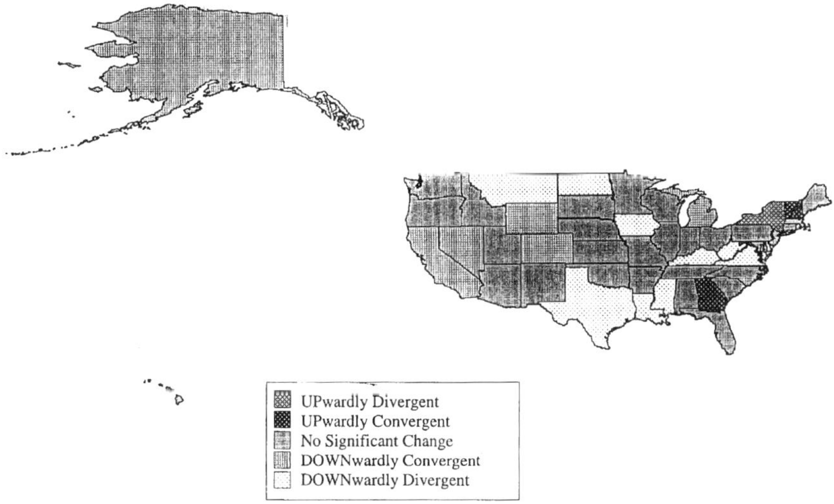

Figure 2. State per capita real income movement with respect to national mean 1979–1990.

TABLE VI

Convergent states: Household real income as a share of national mean

State	Share of national mean (percent)		
	1979	1990	Change
Downward:			
Alaska	127.57	102.07	−25.50
California	107.04	98.01	−9.03
Colorado	102.19	94.90	−7.29
Delaware	122.13	110.89	−11.24
Michigan	107.76	102.71	−5.05
Nevada	116.82	107.76	−9.06
Wyoming	122.05	93.51	−28.54
Upward:			
Georgia	95.78	102.32	6.54
New Hampshire	77.73	83.42	5.69
Vermont	79.71	86.31	6.60

TABLE VII

Divergent states: Household real income as a share of national income

State	Share of national mean (percent)		
	1979	1990	Change
Downward:			
Iowa	99.64	91.63	−8.01
Kentucky	93.27	86.12	−7.15
Louisiana	99.26	89.81	−9.45
Mississippi	84.85	79.53	−5.32
Montana	89.77	82.60	−7.17
North Dakota	100.28	93.93	−6.35
Oklahoma	92.90	83.96	−8.94
Texas	108.60	100.96	−7.64
Virginia	97.03	90.90	−6.13
West Virginia	95.00	79.14	−15.86
Upward:			
District of Columbia	293.24	310.28	17.04
New York	101.33	110.59	9.26

However, the States of Georgia and Vermont replaced the States of Maryland and Virginia.

The results reported in Table VII show that the number of divergent States decreased significantly from 23 to only 12, when household income are adjusted for spatial and temporal price differences. The States of Arizona, Idaho, Indiana, New Mexico, Ohio, Oregon, Utah, and Wisconsin no longer belong to the downwardly divergent group after their incomes were adjusted. That is, the changes in their real incomes were not significant to affect interstate income inequality. It should be noted, however, that the State of Virginia, after income was adjusted, moved from the upwardly convergent group to the downwardly divergent group.

Similarly, the States of California, Connecticut, Massachusetts, and New Jersey were no longer classified as upwardly divergent States after adjusting their incomes. With the exception of the State of California, which as stated earlier, belongs to the downwardly convergent group, the other three States had no significant changes in their real incomes.

The number of States that experienced no significant change in their real household income during the 1979–1990 period was 29. This number is much greater than the 20 States that experienced no significant change in their nominal income (Table VIII).

It is clear from the above reported results that adjusting household income for cost of living differences, and inflation, reduces income interstate inequality and changes the pattern of income distribution among the States.

To examine the effect of broadening the definition of household income on income inequality, we calculated the coefficient of variation for the different components of 1990 real income. When only household earnings were considered, the estimated coefficient of variation amounted to 0.598 (Table IX). Adding the component of 'other labor income' to earnings reduced income inequality by 4.5%, as measured by the coefficient of variation. Broadening the concept of household income to include dividend; interest; and rent in addition to earnings and other labor income, reduced income inequality further by additional 6%. When transfer payments were included in household incomes, income inequality was reduced significantly by an additional 19.9%.

The cumulative reduction in income inequality amounted to 30.4% when household income expanded to include 'other labor income'; dividend, interest, and rent; and transfer payments in addition to earnings. Transfer payments, however, had the greatest effect in this decline.

CONCLUSIONS AND IMPLICATIONS

Much of previous research examining interstate income distribution overlooked key differences in spatial and temporal price levels, an oversight that possibly makes conclusions drawn from these studies as well as resulting policy recommendations very suspect. The results of this study clearly show that adjusting for cost of living differences as well as the rate of inflation reduces interstate household income inequality and alters the pattern of income distribution among the States. The results also show that expanding the

TABLE VIII

States with no significant change: Household real income as a share of national mean

State	Share of national mean (percent)		
	1979	1990	Change
Alabama	85.46	88.43	2.97
Arizona	96.22	94.58	−1.64
Arkansas	85.62	84.60	−1.02
Connecticut	99.07	98.73	−.34
Florida	94.59	99.49	4.90
Hawaii	94.31	93.56	−.75
Idaho	92.30	91.70	−.60
Illinois	112.68	108.98	−3.70
Indiana	96.08	92.96	−3.12
Kansas	93.75	94.12	0.37
Maine	78.74	83.15	4.41
Maryland	89.81	92.43	2.62
Massachusetts	94.87	98.57	3.70
Minnesota	104.02	104.75	0.73
Missouri	99.65	101.35	1.70
Nebraska	98.39	101.18	2.79
New Jersey	90.41	94.33	3.92
New Mexico	90.34	86.23	−4.11
North Carolina	91.20	90.08	−1.12
Ohio	101.20	98.97	−2.23
Oregon	96.99	94.06	−2.93
Pennsylvania	90.74	94.02	3.28
Rhode Island	82.58	84.36	1.78
South Carolina	87.28	92.13	4.85
South Dakota	91.92	95.34	3.42
Tennessee	91.89	93.49	1.60
Utah	95.35	100.07	4.72
Washington	97.58	95.01	−2.57
Wisconsin	97.58	92.61	−4.98

TABLE IX

The effect of broadening the concept of household income on inequality

Component of of income	Coefficient of variation	Cumulative % change
Income I	0.598	
Income II	0.571	4.5
Income III	0.535	10.5

definition of household income to include transfer payments significantly reduces income inequality. At the present time there is no comprehensive developed data set of price indices that is readily available to researchers. The development of such data is crucial to the progress of interstate income distribution research.

REFERENCES

1. Coughlin, C. C. and T. B. Mandelbaum: 1988, 'Why have state per capita incomes diverged recently?', Review of the Federal Reserve Bank of St. Louis 70, pp. 24–36.
2. Abdel-Ghany, M.: 1991, 'Income inequality within the U.S.A.: with emphasis on the "South"', Journal of Consumer Studies and Home Economics 15, pp. 339–345.
3. Abdel-Ghany, M.: 1996, 'Demographic and economic determinants of household income polarization among the states of America', Family Economics and Nutrition Review 9, pp. 14–23.
4. Al-Sammarie, A. and H. P. Miller: 1967, 'State differentials in income concentration', American Economic Review 57, pp. 59–72.
5. Aigner, D. J. and A. J. Heinz: 1967, 'On the determination of income inequality', American Economic Review 57, pp. 175–184.
6. Braun, D.: 1988, 'Multiple measurements of U.S. income inequality', The Review of Economics and Statistics 70, pp. 398–405.
7. Conlisk, J.: 1967, 'Some cross-state evidence on income inequality', The Review of Economics and Statistics 47, pp. 115–118.
8. Frech, H. E. and L. S. Burns: 1971, 'Metropolitan interpersonal income inequality: a comment', Land Economics 47, pp. 104–106.
9. Jonish, J. E. and J. B. Kau: 1973, 'State differentials in income inequality', Review of Social Economy 31, pp. 179–190.

10. Levernier, W., D. S. Rickman and M. D. Partridge: 1995, 'Variation in U.S. state income inequality: 1960–1990', International Regional Science Review 18, pp. 355–378.
11. Nelson, J. I.: 1984, 'Income inequality: the American states', Social Science Quarterly 65, pp. 854–860.
12. Nord, S.: 1984, 'An economic analysis of changes in the relative shape of the interstate Size distribution of family income during the 1960s', The American Economist 28, pp. 18–25.
13. Rice, G. R. and T. S. Sale: 1975, 'Size distribution of income in Louisiana and other southern states', Growth and Change 6, pp. 26–33.
14. Rowley, T. D., J. M. Redman and J. Angle: 1991, 'The rapid rise in state per capita income inequality in the 1980s: Sources and prospects', Staff Report AGES 9104 (USDA, Agriculture and Rural Economy Division, Washington, DC).
15. Ruthenberg, D. and M. Stano: 1977, 'The determinants of interstate variation in income distribution', Review of Social Economy 35, 55–66.
16. Sale, T. S.: 1974, 'Interstate analysis of the size distribution of family income, 1950–1970', Southern Economic Journal 40, pp. 434–441.
17. Slottje, D. J.: 1990, 'Changes in the U.S. income distribution from 1970 to 1980: assessing state and regional impacts', The Journal of Human Resources 25, pp. 267–274.
18. Young, R. and J. Moreno: 1965, 'Economical development and social rigidity: a comparative study of forty-eight states', Economic Development and Social Change 13, pp. 439–452.
19. Fei, J. C. H., G. Ranis and S. W. Y. Kuo: 1978, 'Growth and the family distribution of income by factor components', Quarterly Journal of Economics 92, pp. 17–53.
20. Lerman, R. I. and S. Yitzhaki: 1985, 'Income inequality effects by income source: a new approach and application to the United States', The Review of Economics and Statistics 67, pp. 151–156.
21. Kakwani, N. C.: 1980, Income Inequality and Poverty: Methods of Estimation and Policy Applications (Oxford University Press, London).
22. Kusnic, M. W. and J. Davanzo: 1986, 'Accounting for non-market activities in the distribution of income: an empirical investigation', Journal of Development Economics 21, pp. 211–227.
23. Pyatt, G., C. Chen and J. C. H. Fei: 1980, 'The distribution of income by factor components', Quarterly Journal of Economics 95, pp. 451–473.
24. Shorrocks, A. F.: 1982, 'Inequality decomposition by factor components', Econometrica 50, pp. 193–211.
25. Shorrocks, A. F.: 1983, 'The impact of income components on the distribution of family incomes', Quarterly Journal of Economics 97, pp. 311–326.
26. Bishop, J. A., J. P. Formby and P. D. Thistle: 1994, 'Convergence and divergence of regional income distribution and welfare', The Review of Economics and Statistics 76, pp. 228–235.

27. Deller, S. C., M. Shields and D. Tomberlin: 1996, 'Price differentials and trends in state income levels: a research note', The Review of Regional Studies 26, pp. 99–113.
28. Ram, R.: 1992, 'Interstate income inequality in the United States: measurement, modelling, and some characteristics', Review of Income and Wealth 38, 39–48.
29. Ram, R.: 1995. ' "Nominal" and "real" interstate income inequality in the United States: some additional evidence', Review of Income and Wealth 41, pp. 399–404.
30. Woods and Poole Economics: 1997, Complete 1997 Economic and Demographic Database on CD-ROM: Technical Documentation (Woods and Poole Economics, Inc., Washington, D.C.).
31. McMahon, W. W.: 1991, 'Geographical cost of living differences: an update', Journal of the American Real Estate and Urban Economics Association 19, 426–450.
32. U.S. Department of Labor, Bureau of Labor Statistics (1998). Web site: http://stats.bls.gov/.

The University of Alabama

FORREST B. GREEN and ERIC HATCH

DOES BUSINESS PROCESS REENGINEERING DIMINISH THE QUALITY OF WORK LIFE?

ABSTRACT. This paper examines the development of Business Process Reengineering (BPR). Misconceptions and misapplications of the BPR Concept are discussed using higher education as an example. The authors stress that empowerment and autonomy are the true cornerstones of effectiveness in genuine reengineering efforts. Several examples of BPR's correct applications are then illustrated.

INTRODUCTION

Nothing has characterized the enormity of change in the workplace over the past decade more than the restructuring of business with its emphasis on cost-cutting, down-sizing, and corporate mergers and acquisitions. This combination of intense revision and change resulted in significant disruptions for large numbers of managers and employees who were forced to reconsider their future prospects and careers. Jobs could no longer be taken for granted. For many, the quality of work-life eroded into long hours (for those who still had work), fear, and uncertainty about the future. *Fortune* magazine predicted the "end of the job" in a feature article published in 1994. The radical re-design of business and industry that precipitated these changes is known as Business Process Reengineering (BPR).

Reengineering is defined as "the fundamental rethinking and radical redesign of business processes to achieve dramatic improvements in critical, contemporary measures of performance, such as cost, quality, service, and speed" (Hammer and Champy, 1993: p. 32). By emphasizing the words "fundamental," "radical," and "dramatic," Hammer and Champy emphasize that reengineering isn't about making marginal or incremental improvements, but total reinvention and replacement of existing corporate structures and procedures. They use the term, "heavy blasting." Companies that

Social Indicators Research **60:** 299–307, 2002.

reengineer often challenge the division of labor principle established through scientific management decades ago. Processes that used to be handled in segmented fragments passed from worker to worker are reconnected in logical work-units handled by process teams. Time is spent on work that adds value rather than on work that adds no value. Technology replaces mundane, but necessary, activities and increases the ability of work teams to concentrate on fulfilling requirements rather than performing tasks.

THE DEVELOPMENT OF BPR

The title of this paper suggests that BPR may diminish the quality of work life. The measure of importance here is the degree to which BPR has had an impact on human values. Does business reengineering enhance human values and the quality of work-life, or does it undermine those values by putting competitive drive and corporate zeal ahead of all else? The evolution of BPR, referred to as a "manifesto for business revolution" by Hammer and Champy, began with changes in manufacturing during the 1970's brought about by a recognition that American dominance in a number of industries had given way to a preference for products produced in Japan. Delegations studying the Japanese way of doing business found that their emphasis on quality, continuous improvement, and elimination of waste led to a streamlining of business practices with consequent reductions in cost and improvements in product quality. Although Japan's lifetime employment policy was widely heralded at the time, the significant change noted in work content was the manner by which multiskilled production teams made many improvements on the plant floor without excess supervision. Much of the autonomy exhibited by Japanese workers was said to be a cultural phenomenon that could not be replicated in the United States and other countries.

During the 1980's, Japanese management techniques were adapted and evolved into a new paradigm known as Total Quality Management (TQM). This comprehensive management philosophy, embraced by many corporations worldwide, places primary emphasis on meeting and exceeding customer expectations. The key elements are enhanced leadership, customer focus, emphasis on process as well as product and service improvement, and the empowerment of the workforce through self-directed workteams. Firms began to recognize the value of a committed workforce, cross-trained and motivated to respond at the operational level with an emphasis on continuous improvement. Awards for quality and productivity flourished on several continents as the quality movement gathered momentum.

While many firms and organizations witnessed dramatic results with TQM, others were unable to make the cultural changes necessary to achieve significant advances. Businesses struggling to demonstrate results began looking for more dramatic solutions. At the same time, information technology was making available a vast array of new possibilities which no longer supported corporate hierarchies and tedious step-by-step approval processes. The timing was right for a "business revolution" and a break with old traditions that were no longer effective. However, when BPR emerged in the 1990's, many firms didn't get it. They assumed that reengineering was another name for downsizing, or an excuse for restructuring. Reducing capacity is only doing less with less. Reengineering, according to Hammer and Champy (1993: p. 48) means "doing more with less."

BPR AND THE QUALITY OF WORK LIFE

The questions, then, is this. Does reengineering call for the exploitation of labor and less satisfaction with jobs that remain? Does BRP diminish the quality of work-life? According to Hammer and Champy, it should not and does not when implemented properly. However, the nature of work changes. The first change is that work units become process teams rather than functional departments. Management invests in teams that have the responsibility of completing entire processes. Roles change from control and supervision to challenge and empowerment. Job preparation changes from training to education, and performance measures shift from tasks to results (Hammer and Champy, 1993: pp. 65–82).

Organizational structures after reengineering tend to be flat, with fewer supervisors and middle managers, since work at the operating level is performed by coequal people participating in teams. The role of managers shifts to that of motivation and support, serving as leaders and facilitators, and coordinating resources. With fewer layers of management, executives are closer to customers and employees at the operating level. Although expectations are high, a command and control structure isn't needed. People have a greater degree of autonomy when reengineering is implemented correctly. The attitudes and efforts of empowered people determine the successful accomplishment of work.

Change is always disruptive; there's no doubt about that. But when team based management with self-directed work teams is a consequence of the reengineering effort, there is almost always a higher satisfaction level among the employees who survive the transition. Maslow's hierarchy of needs places self-actualization at the top of the list. An empowered workforce contributes materially to the well-being of the organization, has wide-ranging responsibilities, makes significant decisions, and shares in the rewards. In such an environment, this can and should enhance the quality of work life.

Quality of work life also influences personal adjustment and health. In industry, 65 percent of absenteeism is principally or exclusively due to emotional problems. When a person's life is not going well, work can actually be a refuge, but if the workplace is seen as odious, then the problems are compounded and interwoven. Self-directed work teams give workers some sense of control. Mental health studies have repeatedly shown control to be a major variable in mental health adjustment (Rotter, 1990). These studies validate that internal locus of control, i.e., actually having some influence on outer events, is positively correlated with good mental health.

MIS-APPLICATIONS OF BPR: THE HIGHER EDUCATION EXAMPLE

What has happened, unfortunately, is that many organizations have focused on the "doing more with less" aspect of reengineering and have failed to recognize the human element. The same phenomenon occurred with TQM when it turned out that too many firms were practicing "partial" quality management and merely paid lip service to human resource issues (Kolesar, 1995). Similarly, a large number of firms and organizations used reengineering as excuse to downsize and restructure, leaving the remaining workforce putting in long hours and wondering when the ax would fall again. The deleterious effects of constant downsizing are only now beginning to be understood (Cunniff, 1998). While there are many examples of the mis-application of reengineering, the following is drawn from the experience of higher education in the United States, primarily state institutions across the country. The impetus for change is laudable, but the execution has largely ignored the values that make reengineering a viable concept in the nation's colleges and universities.

Professionals in higher education have been impacted by the so-called "business model" through which legislators, boards of trustees, and academic administrators have called for greater accountability from faculty members. Faculty have been exhorted to increase productivity by doing more with less, and have seen budgets shrink concurrently to force compliance through the elimination of duplicative programs and attacks on tenure. The emphasis, according to the General Secretary of the American Association of University Professors, Mary Burgan, has been on the three C's extolled by the champions of corporate hype: Customers, Competition, and Change. Her reading of Hammer and Champy (1993) observed that "the language has penetrated all sectors of work in our society, creating structures of value which do not conform to human need" (Burgan, 1997). She states that she had to remind herself that she was not in the world of academic satire. The profession is being devalued, she says, in the current effort to measure the cost of goods and services.

What is most remarkable here is that faculty have to a large extent enjoyed the degree of autonomy that Hammer and Champy claim is the appropriate outcome of reengineering. Yet the trend is in the opposite direction. Academic programs are now being micromanaged by trustees, administrators, and legislators to an extent not seen in a long time. Internal governance and collegial responsibility for curriculum matters are being usurped by centralized administrators in the name of flexibility and efficiency. Just a few of the pressures being placed on faculties today are to prepare students for immediate employment, do away with "frivolous" courses, submit to endless evaluations and assessments, spend more time in the classroom, avoid questionable research, and in the words of the University of Minnesota's revision-of-tenure code, "maintain a proper attitude of industry and cooperation" (Burgan, 1997). Higher education is to be a means to an end, a vocational pursuit, a commodity to be delivered rather than a preparation for life. Tenure and academic freedom are seen as inimical to this new world order.

The business model that has been applied to colleges and universities in many cases has been one of command and control, more power to the administration, fewer resources for the faculty, and numerical measures of so-called "productivity." This is a considerable departure from the empowerment and autonomy cited as the cornerstone of effectiveness in genuine reengineering efforts. Moreover, the concept of the "Customer" in higher education is one that cannot be easily identified. While students appear to be the obvious customers, others argue that students attending institutions are participants or partners in educational pursuits, unpaid employees, or (using the beloved terms of industry) work-in-process inventory. Are the real customers then parents, alumnae, employers, or society at large? Just as industries have many stakeholders, so too do colleges and universities have many constituencies. It makes sense for such institutions to service and support all constituencies, but if a business model is going to be applied, let it be the appropriate business model described by Hammer and Champy in which management helps to shape the values and beliefs within an organization: "By values and beliefs, we mean the issues and concerns that people in the organization think are important and to which they pay significant attention" (Hammer and Champy, 1993: p. 81).

A RENEWED EMPHASIS ON PEOPLE

There's already evidence in industry that human resource issues are receiving the attention they should have all along. According to Lancaster (1998), "Companies that once bragged about their reengineered work processes and new quality measurements are now extolling the importance of human beings." Many companies, he says, are encouraging managers to "help rebuild cultures disrupted by mergers and cost cutting." A number of companies, however, never forgot the lessons in the first place. They are among the one-hundred best out of 238 identified by *Fortune* magazine to be featured in their January 12 issue (Levering and Moskowitz, 1998). *Fortune* used to be known primarily for its list of the top 500 companies as determined by annual revenue and financial measures. The more recent article listed and described the best companies to work for. A survey of 55 000 workers was conducted to match employee attitudes with company results. Four attitudes were found to correlate strongly with higher profits. They are:

1. A sense of having the opportunity to do what they do best;
2. A belief that their opinions count;
3. A sense that fellow employees are committed to quality; and
4. A clear connection between their work and the organization's mission (Grant, 1998).

Among *Fortune*'s 100 best companies, eighteen have explicit no-layoff policies, and others go to considerable lengths to avoid layoffs when downsizing (Levering and Moskowitz, 1998: p. 89). As an example, when Minnesota Mining and Manufacturing (3M Co.) went through its biggest restructuring ever in 1996, out of 7000 positions eliminated fewer than 100 persons were terminated involuntarily. Other firms and organizations on the list went through various changes including reorganization, restructuring, and reengineering. All are at least ten years old. Yet the high praise they receive from their own employees clearly indicates that reengineering doesn't have to diminish the quality of work life, and if done properly, will actually enhance it.

SUMMARY AND CONCLUSIONS

There's no doubt that business process reengineering and the resultant fallout (flattening of organizations, turning routine work over to computers, etc.) has made many jobs redundant. Wholesale job cutting had become an accepted technique for streamlining companies. But the evidence now indicates that excessive downsizing leads to moderate cost savings, but low morale, long hours, and minimal productivity improvements from the remaining workforce.

Because BPR, and even TQM to some extent, have been misapplied in many organizations, a reduced level of employee loyalty is the logical consequence. This phenomenon has swept many aspects of corporate life. Thus, an "empowered" response may not be to be a team player within a company structure, but to look to an outside resource for support. Many disenfranchised employees may seek protection from arbitrary personnel actions by joining unions. After decades of declining memberships, unions are embarking on an ambitious organizing drive. In 1977, 23.8 million workers in the United States, almost 24 percent of the work force, belonged to a union. By 1997 unions had 16.3 million members, a 14 percent share of the work force. But things are slowly turning around. For example, after decades of losing members, the AFL-CIO broke even last year. The 13 million member federation's goal is three percent growth a year by 2000.

Thus, as the old saying goes, the more things change the more they are the same. The average worker will continue to respond to deeds, not words, acronyms, or new models. Words like "restructuring" or "reorganization" only have meaning if they are legitimized by actions which are perceived to benefit individuals in the corporation and not just the corporation itself. Already, companies are expressing doubts about the effectiveness of their reengineering efforts. Although Rigby (1998) found in a survey of 224 senior managers that fifteen percent were extremely satisfied with BPR, sixteen percent were dissatisfied, the lowest ranking since its peak in 1995. As BPR is used as the latest excuse for downsizing in a company, it typically leads to reduced productivity on the part of harassed and harried employees who are left. Realization generally comes back to the same thing – human productivity is most linked to stress-reduced environments in organizations where there is a sense of empowerment and belonging.

When implemented properly, BPR does not devastate the quality of work life. Employment trust and empowerment are essential to making reengineering effective. *Fortune* magazine's recent emphasis on the 100 best companies to work for suggests that a dedicated, enthusiastic workforce contributes substantially to organizational viability. Companies that understand this and show respect for human capital contribute to the economy and the quality of work life without sacrificing one for the other.

REFERENCES

Bridges, W.: 1994, September 19, 'The end of the job', Fortune 130(6), pp. 62–68.
Burgan, M.: 1997, Fall, 'Tenure and the management of higher education', Footnotes, a publication of the American Association of University Professors, 2.
Cunniff, J.: 1998, 'Lost amid downsizing: respect for human capital', Roanoke Times, Associated Press Article (exact date unknown).
Grant, L.: 1998, January 12, 'Happy workers, high returns', Fortune 137(1), p. 81.
Green, F. B. and V. B. Waynan: 1996, Summer, 'Viewpoint reengineering: clarifying the confusion', SAM Advanced Management Journal 61(3), pp. 37–39.
Hammer, M., and J. Champy: 1993, Reengineering the Corporation (Harper Business, New York).
Kolesar, P.: 1995, Summer, 'Partial quality management: an essay', Production and Operations Management 4(3), pp. 195–200.
Lancaster, H.: 1998, April 28, 'Will hiring a full staff be the next fashion in management?', Wall Street Journal, B1.
Levering, R. and M. Moskowitz: 1998, January 12, 'The 100 best companies to work for in America', Fortune 137(1), pp. 84–90.
Newark Star Ledger: 1998, August 6, Unions Show a Resurgence, A1.
Rigby, D. K.: 1998, September 7, 'What's today's special at the consultants' café?' Fortune, pp. 162–163.
Rotter, J. B.: 1990, 'Internal vs external locus of control: a case history of a variable', American Psychologist 45, pp. 489–493.
Smith, D.: 1998, May, 'New emphasis on ethics: businesses take a long look at ethics at work', Blue Ridge Business Journal 10(5), pp. 1, 6–10.

Department of Management and Marketing Forrest B. Green
Box 6954
Radford University
Radford, VA 24142
USA
E-mail: fgreen@radford.edu

Department of Psychology Eric Hatch
Appalachian State University
Boone, NC 28607
USA
E-mail: hatchej@appstate.edu

ENRICA AURELI and BARBARA BALDAZZI

UNEQUAL PERCEIVED QUALITY OF LIFE AMONG ELDERLY ITALIANS: DIFFERENT SATISFACTION LEVELS IN SELECTED SPHERES OF LIFE

INTRODUCTION

In Italy recent demographic trends have caused a drop in natality, with Italy being currently one of the countries with the lowest birth levels both in Europe and world-wide. Moreover, considerable gains have also been made in average life expectancy.[1] This combination has led to an absolute and relative increase in the elderly population. Thus in 1995, the elderly population, that is all those aged 65 years and over, comprised 16.6% of the total population.

This has given rise to the need to redefine old age: improved health status, increased economic spending, greater expectations on the part of the elderly has urged for further distinctions to be made among this age group. While it is well known that "registered" age and "biological" age no longer coincide in the same way for everyone, today another factor, "social" age causes further confusion. Retirement no longer coincides with a diminished social importance during the remaining life span. Indeed, this phase, which has steadily lengthened,[2] has been further subdivided into the "young old," the "old," the "old old" and the "oldest old." At each of these stages, people lives are organised differently, bringing to the fore issues relating to individual choices, social organisation, family networks and social assistance.

Moreover, due to increased longevity, the numerical size of the four groups tends to be fairly similar, unlike the past, particularly as far as women are concerned.

Until recently, in Italy, family networks have ensured a stabilising effect, helping to avoid transition crises among the population at different life stages. However, increased social mobility

Social Indicators Research **60:** 309–334, 2002.

TABLE I

Elderly population by age group and gender, in Italy (1995)

Age group	Males	% of males	Females	% of females
65–69 years	1 421 000	36.5	1 784 000	32.5
70–74 years	1 184 000	30.5	1 542 000	28.1
75–79 years	593 000	15.3	850 000	15.5
Over 80 years old	697 000	17.7	1 309 000	23.9
Total	3 885 000	100.0	5 485 000	100.0

Notes: Elaboration on ISTAT data.

and subsequently greater geographical mobility have created a gap between generations and obliged the more elderly to establish greater autonomy with respect to their children, not only economically, but also psychologically. The speed with which this phenomenon has occurred differs according to geographical area and social class, while the role of elderly differs according to gender.

A lengthy stay in a non productive, albeit active, status urges policy makers to have an awareness of the elderly planet and identify destabilising factors which could derive from the failure to satisfy the expectations of such a large population group.

The Italian National Statistical Institute each year performs a Multipurpose Sample Survey focusing on aspects of daily life, with occasional surveys on one or other of these aspects. About 20000 families are involved and their objective status and perceived satisfaction in different spheres of life are studied. In this study data for those aged 65 years and over were used to gain further insight into an unequal perceived quality of life according to satisfaction levels declared in the following areas: economic standing, health status, family, friends, leisure time and work.

An analysis was performed comparing objective indicators relative to different spheres of life and perceived satisfaction, distinct by gender, age, family type, education, work and married status.

INDICATORS USED

Four categories of indicators were used. Subjective-satisfaction indicators obtained from replies to the question, "How satisfied are you with . . .," referring to each of the life aspects mentioned above. Four different replies were foreseen: very, fairly, not very, not at all (Table II).

The second category comprised self-perceived indicators regarding the family's perceived economic status, in absolute terms (very good, acceptable, lacking, totally insufficient resources), and compared with the previous year (improved, unchanged, worse), as well as perceived health status (very poor, poor, fairly good, good, very good) (Table III). A third category referred to more objective indicators, although obtained from statements by the respondents. These indicators were selected on the basis of how important these were for the different life domains. What we are dealing with are options taken regarding free time, relationship networks, economic standing and health status (Table IV). The fourth category comprises explanatory variables for the different satisfaction levels expressed. These also include structural variables such as age, subdivided into four 5-year age groups, the last remaining open-ended, education, the elderly person's family structure, employment and marital status (Table V).

DESCRIPTIVE ANALYSIS

Gender more than any other variable distinguishes the approach taken to old age in light of various considerations, not only demographic, but also psychological and social. In demographic terms women's mortality rates vary according to age group, compared with men, so that the excess female- male ratio gradually increases with age.

Moreover, the age gap in the couple, women being generally younger that men, ensures that there are more widows than widowers. Subsequently, men more often than women liver their old age as part of a couple, whereas women frequently live 10–15 years on their own as widows. These coincide with the tail-end of their lives and thus the worst in terms of health.

TABLE II

Subjective satisfaction indicators: modalities and life domain

Subjective satisfaction indicators	Modalities	Life domains
Economic status: satisfaction	Very	Economic status
	Fairly	
	Not very	
	Not at all	
Health status: satisfaction	Very	Health
	Fairly	
	Not very	
	Not at all	
Leisure time: satisfaction	Very	Leisure time
	Fairly	
	Not very	
	Not at all	
Satisfactory friendship network	Very	Relationship with friends
	Fairly	
	Not very	
	Not at all	
Satisfactory family relationships	Very	Family relationships
	Fairly	
	Not very	
	Not at all	
Satisfactory employment status	Very	Work
	Fairly	
	Not very	
	Not at all	

Psychologically women are better amalgamated into the network of family relationships, while men are more involved in the external world connected to their jobs. Old age acts as an impetus to extend these tendencies. Indeed, on retirement, men more frequently continue with some form of work, while for women domestic and

TABLE III

Subjective perception indicators: modalities and life domains

Subjective perception indicators	Modalities	Life domains
Perceived economic status of the family compared with the past	Improved Unchanged Worse	Economic status
Assessment of family's economic resources	Very good Acceptable Lacking Totally insufficient	Economic status Work
Self-perceived health status	Very good Good Fairly good Poor Very poor	Health

family life become or continue to remain the focal point of their lives.

Socially, women are less well-educated than men and not employed. Thus changes in role with age are less or not at all traumatic.

In light of the above it was decided to perform separate analyses for men and women.

A first stage in the data analysis was to undertake a simple reading of the satisfaction levels declared for the different life spheres. Then, the most significant structural data were used to check the links between perceived satisfaction levels and family structure. A clustering technique was then applied to highlight the different ways of coping with old age. An initial reading of the data provides the stated satisfaction levels (very good, fairly good, not very good, not at all good) for the different life spheres for the four age groups.

Figures 1a and 1b show histograms for the percent frequencies of declared satisfaction levels for each life sphere and by gender. Distinguishing between satisfaction, on the right, and dissatisfac-

TABLE IV

Objective indicators: modalities and life domains

Objective indicators	Modalities	Life domains
Main source of income	Work related income Pension Unanswered	Economic status Work
A five-days holiday in the last year	Never At least once	Leisure time Family relationships Relationship with friends
Listen to the radio	No Yes, sometimes Yes, every day	Leisure time
Watch television	No Yes, less than three hours a day Yes, more than three hours a day	Leisure time
Cinema, theatre attendance during the last twelve month	Never Yes, at least once	Leisure time Family relationships Relationship with friends
Read newspapers	No Yes, sometimes (1–4 days a week) Yes, often (5–7 days a week)	Leisure time
Books read during last twelve months	None Yes	Leisure time
Religious practice	No Yes, sometimes (a few times a year) Yes, once a week Yes, often (5–7 times a week)	Leisure time Family relationships Relationship with friends
Political involvement	No Yes	Leisure time Family relationships Relationship with friends
Member of an associations	No Yes	Leisure time Family relationships Relationship with friends
Voluntary works	No Yes	Leisure time Family relationships Relationship with friends
Own a cash card	No Yes	Economic status
Housing status	Owner Renting	Economic status
Chronic disease	None Only one More than two	Health

TABLE V

Socio-economic, demographic and geographical variables: modalities and life domains

Structural variables	Modalities	Life domains
Age	65–69 years	Demographic variables
	70–74 years	
	75–80 years	
	over 80 years old	
Education	No diploma	Social variables
	Elementary school	
	Junior high	
	High school	
	University	
Family type	Couple with children	Social variables
	Couple without children	Family relationships
	Single parent with children	
	Lone person	
	Other family type	
Status	Employed	Socio-economic variables
	Unemployed	Work
	Housewife	
Married status	Unmarried/separated/divorced	Social variables
	Married	Family relationships
	Widowed	
Geographic regions	North-west of Italy	Geographic variables
	North-east of Italy	Social variables
	Central regions of Italy	
	South of Italy	
	Islands: Sicily and Sardinia	
Type of communes	Center of metropolitan region	Geographic variables
	Periphery of metropolitan region	Social variables
	Less than 2,000 inhabitants	
	2,001–10,000 inhabitants	
	10,001–50,000 inhabitants	
	More than 50,001 inhabitants	

tion, on the left, the four different age groups are specified for each sphere. What immediately emerges, for both genders, is that health and economic status are most frequently found to be dissatisfactory.

Dissatisfaction increases with age for men and women with regard to their health; yet the gap between women and men reduces itself with age. Ageing does not seem to affect women's and men's assessment of their economic situation, but dissatisfaction is more high for "young old women" than for "young old men": then ageing seems to affect women's assessment and men's assessment in different way. The above observation confirms a number of known facts. Indeed, research into poverty in Italy shows that such a risk is greater for women. Psychological studies, on the other hand, show that men are more intolerant of disease and sickness and, thus, the physical decline accompanying oldest age is immediately translated into dissatisfaction.

With age friendships are increasingly unsatisfactory both for elderly men and women, but somewhat assessment of family relationships confirms the continuing existence of a family network in Italy despite changes in family structure and behaviour. Both genders, irrespective of age, clearly state satisfaction with their family relationships.

A second stage consisted of drawing up a graph of the original matrix (AMADO). AMADO (Analyse graphique d'une MAtrice de DOnnées) is part of the SPAD.N software and reorders the data matrix, as a bar graph or histogram, by means of successive permutations, placing columns and rows which are similar near each other. The aim is to obtain a triangular matrix showing trends in the variables in correspondence to the unit groups.

This immediately showed the frequency of choice as well the groups declaring more or less frequently than the average different satisfaction levels. Whether their distribution is linked to all the modalities of a single variable or only to some is also shown.

As stated above, the underlying purpose of this research was to establish what effect family structure has on satisfaction levels in different spheres of life. It is hypothesised that living arrangements influence the elderly person's life and thus their satisfaction levels in all spheres of life. It emerged that only satisfaction with family networks, more so than marital status, was linked to the elderly

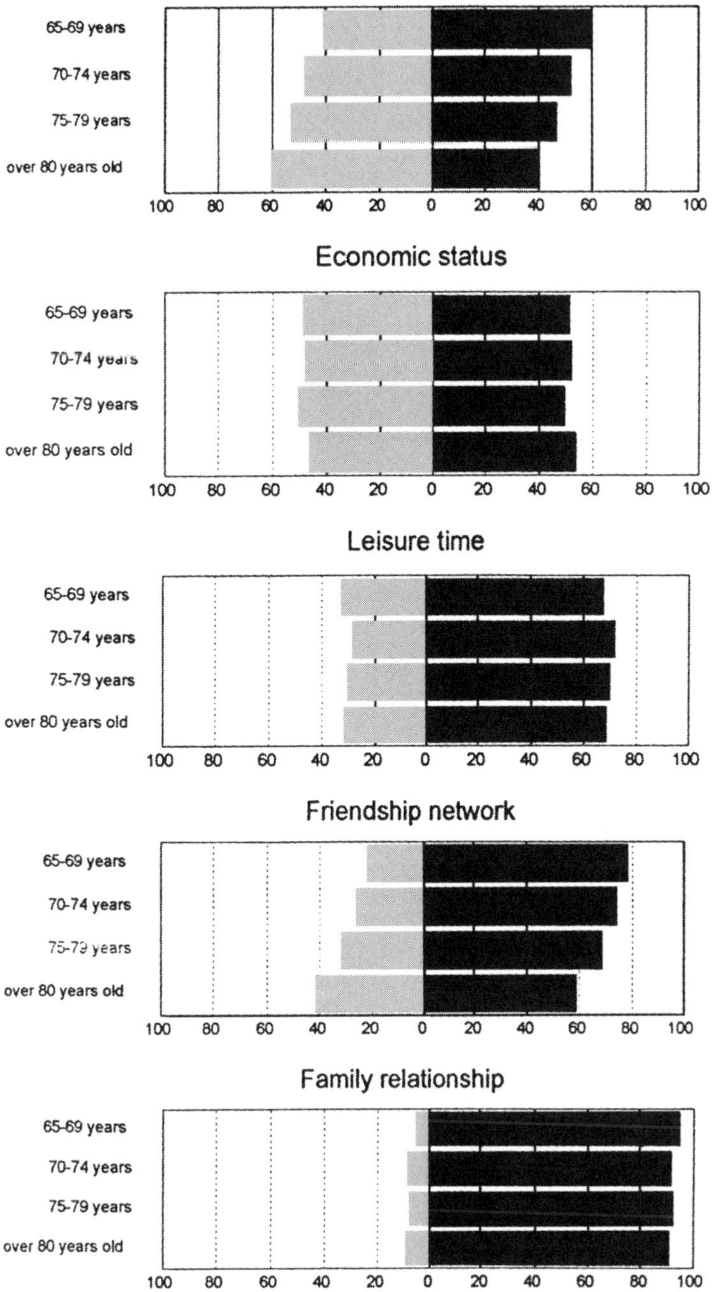

Figure 1a. Satisfaction levels for each life sphere for females.

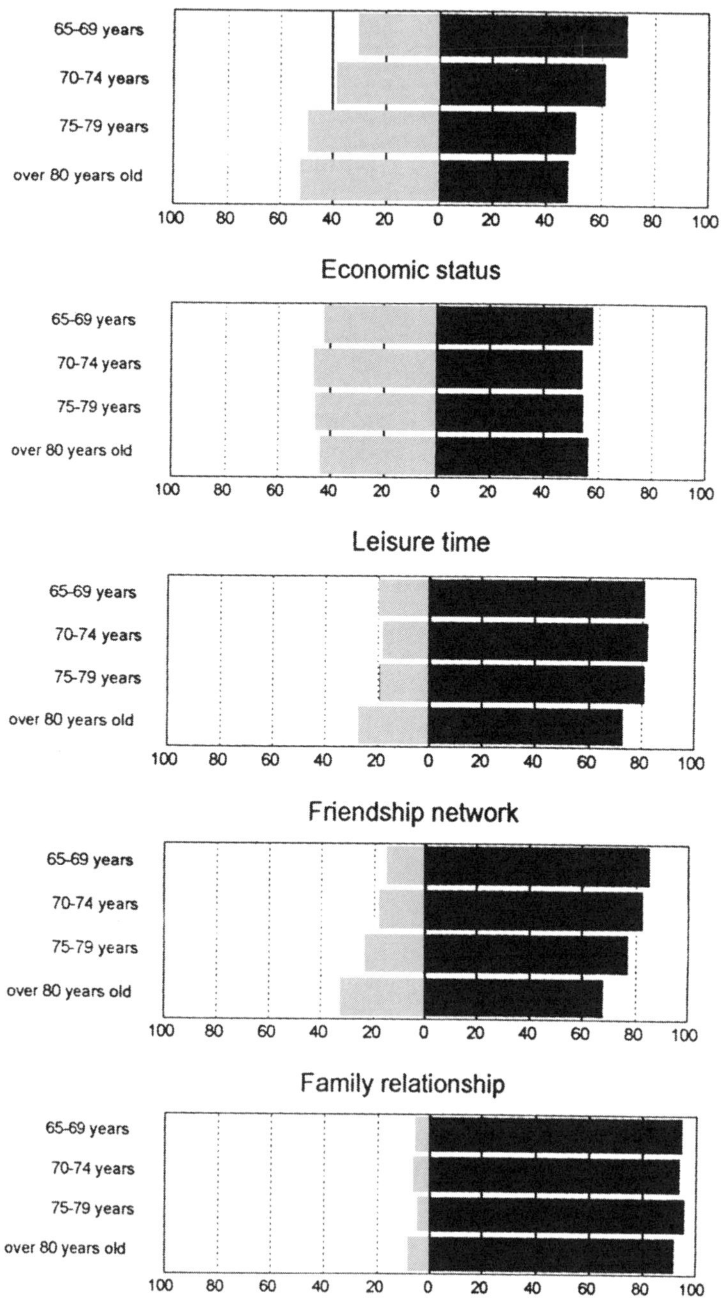

Figure 1b. Satisfaction levels for each life sphere for males.

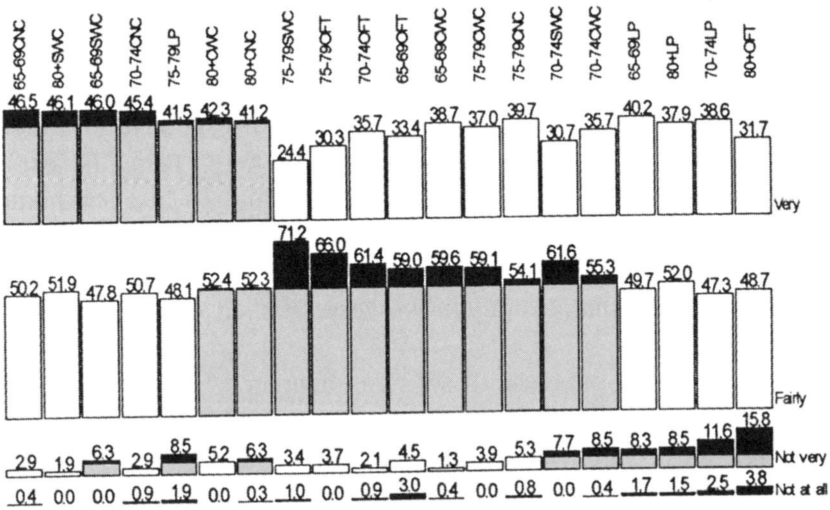

Figure 2a. Satisfaction family relationship – FEMALES.

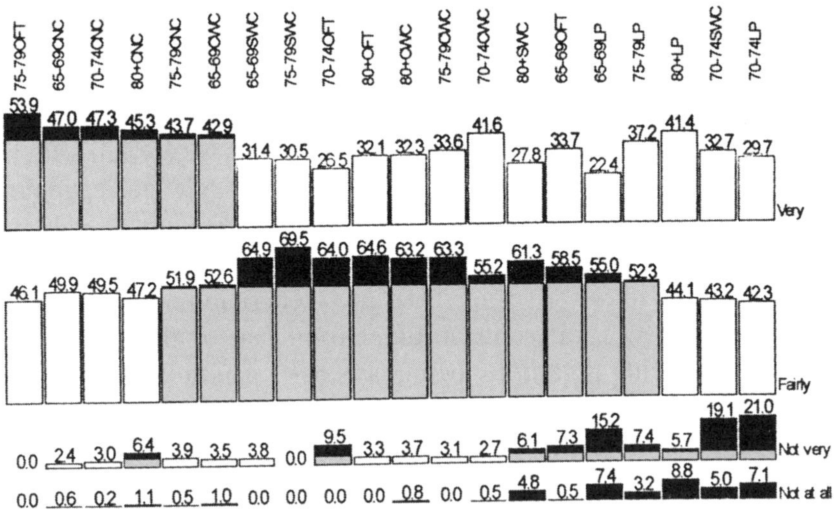

Figure 2b. Satisfaction family relationship – MALES.

person's family structure. The matrix constructed with different family structures (family structures were identified as follows: CNC – Couples without Children, CWC – Couples with children, SWC – Single parent with children, LP – Lone person, OFT – Other family types) and age groups, along with self-perceived satisfaction levels are reordered in Figures 2a and 2b.

Overall 42.1% of over 65-year old men declared that they were very happy with their family network, compared with 40.5% of women of the same age. The figure shows that replies for women were more homogenous than those for men, irrespective of which level of satisfaction was declared. Moreover, for men, the presence of their wives and the fact that their children had left home was essential for them to appreciate their family network. At all ages, men living as part of a couple, without children, declare more frequently than average to be very satisfied with their family network.

The continued presence of sons and daughters[3] still at home for men negatively compromises the quality of their family network. Among those in a couple, with children still at home, only the youngest age group (65–69 years old) expressed satisfaction, slightly more frequently than the average. For other age groups "quite satisfied" was mostly expressed, betraying an evident fall in enthusiasm with this type of living arrangement as they became older. In the absence of a wife, and should they remain a lone parent, the number of very satisfied falls considerably below the average for all ages, and for over 70 year olds, a large number declare that they are not very or not at all satisfied. The impression we are left with is that the continued dependency of children of an adult age is a major source of worry and concern, tingeing on men's psychological and material well-being, particularly in the absence of a wife, a context which appears to further exacerbate inter-generation conflict.

Women show a different attitude from men of the same age, particularly with regard to being a single parent at the oldest extremes (65–69, 80 and over), where they express above average satisfaction with their family network. We could generalise by saying that men are very much dependent on their wives with regard to their family relationships, while elderly women base these more on their children, even more so if cohabiting.

Living alone generates unsatisfactory family relationships. For all age groups, those expressing little satisfaction or total dissatisfaction with this sphere of life were in fact those living alone. It is worth noting that women, albeit with low frequency, stated that they were not at all satisfied much less often than men, thus confirming their known ability to adapt to different circumstances.

Other family living arrangements satisfy men more frequently than women. Dissatisfaction is most often expressed by over 80-year old women compared with the highest frequency of being very satisfied among men aged 75–79 years old. Obviously these living arrangements, which guarantee a measure of protection and assistance, are gratifying. Family relationships for elderly men are viewed positively when obligations regarding their offspring are not involved, and given a context where the presence of a wife or another family member guarantees support.

DIFFERENT APPROACHES TO AGEING

Whether there are different approaches to ageing and, if so, whether these evolve as one progressively ages was the focus of the third phase of the research. A clustering method[4] was applied to pinpoint various types of behaviour in relation to different modalities of the structural variables. Only the most significant modalities were used to interpret the clusters. Significance was considered according to four levels, from one to four asterisks. Significance was taken to be one asterisk if the frequency of the modalities calculated within the group was the highest of those among all the groups, and one to three asterisks if the same relative frequency was greater than the average frequency found in the population, once, twice or three times the squared standard deviation.

Four different types emerged, involving both males and females, although with certain distinguishing features depending on gender, and one type exclusively for males.

Passive Acceptance

This is the largest cluster comprising 74.5% women and 73.4% men. This group includes those who do not pursue any activity outside the home, have no particular interests, do not read or follow political affairs, nor are involved in any voluntary work. These belong to the lowest educated group and mainly reside in Southern Italy.

How are they distinguished by gender?

Women: are mainly married, aged 75–79 years, living in medium sized local authorities or on the outskirts of major cities, pass their free time watching three hours or more television. Although not

TABLE VI

Passive acceptance – FEMALES

Indicators	% in cluster	Significance	Structural variables	% in cluster	Significance
Member of an associations: no	99.4	**	Education: elementary school	52.3	**
Voluntary organizations: no	99.2	**	Geographic region: south of Italy	23.3	**
Own a cash card: no	97.7	**	Type of communes: 10,001–50,000 inhabitants	21.0	**
Books: no	89.0	**	Age: 75–79 years	16.1	**
Political involvement: no	87.2	**	Type of communes: periphery of metropolitan region	8.3	**
Watch television: more than three hours a day	47.2	**	Married status: married	41.8	*
Health status satisfaction: not very	42.4	**	Education: no diploma	34.3	*
Satisfactory friendship network: not very	22.7	**			
Self-perceived health status: poor	22.0	**			
Chronic disease: only one	19.0	**			
Satisfactory employment status: not very	8.7	**			
Cinema, theatre: never	94.6	*			
Holiday: never	79.9	*			
Newspaper: no	67.2	*			
Satisfactory family relationships: fairly	55.9	*			
Leisure time satisfaction: fairly	55.6	*			
Economic status satisfaction: not very	43.7	*			
Health status: fairly good	43.0	*			

suffering from any serious disease, they state that they do not feel well. The declare that they are fairly satisfied in all living domains (Table VI).

For men: live mainly as part of a couple, without children, are found in each elderly age group, reside in small local authorities, pass their leisure time with friends, which they are fairly happy.

New Interests and Commitments

This cluster comprises 17.1% women and 9.7% men. A strong social commitment is the distinguishing feature of this group, which may

TABLE VII

Passive acceptance – MALES

Indicators	% in cluster	Significance	Structural variables	% in cluster	Significance
Voluntary organizations: no	92.5	**	Education: elementary school	53.8	**
Member of an associations: no	91.7	**	Type of communes: less than 2,000 inhabitants	9.8	**
Political involvement: no	66.4	**	Family type: couples without children	57.8	*
Satisfactory friendship network: fairly	64.3	**	Geographic region: south of Italy	23.8	*
Leisure time satisfaction: fairly	63.4	**	Geographic region: islands	12.0	*
Satisfactory family relationship: fairly	61.2	**	Family type: other family type	5.5	*
Religious practice: sometimes	44.1	**			
Watch television: more than three hours a day	42.5	**			
Economic status satisfaction: not very	41.6	**			
Self-perceived health status: fairly good	41.4	**			
Health status satisfaction: not very	36.5	**			
Newspapers: sometimes	30.3	**			
Chronic disease: only one	18.6	**			
Own a cash card: no	90.5	*			
Books: no	85.7	*			
Cinema, theatre: never	83.7	*			
Newspapers: no	42.3	*			
Assessment of family's economic resources: lacking	40.2	*			
Self-perceived health status: poor	17.4	*			
Satisfactory friendship network: not very	15.0	*			

take a traditional form such as religion, or more innovative forms – voluntary works, political involvement, or member of an association. These individuals make quality life choices, are satisfied with how their free time is organized, regularly read newspapers and books, go on holidays and arrange trips (Tables VIII and IX).

In structural terms this is a medium-highly educated group, living in North Italy and in towns with more that 50 001 inhabitants.

TABLE VIII

New interests and commitments – FEMALES

Indicators	% in cluster	Significance	Structural variables	% in cluster	Significance
Voluntary organizations: yes	61.5	****	Geographic region: north-west of Italy	40.5	****
Member of an associations: yes	59.8	****	Education: high school	20.8	****
Holiday: yes, at least once	59.1	****	Education: junior school	18.1	****
Books: yes	56.4	****	Married status: unmarried/ separated/divorced	14.6	****
Cinema, theatre: yes, at least once	48.9	****	Education: university	5.4	****
Political involvement: yes	44.0	****	Status: unemployed	70.3	***
Newsapapers: often	42.2	****	Family type: lone person	36.6	***
Own a cash card: yes	26.2	****	Age: 70–74 years	33.4	***
Economic status satisfaction: fairly	69.7	***	Age: 65–69 years	40.1	**
Watch television: less than three hours a day	56.3	***	Geographic region: north-east of Italy	28.2	**
Religious practice: often	36.7	***	Type of communes: more than 50,001 inhabitants	19.5	**
Self-perceived health status: good	35.1	***	Type of communes: center of metropolitan region	19.5	**
Newspapers: sometimes	32.0	***	Family type: single parent with children	8.5	*
Housing status: owner	74.1	**			
Assessment of family's economic resources: acceptable	71.9	**			
Health status satisfaction: fairly	66.2	**			
Listen to the radio: every day	42.1	**			
Listen to the radio: sometimes	17.7	**			
Main source of income: pension	92.2	*			
Chronic disease: none	75.3	*			
Satisfactory friendship network: fairly	57.5	*			
Satisfactory family relationship: very	49.2	*			
Religious practice: once a week	37.0	*			
Satisfactory friendship network: very	31.4	*			

TABLE IX

New interests and commitments – MALES

Indicators	% in cluster	Significance	Structural variables	% in cluster	Significance
Member of an associations: yes	83.6	****	Education: high school	22.8	****
Voluntary organizations: yes	75.9	****	Type of communes: more than 50,001 inhabitants	22.1	****
Political involvement: yes	70.5	****	Geographic region: north- west of Italy	36.1	***
Cinema, theatre: yes, at least once	63.3	****	Geographic region: north-east of Italy	27.2	***
Newspapers: often	62.7	****	Type of communes: 2,001–10,000 inhabitants	26.3	***
Holiday: yes, at least once	60.7	****	Married status: married	81.3	**
Books: yes	57.4	****	Age: 65–69 years	44.2	**
Listen to the radio: every day	46.4	****	Education: university	14.5	**
Listen to the radio: sometimes	22.4	****	Age: 70–74 years	32.4	*
Religious practice: often	20.2	****	Geographic region: center of Italy	22.6	*
Satisfactory family relationship: very	72.0	***	Education: junior school	16.0	*
Perceived economic status compared with the past: worse	48.1	***	Age: 75–79 years	15.2	*
Self-perceived health status: good	39.7	***			
Own a cash card: yes	38.6	***			
Health status satisfaction: fairly	72.0	**			
Assessment of family's economic resources: acceptable	70.9	**			
Economic status satisfaction: fairly	66.4	**			
Satisfactory friendship network: very	56.4	**			
Leisure time satisfaction: very	50.4	**			
Watch television: less than three hours a day	62.9	*			

A good perception of their economic status was significant, but more so for women than men.

This cluster contains the most gender differences regarding structural features. Women are more concentrated in the first two elderly age groups, that is aged 65–74 years, while for men the 75–79 year old group is also significant. Women are alone by choice – unmarried, separated, divorced.

Men, however, tend to be married and residence in medium-small local authorities (2 001–10 000 inhabitants) was also significant.

Different satisfaction levels were not significant in forming this cluster.

Home and Family

This cluster is quite small, just 2% women and 7,7% men. This gender gap mainly implies that for elderly women their private lives are still firmly neighed down by family burdens. For men, their personal lives offer greater satisfaction with a falling off in commitments related to their working live and subsequently the greater facility with which they can tend to their personal interests.

A distinguishing feature of this group is the high level of satisfaction expressed in all life spheres, a stead, good economic status, and for men, home owner and a clear propensity towards family relationships. Men are interested in politics, associations, voluntary work, reading. Significance levels are however very low (Table XI). Women showed disinterest in all these areas and levels were significant although only slightly so. Education levels were low, and again this was only slightly significant (Table X).

Regarding structural variables, for men residence in the North of Italy, in a medium-big city and belonging to the 70–74 year age group were significant. The only feature exclusive to women was belonging to a young- old age group.

Extended Working Life

This cluster mainly comprises men, representing 5% of the total (table 12). They still have a work-generated income allowing them to judge their economic status as satisfactory. They are quite satisfied with their work, health and economic status. Satisfaction levels regarding family or friendship networks were not significant. They keep informed by reading newspapers and books and watching the television 1–3 hours every day. They go on holidays. Interests and outside commitments were only slightly significant. Employed status, high education levels, and belonging to the young-old age group prevailed among the structural variables.

TABLE X

Home and family – FEMALES

Indicators	% in cluster	Significance	Structural variables	% in cluster	Significance
Satisfactory family relationship: very	97.2	****	Age: 65–69 years	44.0	****
Satisfactory friendship network: very	85.8	****	Education: elementary school	52.2	*
Perceived economic status compared with the past: unchanged	84.6	****			
Health status satisfaction: very	84.1	****			
Leisure time satisfaction: very	74.6	****			
Self-perceived health status: very good	60.0	****			
Listen to the radio: every day	44.2	****			
Economic status satisfaction: very	43.3	****			
Chronic disease: none	87.8	***			
Assessment of family's economic resources: acceptable	79.4	***			
Holiday: yes, at least once	41.7	**			
Voluntary organizations: no	95.5	*			
Member of an associations: no	95.3	*			
Political involvement: no	86.2	*			
Watch television: less than three hours a day	55.1	*			

Extreme Old Age

This cluster comprises 6.4% women and 4.2% men (Table XIII and XIV). Their status is strongly linked to age and the oldest old are usually affected by two or more diseases. Women enter old-old age status earlier than men, the 75–79 age group being significant in assigning women to this group. A negative perception of satisfaction levels is the main distinguishing factor. Moreover, dissatisfaction with their economic status is more urgent for women than men. Lack of independence among older women with regard to home ownership and income aggravate an already negative situation.

TABLE XI

Home and family – MALES

Indicators	% in cluster	Significance	Structural variables	% in cluster	Significance
Satisfactory family relationship: very	93.5	****	Geographic region: north-west of Italy	38.1	****
Chronic disease: none	82.9	****	Geographic region: north-east of Italy	26.4	****
Assessment of family's economic resources: acceptable	78.8	****	Age: 70–74 years	34.9	***
Leisure time satisfaction: very	72.4	****	Type of communes: 10,001–50,000 inhabitants	23.9	***
Health status satisfaction: very	50.0	****	Type of communes: more than 50,001 inhabitants	23.6	***
Self-perceived health status: very good	45.6	****	Education: junior school	17.6	***
Housing status: owner	87.4	***	Status: unemployed	99.8	*
Satisfactory friendship network: very	78.8	***	Education: elementary school	53.6	*
Economic status satisfaction: fairly	71.9	***	Type of communes: 2,001–10,000 inhabitants	24.8	*
Listen to the radio: every day	42.8	***			
Perceived economic status compared with the past: unchanged	70.4	**			
Newspapers: often	57.2	**			
Religious practice: once a week	35.6	**			
Main source of income: pension	97.0	*			
Watch television: less than three hours a day	65.1	*			
Political involvement: yes	43.9	*			
Holiday: yes, at least once	41.6	*			
Books: yes	33.8	*			
Cinema, theatre: yes, at least once	33.7	*			
Self-perceived health status: good	31.2	*			
Own a cash card: yes	19.0	*			

CONCLUSIONS

The positions of the points-group on the factorial graphic derived from the multiple correspondence analysis show differences between women and men (Figures 3a and 3b). Women's group presents more variability than men's one. Indeed women's answers are more extreme than men's answers. The age has a different posi-

TABLE XII

Extended working life – MALES

Indicators	% in cluster	Significance	Structural variables	% in cluster	Significance
Main source of income: work	97.8	****	Status: employed	98.6	****
Watch television: less than three hours a day	77.2	****	Age: 65–69 years	70.4	****
Perceived economic status compared with the past: unchanged	72.2	****	Family type: couples with children	39.0	****
Satisfactory employment status: fairly	57.6	****	Education: university	31.4	****
Own a cash card: yes	41.3	****	Type of communes: 10,001–50,000 inhabitants	23.7	**
Leisure time satisfaction: not very	28.6	****	Geographic region: north-west of Italy	29.3	*
Assessment of family's economic resources: acceptable	78.4	***			
Health status satisfaction: fairly	72.4	***			
Cinema, theatre: yes, at least once	60.8	***			
Newspapers: often	60.1	***			
Holiday: yes, at least once	56.2	***			
Books: yes	45.9	***			
Housing status: owner	81.2	**			
Economic status satisfaction: fairly	71.8	**			
Chronic disease: none	70.9	**			
Political involvement: yes	53.2	**			
Self-perceived health status: good	36.0	**			
Self-perceived health status: very good	26.2	**			
Religious practice: sometimes	43.8	*			
Religious practice: once a week	33.6	*			
Member of associations: yes	33.3	*			
Voluntary organizations: yes	27.1	*			

tion on two graphics, because, for males, the work brings high satisfaction among "old men" aged 70–74 years old (work seems to be for them a choice) and not among "young old men" aged 65–69 years old. Nevertheless, high satisfaction comes from good family relationship; on the other hand, low satisfaction comes from sickness and lack of economic resources.

TABLE XIII

Extreme old age – FEMALES

Indicators	% in cluster	Significance	Structural variables	% in cluster	Significance
Health status satisfaction: not at all	78.2	****	Married status: widowed	56.3	****
Self-perceived health status: very poor	62.0	****	Age: over 80 years old	43.9	****
Perceived economic status compared with the past: worse	57.9	****	Education: no diploma	42.3	***
Leisure time satisfaction: not at all	53.5	****	Status: housewife	36.3	***
Satisfactory friendship network: not at all	50.5	****	Type of communes: center of metropolitan region	32.7	***
Chronic disease: more than two	49.2	****	Geographic region: center of Italy	21.7	***
Religious practice: no	49.1	****	Type of communes: more than 50,001 inhabitants	20	***
Housing status: renting	45.2	****	Family type: couples with children	15.7	***
Economic status satisfaction: not at all	44.4	****	Geographic region: islands	14.1	***
Watch television: no	26.6	****	Family type: lone person	36.5	**
Satisfactory employment status: not at all	23.2	****	Geographic region: south of Italy	22.9	*
Assessment of family's economic resources: totally insufficient	18.9	****	Age: 75–79 years	15.7	*
Satisfactory family relationship: not very	12.0	****			
Holiday: never	88.5	***			
Listen to the radio: no	70.3	***			
Newspapers: no	75.3	**			
Assessment of family's economic resources: lacking	51.2	**			
Own a cash card: no	96.6	*			
Cinema, theatre: never	96.5	*			
Books: no	88.0	*			
Political involvement: no	86.6	*			

The fact that almost three quarters of our population expressed a similar type of behavior, labeled, "passive acceptance of old age" would appear to belie the hypothesis that, once having retired, the remaining life span could be divided into different stages corresponding to different approaches to old age. What emerges from

TABLE XIV

Extreme old age – MALES

Indicators	% in cluster	Significance	Structural variables	% in cluster	Significance
Health status satisfaction: not at all	79.7	****	Age: over 80 years old	49.9	****
Listen to the radio: no	78.8	****	Education: no diploma	46.5	****
Newspapers: no	67.8	****			
Leisure time satisfaction: not at all	65.2	****			
Self-perceived health status: very poor	62.4	****			
Satisfactory friendship network: not at all	59.3	****			
Religious practice: no	58.6	****			
Chronic disease: more than two	43.3	****			
Economic status satisfaction: not at all	33.6	****			
Housing status: renting	31.5	****			
Cinema, theatre: never	97.3	***			
Holiday: never	90.5	***			
Political involvement : no	83.7	***			
Own a cash card: no	94.2	**			
Books: no	89.8	**			
Perceived economic status compared with the past: worse	46.1	**			
Assessment of family's economic resources: lacking	43.4	*			
Economic status satisfaction: not very	41.1	*			

our results is that only the oldest-old are clearly distinguished by a negative life attitude, which however is related to disease and illness rather than age. Indeed, the size of the group described as "extreme old-age" is less than a quarter of all those aged 80 and over, a significant but not exclusive feature of this group.

However, what is a major differential in the approach to old age is education. Those who do not passively accept old age and who are not conditioned by poor health are divided into two groups: the better educated who opt for new interests and commitments and the less well- educated who freely choose home and family.

Well-educated men are further subdivided into those who continue to work and those who do not. Age also pinpoints a time

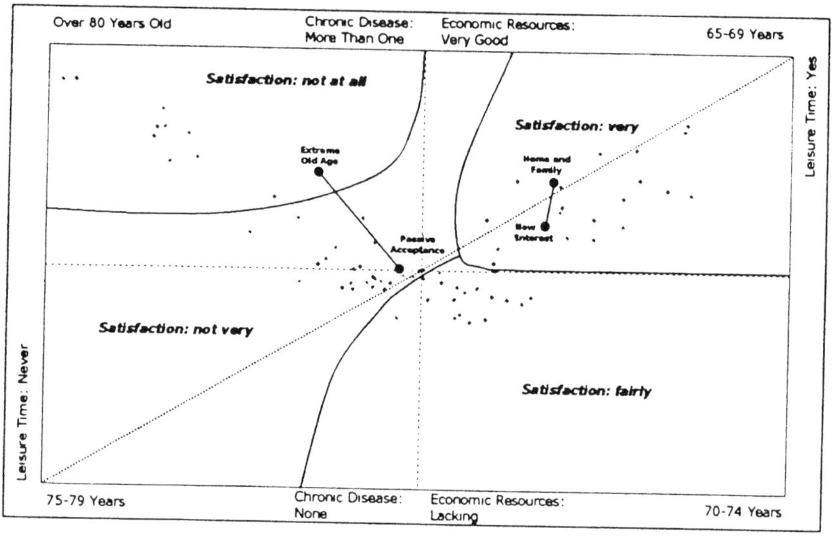

Figure 3a. Representation of groups on multiple correspondence graphic – Females.

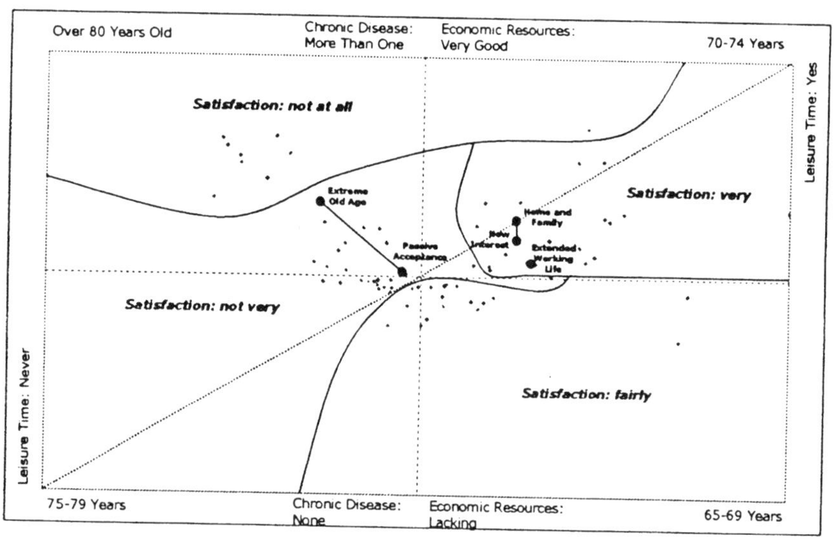

Figure 3b. Representation of groups on multiple correspondence graphic – Males.

lag between men and women. Women put off the passive acceptance of old age, so that while found in all elderly age groups, this is only significant among 75–79 year old.

Women put a stop to outside interests and commitments earlier than men, continuing these only during the two younger elderly stages, while men continue until they are 75–79 years old.

A time lag also occurs regards opting for home and family, this being significant for men in the 70–74 year old group, and for women in the 65–69 year old group.

The hypothesis that family structure influences satisfaction with all life spheres is contradicted by the multivariate analysis. This hypothesis is only confirmed for the cluster which approached old age by taking up new interests and commitments. This approach was only possible for women who are alone by choice. Such an option for married men is more straight forward, their wives facilitating rather than hindering such an approach.

NOTES

[1] Life expectancy in Italy for men in 74.7 years and for women 81.2 years (1994).

[2] Life expectancy at 65 years, is 15.6 years for men and 19.4 years for women (1994).

[3] Of all the developed countries, Italy is that in which children tend to live longer at home. The "extended family" depends on structural factors: length of studies; economic – difficult in finding a first job; cultural – whereby leaving the family of origin coincides with creating a new family, there being no gap in between.

[4] The Ward method was used which constructs groups minimising the distances among the units within the groups themselves. This method was not applied to the original variables but rather to factors obtained from a multiple correspondence analysis, following the French statistical school (Benzecri, 1973). Using this technique the representation of a space sized k may be reduced to a space sized k^*, where $k^* < k$, proceeding by a linear combinations of variables, with the minimum loss of variability possible being the aim. The k^* dimensions form factors each of which synthesises one aspect of the multivariate data obtained, while eliminating the redundant data.

The multiple correspondence analysis (MCA) calls for the definition of a matrix $M\{\delta_{ij}\}$ whose elements are $\delta_{ij} = 1$ presence of a phenomenon, $= 0$ other wise, as this was designed to be applied to variables regardless of scale (even nominal) and the Euclidean metric is used. Thus multiple correspondence analysis is particularly useful when dealing with qualitiative data and even mixed component multiple variables (both quantitative and qualitative) as is our case.

REFERENCES

Andrews, F. M.: 1974, 'Social indicators of perceived life quality', Social Indicators Research 1.

Arber, S. and J. Ginn: 1995, Connecting Gender and Ageing (A Sociological Approach, OUP).

Aureli Cutillo, E.: 1996, Indicatori della qualità della vita, Workshop (Terza Conferenza Nazionale di Statistica, Istat, Roma).

Baldazzi, B., L. Quattrociocchi and R. Ranaldi: 1998, 'L'autovalutazione della salute nella popolazione anziana', in C. Palagiano, G. de Santis, D. Castagnoli (a cura di), Atti del Sesto Seminario Internazionale di Geografia medica – Metodi di raccolta dati e percezione della salute – (Roma, 4–6 dicembre 1997) (Ed. Rux, Perugia).

Benzecri, J. P.: 1973, L'analyse des données (Dunod, Paris).

ISTAT: 1997, Gli anziani in Italia (Il Mulino, Bologna).

ISTAT: 1997, 'La vita quotidiana nel 1995 – Indagine multiscopo sulle famiglie', Informazione (46).

Medley, M. L.: 1976, 'Satisfaction with life among persons sixty-five years and older', Journal of Gerontology 31(4).

McNeil, J. K., M. J. Stones and A. Kozma: 1986, 'Subjective well-being in later life: issues concerning measurement and prediction', Social Indicators Research 18.

Michalos, A. C.: 1986, 'An application of multiple discrepancies theory (MDT) to seniores', Social Indicators Research 18.

Schifini D'Andrea, S.: 1998, 'Italian quality of life', Social Indicators Research – Studies on the Quality of Life in Italy (May) 44(1).

Schifini, D'Andrea, S.: 1997, 'Indicatori della qualità della vita percepita', in Atti della giornata di studio in memoria di Bruno Grazia-Resi, a cura di E. Aureli Cutillo e E. Koch-Weser Ammassari (SIAE, Roma).

Shen, S. M. and Y. L. Lai: 1998, 'Optimally scaled quality of life indicators', Social Indicators Research 44(2).

Veenhoven, R.: 1993, 'Happiness in nations: subjective appreciation of life', 56 Nations 1946–1992 (RISBO, Rotterdam).

Department of Statistics
Probability and Applied Statistics
University of Rome
Italy

Enrica Aureli

ISTAT
Italian National
Statistical Institute

Barbara Baldazzi

INDEX OF AUTHORS
VOLUME 60, 2002